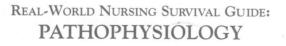

REAL-WORLD NURSING SURVIVAL GUIDE:
PATHOPHYSIOLOGY

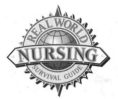

REAL-WORLD NURSING SURVIVAL GUIDE SERIES

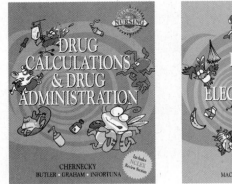

DRUG CALCULATIONS & DRUG ADMINISTRATION

CHERNECKY
BUTLER • GRAHAM • INFORTUNA

Includes NCLEX Review Section

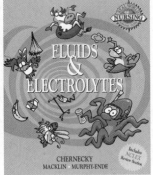

FLUIDS & ELECTROLYTES

CHERNECKY
MACKLIN • MURPHY-ENDE

Includes NCLEX Review Section

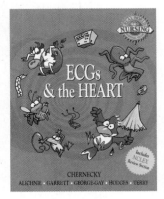

ECGs & the HEART

CHERNECKY
ALICHNIE • GARRETT • GEORGE-GAY • HODGES • TERRY

Includes NCLEX Review Section

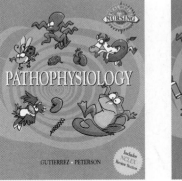

PATHOPHYSIOLOGY

GUTIERREZ • PETERSON

Includes NCLEX Review Section

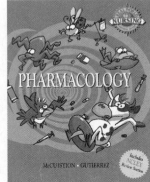

PHARMACOLOGY

McCUISTION • GUTIERREZ

Includes NCLEX Review Section

REAL-WORLD NURSING SURVIVAL GUIDE:
PATHOPHYSIOLOGY

KATHLEEN JO GUTIERREZ, PhD, RN, ANP, CNS

Independent Practice, Internal Medicine
Littleton, Colorado
Affiliate Faculty
Regis University
Denver, Colorado

PHYLLIS GAYDEN PETERSON, RN, MN, APRN

Assistant Professor, Division of Nursing
Our Lady of Holy Cross College
New Orleans, Louisiana

W. B. SAUNDERS COMPANY

Philadelphia London Montreal Sydney Tokyo Toronto

W.B. Saunders Company

The Curtis Center
Independence Square West
Philadelphia, Pennsylvania 19106-3399

Library of Congress Cataloging-in-Publication Data

Pathophysiology / [edited by] Kathleen Jo Gutierrez, Phyllis Gayden Peterson.
    p. ; cm. — (Real world nursing survival guide)
  Includes bibliographical references and index.
  ISBN 0-7216-9046-7 (pbk.)
    1. Physiology, Pathological. 2. Nursing. I. Gutierrez, Kathleen. II. Peterson, Phyllis Gayden.
  III. Series.
    [DNLM: 1. Disease—etiology—Nurses' Instruction. QZ 40 P297 2002]
  RB113 .P3572 2002
  616.07—dc21

                                                                          2001049985

Vice President and Publishing Director, Nursing: Sally Schrefer
Acquisitions Editor: Robin Carter
Developmental Editor: Gina Hopf
Project Manager: Catherine Jackson
Designer: Amy Buxton
Cover Designer and Illustrator: Chris Sharp, GraphCom Corporation

NOTICE

Nursing is an ever-changing field. Standard safety precautions must be followed, but as new research and clinical experience broaden our knowledge, changes in treatment and drug therapy may become necessary or appropriate. Readers are advised to check the most current product information provided by the manufacturer of each drug to be administered to verify the recommended dose, the method and duration of administration, and the contraindications. It is the responsibility of the licensed prescriber, relying on the experience and knowledge of the patient, to determine dosages and the best treatment for each individual patient. Neither the publisher nor the editor assumes any liability for any injury or damage to persons or property arising from this publication.

The Publisher

REAL-WORLD NURSING SURVIVAL GUIDE:

PATHOPHYSIOLOGY   ISBN 0-7216-9046-7

Printed in the United States of America

Last digit is the print number: 9 8 7 6 5 4 3 2 1

About the Authors

Dr. Kathleen Jo Gutierrez completed an associate degree in nursing from the Community College of Denver, a bachelor of science degree in nursing from Metropolitan State College of Denver, and a master of science degree from the University of Colorado Health Sciences Center. She also completed a post-master's program as an adult nurse practitioner through Beth El College in Colorado Springs. Her interest in education and professional development compelled her to obtain a doctorate degree in education from the University of Denver.

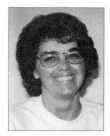

Dr. Gutierrez is currently a primary health care provider in an internal medicine office in the Denver area. During the 15 years before entering private practice, she was an associate professor with the Department of Nursing at Regis University in Denver. She remains active with the National League for Nursing Accreditation Commission as a program evaluator and member of the program review panel.

In addition to her work on *Real-World Nursing Survival Guide: Pathophysiology*, Dr. Gutierrez is the author and editor of *Pharmacotherapeutics: Clinical Decision-Making in Nursing* and a co-author for the *Real-World Nursing Survival Guide: Pharmacology*. She has published numerous journal articles, the latest of which is a research article describing the prescribing behaviors of Colorado's advanced practice nurses.

Dr. Gutierrez has been named in "Who's Who in American Nursing," "Who's Who in American Education," and "Who's Who in Medicine and Health Care." She is board certified as both an adult nurse practitioner and medical-surgical clinical nurse specialist. She is a member of the American Nurses Association, the National Organization of Nurse Practitioner Faculties, American Academy of Nurse Practitioners, and Sigma Theta Tau, the International Honor Society of Nursing.

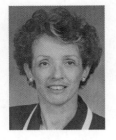

Phyllis Gayden Peterson has been a nurse for 21 years. Most of her nursing practice has been in adult medical oncology, with a special emphasis on the care of patients receiving chemotherapy and those undergoing bone marrow transplantation. She has extensive experience as a staff nurse and in nursing administration. She holds a bachelor of arts degree in French and Spanish from Michigan State University. She earned a diploma in nursing from Charity Hospital School of Nursing in New Orleans in 1980 and a bachelor of science degree in nursing from Loyola University of the South in 1985. She completed her master's degree in adult health nursing at Louisiana State University Medical Center in 1990. She has been a member of the nursing faculty of Our Lady of Holy Cross College in New Orleans, Louisiana, since 1991. She is a chemotherapy trainer for the Oncology Nursing Society and has been a featured guest speaker at international oncology conferences.

Contributors

Tracey D. Allen, BSN, BS, Certified Gerontological Nurse
Nurse Consultant
New Orleans, Louisiana

Leslie S. Arceneaux, FNP, MAFN
Family Nurse Practitioner, Board Certified
Endocrinology
Ochsner Foundation Clinic
New Orleans, Louisiana

Sheila A. Arrington, MSN, RN, GNP, CS, OCN
Nurse Practitioner
Hematology/Oncology Department
Wake Forest University Baptist Medical Center
Winston-Salem, North Carolina

Joanne M. Bullard, BSN, MN, APRN
Assistant Professor of Nursing
Our Lady of Holy Cross College
New Orleans, Louisiana

Karen L. Beard-Byrd, MSN, RN, GNP, OCN
Nurse Practitioner
Hematology/Oncology Department
Wake Forest University Baptist Medical Center
Winston-Salem, North Carolina

Charlotte M. Cline-Taylor, MSN, RN, CNS, C-FNP
Nurse Practitioner Associates, Inc.
Franklin, Louisiana

Kathleen Jo Gutierrez, PhD, RN, ANP, CNS
Independent Practice, Internal Medicine
Littleton, Colorado
Affiliate Faculty
Regis University
Denver, Colorado

Linda Eilee Schmidt McCuistion, PhD, RN
Associate Professor, Division of Nursing
Our Lady of Holy Cross College
New Orleans, Louisiana

Margaret M. Mulhall, MSN, RN
Assistant Professor of Nursing
Regis University
Denver, Colorado

Mary Ann Nemcek, DNS, RN
Assistant Professor of Nursing
Loyola University
New Orleans, Louisiana
Continuing Education Coordinator
Home Care Services
Egan Health Care Services
Metairie, Louisiana

Phyllis G. Peterson, RN, MN, APRN
Assistant Professor
Division of Nursing
Our Lady of Holy Cross College
New Orleans, Louisiana

Karen L. Rice, MSN, APRN
Adult Nurse Practitioner and Geriatric Resource Nurse
Division of Nursing
Alton Ochsner Foundation Hospital
New Orleans, Louisiana

Susan M. Sciacca, RN, BSN
Staff Nurse
Craig Hospital
Englewood, Colorado

Gwen Pfeffer Skaggs, BSN
Staff Nurse/Registered Nurse
Pediatric Emergency Room, Medicine Clinic
University Hospital, Medical Center of Louisiana
New Orleans, Louisiana

Eileen H. Stoll, MSN, CCRN
Assistant Professor
Division of Nursing
Our Lady of Holy Cross College
New Orleans, Louisiana

Lynn C. Wimett, EdD, MSN, RN, BSN, ANT
Assistant Professor of Nursing
Regis University
Denver, Colorado

Faculty & Student Reviewers

FACULTY

Nancy Henne Batchelor, MSN, RNC, CNS
Northern Kentucky University
Highland Heights, Kentucky

Stephanie Lynn Boots, RN, BSN

David Derrico, MSN, RN, OCN
Assistant Clinical Professor
College of Nursing
University of Florida
Gainesville, Florida

Margaret H. Doherty, MSN, RN, CCRN
Instructor, Department of Nursing
Sonoma State University
Rohnert Park, California

Diane Marie Ford, RN, MS, FNP, CS, CCRN
Andrews University
Berrien Springs, Michigan

Margaret M. Gingrich, MSN, RN
Harrisburg Area Community College
Harrisburg, Pennsylvania

Margie J. Hansen, PhD, RN
Clinical Associate Professor of Nursing
University of North Dakota
Grand Forks, North Dakota

Joan Klemballa, PhD, RN, FNP-C
The College of West Virginia
Beckley, West Virginia

Sharon Mitchell, LPN, BS
Canadian Valley Technology Center
El Reno, Oklahoma

Mary Ellen Mitchell-Rosen, RN, BSN
RTM Star Center
Dania Beach, Florida

Harry Peery, RN, MS, BS
Lecturer, Departments of Pharmacology, Toxicology, and Medical Chemistry
Division of Nursing Practice, College of Nursing
College of Pharmacy
University of Arizona
Tucson, Arizona

Kimberly R. Pugh, MSEd, RN, BSN
Nurse Consultant
Baltimore, Maryland

Dottie Roberts, MSN, RN, C, MACI, ONC CNS
Penrose—St. Francis Health Services
Colorado Springs, Colorado

Susan B. Stillwell, MSN, RN
Clinical Associate Professor
Arizona State University
Tempe, Arizona

Christine L. Vandenhouten, MSN, RN, CNOR
Bellin College of Nursing
Green Bay, Wisconsin

Janis Waite, EdD, MSN, RN
Associate Professor
St. Francis Medical Center College of Nursing
Peoria, Illinois

James Joseph Wojcik, BA, BSN, MBA
Instructor
Virginia College of Huntsville
Huntsville, Alabama

STUDENTS

Evelyn DeMoss, ADN
Austin Community College
Austin, Texas

Mary Jo Lampart, RN, BSN
Geisinger Medical Center
Danville, Pennsylvania
Former Student
Bloomsburg University
Bloomsburg, Pennsylvania

Clifford (Troy) Shaffer Jr., EMT
Medical College of Georgia
School of Nursing
Augusta, Georgia

The following students from Our Lady of Holy Cross College and Charity Delgado School of Nursing, New Orleans, Louisiana, helped the editors shape the vision of this reference through focus group reviews and breakout sessions:

Kenya Michelle Alexander
Brian Badeaux
Deana Bell
Cynthia G. Bienvenu
Anastasia Erb
Bernard Fernandes
Faith A. Fray
Bridgette Rowena Gasaway
Elizabeth Gonzalez
Heather G. Herbert

Thomas J. Higgins, Jr.
Joy Jones
Mae Crovetto Juan
L. Michelle Keller
Jana Kellogg
Ronni McCaskill
Amy E. McDonald
Kimberly A. Palmisano
Shawn R. Passons
Shanny M'Lee Pierce

Robin Richoux
Francine S. Ricks
Catherine Roark
Gretchen Rothenberger
Erica Saia
Melissa Tefft
Rachel Till
Sharon Nance Vincent

Series Reviewers

FACULTY

Edwina A. McConnell, PhD, RN,
   FRCNA
Professor
School of Nursing
Texas Technical University Health
   Sciences Center
Lubbock, Texas
Consultant
Gorham, Maine

Judith L. Myers, MSN, RN
Health Sciences Center
St. Louis University
School of Nursing
St. Louis, Missouri

FEATURED STUDENTS

Shayne Michael Gray, RN, was born in Little Rock, Arkansas, and graduated with a BSN degree from the University of Arkansas for Medical Sciences (UAMS) in 1999. He has spent a year working at the University as an Intensive Care Nurse and has also applied for a medical commission in the Naval Reserve. Future plans include becoming a CRNA. Before nursing school, Shayne played drums in a band that eventually signed with a record label and was distributed by Polygram and Phillips Multimedia; this afforded him the opportunity to tour the United States and Canada for 3 years. Following that, he left the band and earned a leading role in an independent film that was shown at the prestigious Sundance Film Festival. It is the earnings from this movie role that Shayne credits with helping him finish his nursing school prerequisites at the University of Arkansas at Little Rock, and he married his wife Michelle in 1996, just as he was being accepted into the nursing program. He spent 2 years serving as a volunteer for the Arkansas Lung Association, speaking about the dangers of smoking to local school children, and has also been a volunteer for many of UAMS's fundraisers and community clean-up projects. A former Helicopter Flight Medic in the Army National Guard, Shayne is a certified scuba diver and loves the outdoors, playing guitar, and writing. He is also ACLS qualified and hopes to participate in nursing/medical research in the future.

For **Jill Hall,** attending nursing school has been the fulfillment of a childhood dream. Before that opportunity, she served an apprenticeship as a Mechanical and Production Engineer with British Aerospace. She then spent 2 years as a stay-at-home mother for her two children. When her husband accepted a job in California, the family moved from northern England to Huntington Beach, where Jill began taking prerequisite nursing classes at Golden West College. Once into the nursing program, she knew she had found what she was meant to do. She became involved in the Student Nurses' Association, and a trip to the mid-year NSNA convention in Dallas sparked her enthusiasm to run for national office. At the annual convention in Pittsburgh, she was elected to the Nominations and Elections Committee, and her year in office involved conventions in both Charlotte and Salt Lake City. In her own community, she is a member of the United Methodist Church and the high school PTO. She has been a Girl Scout leader, Sunday school teacher, soccer coach, and soccer camp coordinator, as well as a volunteer in the emergency room of a local hospital. She is currently employed in the Pediatric ICU at Miller Children's Hospital in Long Beach, California. She also plans to pursue both BSN and MSN degrees. She offers special thanks to two instructors who have served as mentors during her time in the nursing program at Golden West College, Nadine Davis and Marcia Swanson: "Their standards of excellence have inspired me to achieve more than I ever thought I could. Gracious thanks for all they have done for me."

Elizabeth J. Hoogmoed, RN, BSN, recently graduated from William Paterson University and is currently a neurological nurse at Valley Hospital in Ridgewood, New Jersey. She serves on the Executive Board of Sigma Theta Tau as Corresponding Secretary for the Iota Alpha chapter. She also served as Membership and Nominations Chair for New Jersey Nursing Students from 1998 to 1999 and continues to be a sustaining member of the organization. She has also been a volunteer for her local ambulance corps for 7 years. She has been accepted into the program at New York University, where she will complete her Masters degree to become a Nurse Practitioner. Her hope is to promote the profession of nursing and show its importance to the future of health care. In this era of computers and technology, she believes it is reassuring to know that a select number of individuals continue to follow the inner call to care for people and promote wellness in society: "These are the nurses."

Katie Scarlett McRae, BA, BSN, says that if you talk to her for more than a few minutes, you'll be sure to hear her say, "I love my job." She serves as a staff RN on the cardiovascular/telemetry floor at Oregon Health Sciences University (OHSU) in Portland, caring for patients who have had heart transplants or other cardiac/vascular surgeries or who suffer from congestive heart failure, diabetes, or arrhythmias. Working with many experienced nurses "great at sharing their insights and knowledge," Katie loves the teaching hospital environment and jokes that nursing is her "second career"; when she graduated from the OHSU nursing program in 1999, it was actually her second Bachelor's degree, but "the two degrees were 24 years apart!" Katie credits the rigorous OHSU program with giving her the confidence to know she could practice nursing safely. During nursing school, she was active in student government, and she is also a current member of the Oregon Nurses' Association, the ANA, and the AACN. She plans to return to OHSU soon to begin work on a Master's degree in Adult Health and Illness, with a focus on diabetes, and her ideal career would be to create and manage a comprehensive diabetes management for the state of Oregon.

STUDENTS

Angela M. Boyd, AS
University of Tennessee at Martin
Martin, Tennessee

Jennifer Hamilton
University of Virginia
Charlottesville, Virginia

Joy Kutlenios Amos, RN, BSN
Piedmont Medical Center
Rock Hill, South Carolina
Former student
Wheeling Jesuit University
Wheeling, West Virginia

Preface

Nursing is an art, as well as a science. To assess, plan, and implement a successful plan of care for patients, nurses must possess at least a basic understanding of pathophysiology. Knowledge of pathophysiology will help you anticipate and prevent or at least minimize complications of disease processes. This book is intended to serve as a resource, offering easy-to-read information on common diseases and helping you understand the role of nursing interventions in your patients' plans of care.

This text is one book in a series that was created with direct input from nursing students. Focus groups held at the meeting of the National Student Nurses Association were asked to identify what they found helpful when trying to master new material. Their responses have been used in the creation of the basic structure and approach behind the *Real-World Nursing Survival Guide Series*. *Pathophysiology* includes chapters devoted to specific body system disorders and a section with NCLEX review questions to reinforce what you learn.

We have included many features in the margins to help you focus on the most important information you will need to succeed in the classroom and in the clinical setting. TAKE HOME POINTS 🏠 are composed of both study tips for classroom tests and "pearls of wisdom" to assist you in caring for patients. Both study tips and pearls are drawn from our many years of combined academic and clinical experience. Content marked with a caution icon ⚠️ is vital and usually involves nursing actions that may have life-threatening consequences or those that may significantly affect patient outcomes. The lifespan icon 🌼 and the culture icon ☯️ highlight variations in treatment that may be necessary for specific age or ethnic groups. A calculator icon 📱 is designed to draw your eye to important equations and examples that will help you calculate proper medication dosages. A web links icon 💻 will direct you to sites on the Internet that will give more detailed information on specific topics. Each of these icons will specifically help you focus on "real-world" patient care, the nursing process, and positive patient outcomes. Finally, we have created a special icon for use in *Pathophysiology*. A cross-reference icon 🐂 will refer you to drug treatment regimens in the *Real-World Nursing Survival Guide: Pharmacology* that correspond to the pathophysiologic disorders. This information is not absolutely necessary to your understanding of the pathophysiology of a given disorder or its associated nursing responsibilities; however, it will give you a more rounded view of the disorders' treatments.

We have also used consistent headings that emphasize specific nursing actions. What It IS provides a brief definition of the disease, along with a summary of the physical changes that take place as a result of the disease process. When applicable, at-risk populations are also specified. What You NEED TO KNOW summarizes signs and symptoms of the disease (clinical manifestations), as well as prognoses and treatment regimens. What You DO includes bulleted lists of nursing interventions and responsibilities. As professionals, we are *responsible* for providing expert, comprehensive care for our patients. Under this heading you will find special *green apple bullets* that highlight the necessary patient teaching points of the care plan for a disorder. Finally, Do You UNDERSTAND? provides questions and exercises that are both entertaining and useful to reinforce the topic's concepts. This four-step approach provides information and helps you learn how to apply it in the clinical setting.

We hope this book will make a difficult topic easier and provide you with new insights and understanding of the affects of illness and disease. Please share the knowledge you gain with others; most of all, use this information to make a positive difference in the lives of your patients.

Kathleen J. Gutierrez, PhD, RN, ANP, CNS
Phyllis G. Peterson, RN, MN, APRN

My heartfelt appreciation, gratitude, and thanks to my husband and soul mate, Pat, and to our children, Mike, Pam, and Brad, for their undying support and understanding.

Blessed are those who have learned to admire without envy, to follow without mimicking, to praise without flattery, and to lead without manipulation.

Kathleen J. Gutierrez

This book is dedicated to everyone who has inspired and challenged me to read, to study, and to learn—particularly my parents, my husband, and my students.

"When I get a little money I buy books and if any is left I buy food and clothes."—*Erasmus*

Phyllis G. Peterson

Acknowledgments

Special thanks are due to many people who participated in the preparation of this book. Comments and suggestions from students in the original focus group provided the initial concept for this series and valuable insights from the perspective of the students of nursing education. Student nurse reviewers from Our Lady of Holy Cross College and Charity Delgado School of Nursing generously gave their time to scrutinize and critique the chapters while still in draft form and helped make the text more "student friendly."

The content in this book was provided by many different nurse experts from across the country. Without the help of our contributors, this book would not have been possible. Cynthia Chernecky, PhD, RN, CNS, AOCN, played an important role in the early stages of this project and helped establish content and format.

Last, we extend our appreciation to Robin Carter and Gina Hopf, editors in the nursing division of W.B. Saunders, for their patience and persistent guidance in all aspects of the publishing process.

Kathleen J. Gutierrez
Phyllis G. Peterson

Contents

Immune System

HYPERSENSITIVITY REACTIONS

This section provides information on the body's immune system and related diseases and disorders that can adversely affect this protective mechanism.

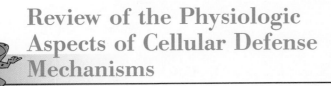

Review of the Physiologic Aspects of Cellular Defense Mechanisms

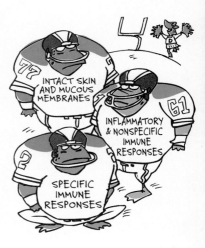

The body has three main lines of defense that provide protection against injury and disease. These defenses include intact skin and mucous membranes, the inflammatory and nonspecific immune responses, and specific immune responses by antigens and activated cells.

When properly functioning, immunity is both specific and nonspecific. The immune system must recognize an invading organism as a threat and mount an appropriate response. Additionally, the immune system must distinguish between foreign substances and those of our own bodies, otherwise autoimmune disorders can result.

Inflammation is a mechanism that allows cells to be repaired when subjected to stress or damage. The body has a two-pronged response to injury that is both vascular and cellular in nature. During the vascular phase, the body causes an increase in blood flow and capillary permeability in the damaged area.

Certain agents secreted by the body are responsible for regulating the inflammatory response (mediators). These agents cause dilation of blood vessels, fever, and narrowing of the airways in the lungs. Additionally, these agents affect the activity and effectiveness of a wide variety of white blood cells in the event of tissue damage.

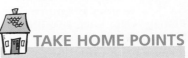

Kuby's Immunology
http://www.whfreeman.com/kuby/index.htm

Anatomy of the Immune System
http://www-micro.msb.le.ac.uk/MBChB/2b.html

TAKE HOME POINTS

The vascular phase results in three cardinal signs of inflammation—redness, warmth, and swelling—that are frequently observed in an area of tissue damage.

During the cellular response phase, specialized white blood cells move out of the circulatory system and into the tissues in which they clean up debris and deactivate potentially dangerous foreign organisms, such as bacteria and viruses. Some of these specialized white cells "remember" invading organisms, a process that helps them launch a response that is significantly more rapid and aggressive, if a similar attack occurs in the future.

Immune Cell Review

CELL TYPE	FUNCTION
Macrophages	Engulf cellular debris, present foreign proteins or antigens to lymphocytes. Phagocytic cells can be found throughout the body.
Neutrophils	Move to areas of tissue damage. Important defenders against bacterial colonization and infection.
Eosinophils	Important in preventing parasitic infections. Active in adaptive immunity.
Basophils	Protect mucosal surfaces. Release cell mediators that promote the inflammatory response.
Mast cells	Provide cellular mediators that support and maintain the immune response.
B lymphocytes	Produce antibodies. Provide specific immunity for antigens found outside of the host cells. Most humoral immunity requires interaction with T lymphocytes.
Antibodies (immunoglobulins)	Bind to specific antigens and promote inflammation by attracting phagocytic cells. IgG: Most common antibody to respond to infection. IgA: Prevents germs from entering through external openings. IgM: Active in primary responses; mediates cytotoxic responses. IgE: Active in allergic responses. IgD: Function unknown.
T lymphocytes	Have three main functions: helper, killer, and suppressor. Able to destroy antigens and regulate the activity of other immune cells.

⚠ **In some cases, an exaggerated inflammatory response damages the host, resulting in chronic inflammatory diseases and even life-threatening complications, such as septic shock.**

Chronic or recurrent infections frequently trouble patients with defects in cellular immunity. Genetic disorders, disease processes, malnutrition, and abuse of alcohol and certain drugs (e.g., steroids) can adversely affect white cell function.

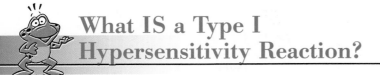

What IS a Type I Hypersensitivity Reaction?

Hypersensitivity reactions are the result of an extreme response of the immune system to an antigen (allergen). An antigen is a foreign protein that stimulates an immune response in a susceptible individual. Type I reactions are noted for their rapid and occasionally dramatic onset of symptoms. Symptoms of Type I reactions range from sniffling and runny nose commonly present with hay fever, to the respiratory distress, generalized edema, and cardiopulmonary arrest commonly observed with anaphylaxis. Atopic symptoms affect the skin, respiratory, and gastrointestinal systems because these tissues contain a large number of mast cells.

Pathogenesis

Type I reactions are the result of an excessive or inappropriate production of IgE antibodies after exposure to some type of environmental antigen. With initial exposure to the allergen, IgE (an immunoglobulin) forms, attaches to mast cells, and forms a complex. The individual is now sensitized to the allergen. With subsequent exposure to the allergen, tiny sacs in the mast cells called granules break open and release a vasoactive substance known as histamine, which then triggers the inflammatory response.

At-Risk Populations

Allergies tend to be hereditary. The children of allergic mothers are likely to have allergies. When both parents have allergies, the likelihood that their offspring will be allergic is at least 80%.

 TAKE HOME POINTS

A Type I reaction results from exposure to an environmental allergen. Common environmental allergens include animal dander, dust, dust mites, bee stings, certain drugs (particularly penicillin), molds, fungi, pollen, feathers, wheat, eggs, peanuts, chocolates, shellfish, and dairy products. Typically, the patient must be exposed repeatedly to the allergen to cause sufficient production of IgE to sensitize and produce an allergic response.

Native Americans and African Americans are more likely to be allergic to foods containing lactose than are those of Middle European ancestry.

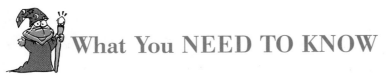

What You NEED TO KNOW

Clinical Manifestations

Allergic reactions vary. Type I hypersensitivity reactions typically have a sudden onset. The signs and symptoms may include watery, reddened eyes, runny nose, sneezing, wheezing, itching, shortness of breath, rashes, swelling of the face and hands, diarrhea, stomach cramps, and abdominal pain. In some individuals, these symptoms are merely a nuisance that is easily treated with over-the-counter medicines and removal of the offending agent.

Prognosis

In most cases, Type I hypersensitivity reactions can be reversed with prompt treatment and removal of the offending agent.

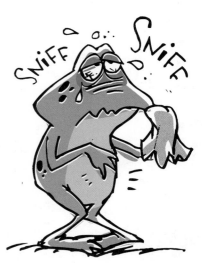

For some individuals, initial hypersensitivity symptoms rapidly progress to acute respiratory distress and, ultimately, cardiopulmonary arrest. Recognizing the signs and symptoms of hypersensitivity reaction is important.

See Chapters 2A, 6B, and 7B in RWNSG: *Pharmacology*

 Patients with severe respiratory failure who fail to respond to drug therapy may require supportive measures, including endotracheal intubation or a tracheostomy, to maintain their airway. Respiratory support with a mechanical ventilator may also be required to help these patients breathe, in addition to further drug therapy to support their heart and vascular system.

 Be mindful of substances that are likely to cause allergies, and monitor patients accordingly.

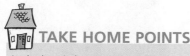 **TAKE HOME POINTS**

In the hospital setting, the most common drugs that produce Type I hypersensitivity reactions are penicillin and cephalosporin antibiotics. Patients who have experienced allergic reactions to one class of antibiotics are likely to react to other drugs in the same category.

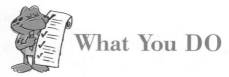 # What You DO

Treatment

Treatment for hypersensitivity reactions varies depending on the severity of the symptoms involved. In mild cases, removing the offending agent from the patient's environment may be the only requirement. When this is impossible, the patient may benefit from over-the-counter antihistamines and decongestants. If symptoms continue, then the patient may need to consult a health care provider.

In severe cases, the patient requires emergency intervention and cardiopulmonary resuscitation. Various drugs may be given, typically intravenously, to treat severe reactions. These drugs include methylprednisolone—a glucocorticoid that is given to decrease the inflammation associated with the allergic reaction.

Diphenhydramine hydrochloride is given for its antihistaminic effect, which then leads to decreased edema formation and decreased constriction of smooth muscles in the respiratory tree and blood vessels. Epinephrine can be given via various routes to open airways and constrict blood vessels to maintain the patient's blood pressure.

Nursing Responsibilities

All patients should be asked about possible allergies as a part of the initial assessment or before administering medications. The patient should also know the difference between allergic and adverse reactions. Many patients believe that they are allergic to a drug when, in reality, they are experiencing a side effect or adverse reaction caused by a drug.

The nurse should:
- Ask the patient about allergic reactions as part of the health history assessment.
- Report allergic reactions to the appropriate health care provider immediately, and document the allergy in the patient's medical record. Take special note of rashes, watery eyes, runny noses, or itching, particularly in the absence of fever.
- Be alert to your patient's complaints. Rash and itching are frequently the earliest signs of an allergic reaction. When a reaction occurs, carefully inspect your patient's environment and treatment plan for any possible causes, such as new drugs, a change in diet, or the environment. Obtain orders to treat the allergic symptom when indicated.
- After the source of the allergy is identified, clearly label the patient's chart accordingly, and note the allergy in the patient's medical record.
- Educate your patients to help them eliminate potential causes from the environment and assist them in changing their lifestyle to avoid exposure to the cause of the allergy.

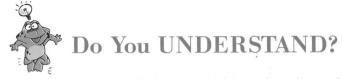

Do You UNDERSTAND?

DIRECTIONS: Write the letter that corresponds to the words that correct-ly completes each of the following statements.

_____ 1. An antigen is:
    a. A foreign protein capable of stimulating an immune response in anyone with a healthy immune system. ,
    b. A foreign protein capable of stimulating an immune response in a susceptible individual.
    c. A protein that binds with an antibody.
    d. A protein that is released by the immune system.

_____ 2. An anaphylactic reaction is an example of:
    a. Type I hypersensitivity.
    b. Type II hypersensitivity.
    c. Type III hypersensitivity.
    d. Type IV hypersensitivity.

_____ 3. Histamine is released by:
    a. T lymphocytes.
    b. B lymphocytes.
    c. Monocytes.
    d. Mast cells

_____ 4. Signs and symptoms of a Type I reaction usually appear
    a. After repeated chronic exposure to the allergen.
    b. 12 to 24 hours after exposure to the allergen.
    c. After only one exposure to the allergen.
    d. Soon after exposure to the allergen.

What IS a Type II Hypersensitivity Reaction?

In this type of reaction, an antibody reacts with an antigen on the surface of a cell. In most cases, the antibodies are IgG and IgM type. The antigen can be found on the membranes of red blood cells received during a transfusion, result-ing in a transfusion reaction. The antigen may be from a drug that adheres to the surface of the patient's own cells. Antibodies produced by the patient's own cells may then cause an autoimmune hemolytic anemia.

Pathogenesis

Type II reactions involve the activation of complement by antibodies, which, in turn, results in destruction of cells. Complement is a series of proteins that controls the immune response. In the healthy individual, complement distinguishes the individual's own cells from foreign substances (self-tolerance or self-recognition). When this ability is lost, the individual is susceptible to autoimmune diseases.

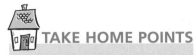
TAKE HOME POINTS

- After an allergen has been identi-fied, inform the patient of the allergy, and make certain that the patient understands the ways to avoid the allergy in the future. This knowledge is particularly impor-tant, because repeated exposure to an allergen can leave a patient at risk for anaphylaxis, a potential-ly life-threatening reaction.
- Advise highly susceptible patients to obtain a MedicAlert armband or pendant to wear after discharge.
- Suspect an allergic reaction when itching and rash are present. Remember that cross-sensitivities can occur between related cate-gories of drugs.
- Be prepared to initiate emergency measures for severe reactions.

Be prepared to monitor your allergic patient for potentially life-threatening progression of symptoms. Be certain that emergency resuscitation equipment and rescue drugs such as diphenhydramine hydrochloride, methylpred-nisolone and epinephrine are readily available.

Answers: 1. b; 2. a; 3. d; 4. d.

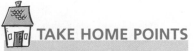 In the case of pregnancy, a condition called ery-throblastosis fetalis (hemolytic disease of the newborn) can occur when there is an Rh or ABO incompatibility between the blood of the mother and her fetus. As a result of the hemolytic process, the red blood cells of the fetus are destroyed.

TAKE HOME POINTS

- Type II hypersensitivity reactions result from the interaction of an antigen with an antibody.
- Type II reactions are observed primarily as the result of blood transfusions or mismatches between the blood of a mother and her fetus.
- Drugs can occasionally cause Type II reactions that result in hemolysis and anemia.

⚠ **Patients with severe reactions can have damage to the renal tubules because of precipitation of hemoglobin in the urine. As a result of the decreased blood flow to the kidneys, circulatory shock associated with a severe reaction can also contribute to renal failure.**

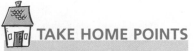 When a pregnant woman who is Rh⁻ becomes sensitized to the red blood cells of her Rh⁺ fetus, *Erythroblastosis fetalis* occurs in second or third pregnancies.

Type II hypersensitivity reactions result primarily from blood transfusions and mismatches between the blood of a mother and her fetus. After receiving a transfusion, antibodies are produced to the recipient's own blood cells, which then trigger the process of hemolysis.

In some cases, disease can cause hemolytic anemia. Patients with chronic lymphocytic leukemia tend to have small, ineffective lymphocyte cells. When these cells produce antibodies, they tend to attach to the patient's red blood cells. Hemolytic anemia has also been associated with systemic infection.

At-Risk Populations

Anyone receiving transfusion or drug therapy is at risk for a Type II hypersensitivity reaction. Banking the patient's own blood before surgery and using donated blood only when absolutely necessary reduces the degree of risk.

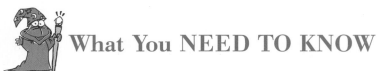

What You NEED TO KNOW

Clinical Manifestations

Signs and symptoms of Type II reactions vary depending on the overall physical status of the patient and the nature of the precipitating factors. In the case of transfusion-associated hemolytic anemia, symptoms can range from mild to life threatening. Mild symptoms include chills, fever, and headache. Other symptoms include apprehension, chest pain, flank pain, elevated heart and respiratory rates, hypertension, and hemoglobinuria. Severe cases can progress to disseminated intravascular coagulation, renal failure, and circulatory collapse.

A 10% mortality rate is common when large amounts of incompatible blood are transfused.

When a pregnant woman who is Rh⁻ becomes sensitized to the red blood cells of her Rh⁺ fetus, *Erythroblastosis fetalis* occurs in second or third pregnancies. Ultimately, the mother's antibodies cross the placenta and attack the red cells of the fetus. Infants of mothers with toxemia, mothers who have undergone manual removal of the placenta, or mothers who have had caesarean deliveries are at additional risk for developing hemolytic anemia because these events tend to mix fetal and maternal blood. Jaundice usually appears in the neonate within 24 hours after birth. An enlarged spleen and liver can be detected through a clinical examination. The blood may have varying degrees of anemia, ranging from mild to severe.

Autoimmune hemolytic anemia associated with disease in the adult will have a wide range of symptoms depending on the severity of the anemia. In mild cases, the patient will be pale and complain of fatigue and weakness. In severe cases, the patient may be hypoxic, breathless, and have other symptoms of heart failure.

Prognosis

The prognosis is highly individual and depends on the patient's underlying state of health and the severity of the reaction. Vulnerable or otherwise compromised patients are much less likely to survive an acute event.

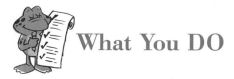

What You DO

Treatment

In most cases, patients who have experienced a mild reaction may require only monitoring and supportive care. Transfusion-associated hemolytic transfusion reactions can be treated with acetaminophen, antiinflammatory drugs, and intravenous fluids. Whenever a transfusion reaction is suspected, the infusion of blood should be stopped immediately and the health care practitioner notified. Patients with severe reactions may require aggressive measures, supportive care, and hemodialysis to survive.

Hemolytic anemia associated with disease or infection usually is refractory to treatment until the underlying cause of the problem is corrected. These patients will require supportive care, including transfusions, until they can complete appropriate treatment for their disease or illness. Hemolytic anemia is an indication for discontinuing drug therapy. In most cases, when the drug is discontinued, the hemolytic process resolves without requiring further intervention.

Nursing Responsibilities

In the instance of transfusion-associated hypersensitivity reactions, the nurse's most important function is preventive. When blood is drawn for a type and crossmatch for the transfusion, the nurse must be *absolutely certain* that the blood is drawn from the correct patient and labeled appropriately.

Patients who have been heavily transfused or those who have certain forms of cancers are at risk for hypersensitivity reactions and may require premedication with acetaminophen and diphenhydramine before the transfusion. When blood products arrive from the blood bank, nurses must take special precautions to ensure that the correct blood product is given to the patient for which it is intended.

After the transfusion is initiated, the nurse must:
- Carefully monitor patients for evidence of a transfusion-associated hypersensitivity reaction.
- Take vital signs every 15 to 30 minutes during the transfusion. A decrease in blood pressure and an increase in heart rate or body temperature may indicate an early transfusion reaction.
- Observe for the presence of early symptoms such as fever and chills. These mild symptoms may indicate a need to discontinue the transfusion.
- Evaluate abnormal symptoms and patient complaints associated with transfusions and report these findings to the health care provider.

 Many potentially fatal complications can result from hemolytic disease; infants who are severely affected can have hypoxia, brain damage, heart failure, and abnormal accumulations of fluid (effusions) in the heart, lungs, and abdomen.

Treatment for erythroblastosis fetalis may include intrauterine transfusions and phototherapy following birth to decrease jaundice. Phototherapy involves exposing the infant to fluorescent light to promote the excretion of bilirubin. When phototherapy fails, a series of exchange transfusions can be performed to replace the infant's blood with compatible blood.

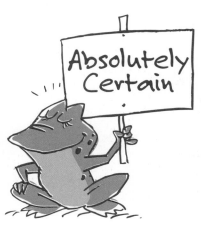

Erythroblastosis fetalis can be prevented with appropriate obstetric care. Shortly after their first delivery, women who do not have the Rh antigen in their blood should receive the drug RhoGAM to prevent sensitization of the mother to the Rh factor.

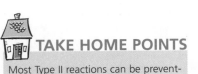

TAKE HOME POINTS

Most Type II reactions can be prevented with appropriate nursing and medical care.

Do You UNDERSTAND?

DIRECTIONS: Write the letter that corresponds to the words that correctly completes each of the following statements.

_____ 1. Type II reactions can be the result of:
   a. Drug therapy
   b. Blood transfusions
   c. Disease
   d. All of the above

_____ 2. While monitoring a patient receiving a blood transfusion, the nurse notes that the patient's blood pressure has fallen from 140/90 to 116/70, and the heart rate has increased from 84 to 110 beats per minute. The nurse's most immediate action should be to:
   a. Decrease the rate of the transfusion.
   b. Increase the rate of the transfusion.
   c. Stop the transfusion.
   d. Call the physician.

_____ 3. To prevent a hemolytic transfusion reaction, it would *not* be helpful to give _____ and _____.
   a. Morphine
   b. Meperidine
   c. Diphenhydramine
   d. Acetaminophen

_____ 4. Erythroblastosis fetalis is the result of:
   a. ABO incompatibility between the blood of the fetus and the blood of the mother.
   b. Rh incompatibility between the blood of the fetus and the blood of the mother.
   c. Drug therapy given during pregnancy.
   d. Sensitization to foreign antibodies.
   e. Both b and d.

_____ 5. RhoGAM is given after childbirth to:
   a. Treat jaundice in the neonate.
   b. Decrease hemolysis of the red blood cells in the neonate.
   c. Revent hyperbilirubinemia in the mother.
   d. Prevent sensitization of the mother to the Rh factor.

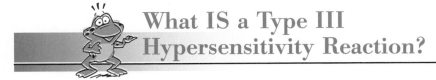

What IS a Type III Hypersensitivity Reaction?

Type III hypersensitivity reactions are the result of the body's failure to rid itself of antigen-antibody immune complexes. Immune complexes are large molecules that form when antibodies attach to antigens. The size of the complexes influences whether they remain in plasma or lodge in tissues, in which they set up an inappropriate immune response that eventually results in tissue damage. Type III reactions can produce local manifestations or be systemic.

Pathogenesis

Persistent immune complexes in the circulation set up a cascade of abnormal immune responses. While in the circulation, the immune complexes may cause damage to the walls of veins, arteries, and capillaries. Eventually, these complexes deposit in areas of the body in which increased vascular permeability exists, increasing the likelihood of disruptions in blood flow that result from increased pressure and turbulence within the vascular system. As a result, complement is released. Complement attracts macrophages and neutrophils to the area, which release cytokines and activate the inflammatory response. This inappropriate inflammatory response can damage and destroy healthy tissue. Tissue destruction then leads to further activation of the immune response, and a vicious cycle begins. Histamine is released from mast cells, which results in increased capillary permeability and vasodilation. Increased capillary wall permeability causes edema, which then permits greater activity of inflammatory components.

The exact mechanism that causes this damaging reaction is not fully understood. Two possible causes include the formation of the antigen from a foreign protein, such as a virus or bacteria, or the formation of antibodies against self-components (endogenous antigens). Because autoimmune disorders tend to occur in families, a genetic link may exist for many of these disorders. Three common illnesses thought to be the result of Type III reactions are glomerulonephritis, lupus, and rheumatoid arthritis.

At-Risk Populations

Patients with a family history of hypersensitivity reactions should be monitored carefully for the development of these disorders. Additionally, patients with persistent infections from bacterial, viral, fungal, or protozoan organisms, or people who are receiving treatment with allergenic drugs, should be evaluated carefully for the development of hypersensitivity reactions. Prompt detection and treatment can minimize complications from tissue damage.

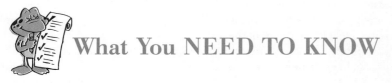

What You NEED TO KNOW

Clinical Manifestations

Symptoms of Type III hypersensitivity reactions vary depending on the organ that is affected by the abnormal accumulation of immune complexes. Because many symptoms are vague and nonspecific, an individual with an autoimmune disorder may be ill for quite some time before a diagnosis is established.

TAKE HOME POINTS

- Type III reactions are the result of persistent antigen-antibody complexes that set up an inappropriate immune response. This faulty immune response leads to destruction of normal healthy tissue.
- Causes of Type III reactions include low-grade infections, inhalation of antigens in the environment, and the formation of autoantibodies.

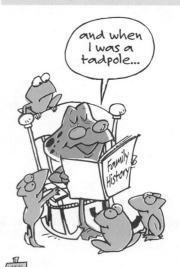

TAKE HOME POINTS

- Untreated, glomerulonephritis may eventually lead to chronic renal failure requiring dialysis.
- Systemic lupus erythematosus (SLE) can affect almost any organ in the body and can cause arthritis, anemia, coagulopathies, and disturbances in central nervous system function, to name a few. Approximately 15% of people with SLE die within the first 5 years after diagnosis.
- Because of damage to the cartilage and joints by immune complexes, rheumatoid arthritis causes chronic severe pain and disability. This disease also affects arteries, which may then lead to damage to major organs, including the heart, lungs, skin, and eyes.

Prognosis

The outcome of Type III hypersensitivity reactions is highly variable and is a function of the nature of the reaction and whether major organs are damaged. Other factors that affect the outcome include the ability of the individual to seek and comply with medical care, as well as the existence of other diseases and conditions.

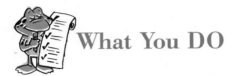 # What You DO

Treatment

Therapy involves the use of antiinflammatory agents, antihistamines, and glucocorticoids to suppress the inflammatory response thereby protecting healthy tissues from damage and preserving normal function. Severe cases may require the use of immunosuppressants, which can leave the individual prone to infections. The following drugs are commonly used in the treatment of hypersensitivity reactions.

- Aspirin
- Salsalate
- Ibuprofen
- Imuran
- Cyclophosphamide
- Hydroxychloroquine
- Hydrocortisone Sodium Succinate
- Methylprednisolone
- Dexamethasone

See Chapters 6B, 7B, and 11 in RWNSG: *Pharmacology*

Nursing Responsibilities

Nursing care begins with a careful assessment and evaluation of the needs of the individual. Special attention should be paid to the individual with a medical history or family history of allergies. Whenever possible, ask the person to discuss in detail the nature of the reaction. What many consider as an allergic reaction, particularly when dealing with drugs, may actually be an adverse reaction (e.g., nausea and vomiting) that is commonly observed with oral antibiotic therapy.

- Educate patients with autoimmune diseases on the ways to cope with their disease. Include the causes of the disease, factors that may lead to an exacerbation of the symptoms, treatment regimens, and lifestyle adjustments that will help the patient minimize distressing symptoms and associated problems.
- Tell patients that they must adhere to a medication regimen to avoid more severe consequences, up to and including organ damage and death. Many medications prescribed for hypersensitivity reactions and associated autoimmune disorders have side effects and toxicities. You must encourage patients to adhere to the medication regimen despite uncomfortable side effects and toxicities.
- Teach patients about symptoms that indicate a need to seek medical intervention immediately to prevent the advent of severe illness.

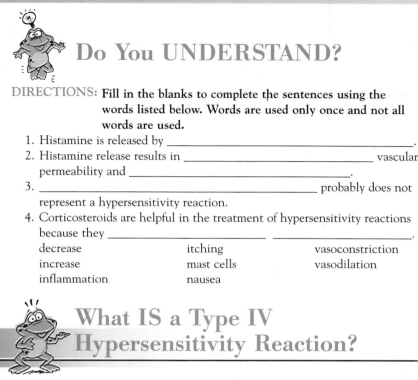

Do You UNDERSTAND?

DIRECTIONS: Fill in the blanks to complete the sentences using the words listed below. Words are used only once and not all words are used.

1. Histamine is released by _____.
2. Histamine release results in _____ vascular permeability and _____.
3. _____ probably does not represent a hypersensitivity reaction.
4. Corticosteroids are helpful in the treatment of hypersensitivity reactions because they _____ _____.

decrease	itching	vasoconstriction
increase	mast cells	vasodilation
inflammation	nausea	

What IS a Type IV Hypersensitivity Reaction?

Type IV hypersensitivity reactions differ from other hypersensitivity responses in that cells mediate the reaction, not antibodies. This reaction is delayed, typically occurring within 24 to 72 hours after exposure to the offending antigen.

Pathogenesis

Type IV hypersensitivity is regulated by T lymphocytes that are damaging to cells (cytotoxic). T lymphocytes secrete lymphokines that release inflammatory cytokines, which, in turn, attract monocytes, neutrophils, and basophils. Cytokines also activate macrophages. These cells and substances augment the inflammatory response, which is designed to inactivate and destroy foreign substances. This type of reaction is a protective form of defense against certain pathogens, including mycobacteria, fungi, and parasites. In some circumstances, however, this protective mechanism can backfire and result in disease, particularly when exposure to the offending antigen is over a prolonged period.

Delayed hypersensitivity reactions tend to be present in response to exposure to large antigens that are poorly soluble and difficult for the body to attack and destroy. Type IV reactions are initiated when a sensitized individual is exposed to this type of antigen. Various conditions and disorders can result from Type IV reactions, including contact dermatitis, positive reactions to tuberculin tests, and transplant rejection.

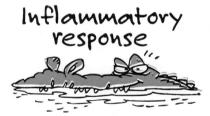

Inflammatory response

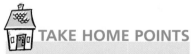

TAKE HOME POINTS

- Type IV hypersensitivity reactions are delayed reactions that are mediated by T lymphocytes.
- Common causes of Type IV reactions include chemicals, cosmetics, plant toxins, drugs, and dyes.

At-Risk Populations

Even normal, healthy individuals can experience a Type IV reaction if they have been previously sensitized to an antigen. Tuberculin skin testing is an example of a way in which this reaction can be used for diagnostic purposes. Contact dermatitis is another example of a common Type IV reaction. For susceptible individuals, other sensitizing agents include chemicals, cosmetics, and plant toxins, such as poison ivy and poison sumac.

Certain chronic diseases and autoimmune conditions can also be the result of cell-mediated hypersensitivity reactions. Allergic alveolitis occurs in response to inhaled organic dusts or antigens that may be found in the home or work environment. When exposure to the antigenic substance is prolonged, chronic irreversible lung disease can result. Other disorders thought to result from Type IV reactions include type I diabetes mellitus and multiple sclerosis. In both cases, T cells react with normal host antigens to launch an inflammatory response that results in destruction of normal tissue.

Organ transplantation is also associated with Type IV reactions. T lymphocytes of the organ recipient recognize foreign antigens on the cells of the donated organ. CD8 cells mature into cytotoxic T lymphocytes and initiate the release of cytokines that mediate the inflammatory response. CD4 cells release cytokines that lead to increased vessel permeability and promote the local accumulation of lymphocytes and macrophages, all of which begin the process of breaking down the foreign grafted tissue. When uncontrolled, the tissue damage will lead to eventual rejection of the grafted or transplanted organ.

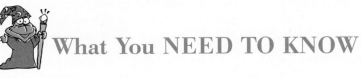

What You NEED TO KNOW

Clinical Manifestations

Symptoms of a Type IV reaction are highly variable depending on the body system that is affected and the nature of the exposure. Because this reaction is delayed, identifying the triggering factor can be difficult.

Sensitizing agents that are inhaled by susceptible individuals can cause respiratory and upper airway symptoms, such as wheezing, coughing, and shortness of breath. Repeated, prolonged exposures can lead to chronic respiratory symptoms.

Prognosis

The prognosis for recovery from a Type IV reaction depends on the nature of the exposure and the severity and duration of the damage imposed to organs by the reaction. Contact dermatitis, one example of this type of reaction, is usually readily treated through the removal or avoidance of the causative agent.

Hypersensitivity involving the respiratory system is more problematic. Particularly after prolonged exposure, patients can develop chronic, disabling lung disease that leaves them unable to work, dependent on others for care, and with a shortened life expectancy because of eventual respiratory failure.

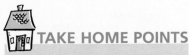

TAKE HOME POINTS

Prolonged exposure to the causative substance can cause irreversible structural changes in an organ, resulting in diseases such as "black lung," pneumoconiosis, or farmer's lung.

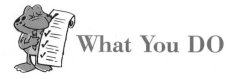

What You DO

Treatment

Treatment modalities for Type IV hypersensitivity reactions are directed toward identifying and removing the causative agent or agents and using pharmacologic measures when necessary to speed the patient's recovery. Antihistamines such as diphenhydramine (Benadryl) and topical and systemic corticosteroid therapy may be indicated.

See Chapters 6B and 7B in RWNSG: *Pharmacology*

Nursing Responsibilities

When dealing with a patient who is experiencing a delayed hypersensitivity reaction, the nurse should:

- Obtain an accurate, detailed history to help identify the source of the problem. Possible sources of the reaction include chemicals, aerosolized cleaning compounds, cosmetics, and plant toxins.
- Implement treatment modalities that may include soothing baths, lotions, and ointments for skin involvement, as well as the administration and management of pharmacologic therapy, such as corticosteroids.
- Educate the patient regarding the nature of the allergic reaction. Help the patient develop strategies to avoid the allergic triggers and understand the ways to treat reactions if they occur in the future.

Do You UNDERSTAND?

DIRECTIONS: Unscramble the letters to form diseases or situations related to type 3 hypersensitivity reactions.

_____   _____

(ontcatc istredamti)

_____   _____

(brecluntui etts)

_____   _____

(jircteneo splartnat)

IMMUNODEFICIENCY DISORDERS

This section provides an overview of immunodeficiency diseases, specifically human immunodeficiency virus (HIV) disease, acquired immunodeficiency syndrome (AIDS), and B- and T-cell disorders. Since the identification of the virus that causes AIDS, medical research has made significant strides in understanding of the immune system and its role in maintaining health and normal function.

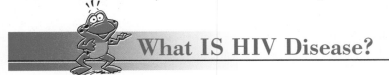

What IS HIV Disease?

AIDS is the result of infection by one of two retroviruses: HIV Type 1 or HIV Type 2. These viruses selectively attack and destroy cells within the immune system. A person infected with either of these viruses is said to be "HIV positive," meaning that they have contracted the virus. HIV disease is a chronic illness that can either be asymptomatic or manifest itself with a wide variety of symptoms. Characteristics of this disease include profound immunosuppression, opportunistic infections, cancers, and neurologic dysfunction. Patients who are infected with HIV experience the gradual destruction of their immune system. New drug therapies have delayed the progression of the disease and offer hope of an eventual cure.

See Chapter 1B in
RWNSG: _Pharmacology_

Pathogenesis

HIV tends to gravitate to certain types of cells within the body, including a type of lymphocyte called CD4 cells and macrophages **(helper-inducer cells or T4 lymphocytes)**. These cells play a vital role in maintaining normal immune function. In the healthy individual, these cells are responsible for initiating the immune response. After these helper-inducer cells recognize foreign antigens and infected cells, they stimulate B lymphocytes to produce antibodies, mobilize phagocytic cells, and influence cell-mediated immunity.

HIV is attracted to protein molecules on the surface of CD4 cells and is also capable of infecting macrophages, monocytes, and dendritic cells. HIV is covered with a protein called gp120. This protein envelope binds to the CD4 receptor. The virus then enters the host's cells and uses an enzyme to copy its own RNA into the host cell's DNA. Depending on the type of cell infected, the infected cell may then enter a dormant phase or release the virus into the blood stream where it infects other cells. Early in the disease process, HIV colonizes lymphoid tissue, particularly the spleen and lymph nodes. These areas are reservoirs for infected cells. The virus may then continue to replicate, killing the CD4 cells, thereby promoting the spread of the infection.

Patients with HIV also suffer from abnormal B-cell function and are unable to mount an antibody response to a new antigen. Impairments in humoral immunity cause people with HIV to be at risk for infections caused by *Streptococcal pneumoniae* and *Haemophilus influenzae*. Overall, patients with HIV are susceptible to a wide variety of infections, many of which cause no significant mortality or morbidity in patients with normal immune systems. Because these infections rarely occur in the healthy population, but are relatively common in patients with HIV, many of these infections are considered to be diagnostic indicators.

Because HIV generates billions of viral particles on a daily basis, the virus ultimately wins the battle against the host's immune defenses. In most cases, the CD4 count will gradually decline and the viral load in the host's blood gradually increases. As the CD4 count decreases and virus count rises, patients experience more symptoms associated with AIDS.

In nearly all cases, the progression of HIV infection is a reflection of the host's immunologic status. Most individuals infected with HIV experience phases of the infection, as summarized in the following table.

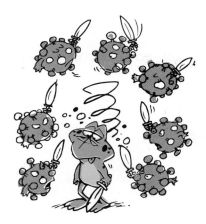

Phases of HIV Infection

PHASE	SYMPTOMS	PHYSIOLOGIC EVENTS	CD4 COUNT
Early	Fever, sore throat, myalgias, fatigue, weight loss, enlargement of cervical lymph nodes	Increased levels of viral production, viremia, seeding of lymphoid tissues	Normal
Middle	May be asymptomatic or have minor troublesome opportunistic infections May also develop persistent generalized lymphadenopathy	Immune system intact, especially when virus is clinically latent	Normal
Crisis	Persistent fever, fatigue, weight loss, diarrhea Onset of opportunistic infections, cancers, and neurologic disorders	Failure of host defenses against virus	< 500

Some individuals with HIV disease appear to have a nonprogressive form and remain asymptomatic for 10 years or more with stable CD4 counts. Untreated, most individuals with HIV infection progress to AIDS within 7 to 10 years.

At-Risk Populations

Transmission of HIV has been clearly proven to be via the exchange of body fluids. High-risk behaviors include:

- Unprotected sexual intercourse with multiple partners, or with one partner who has engaged in high-risk behavior, such as sharing needles for intravenous drug use, or unprotected sexual intercourse with others. Studies indi-

Risk of contracting HIV is not limited to any specific socioeconomic group or ethnic population, but rather by high-risk behaviors and situations.

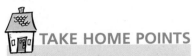

Perinatal transmission occurs from an infected mother to her fetus. Transmission is thought to occur either in utero, during labor and delivery, or by breast-feeding after birth.

TAKE HOME POINTS

- Overall, people with coexisting sexually transmitted diseases (STDs) are at an increased risk for transmitting HIV, particularly when the STD causes genital ulceration.
- Tears and saliva have not been proven to transmit the virus.
- In the United States, 58% of AIDS cases are among homosexual men, 6% are traced to heterosexual contact, and 32% are among people who inject drugs.

⚠ **All patients must be treated as potential carriers of HIV.**

cate that rectal intercourse conveys a greater risk of transmission to the receptive partner, likely because of the increased probability of damage to the rectal mucosa. In heterosexual intercourse, male-to-female transmission is more common than is female-to-male transmission.

- Transfusions of blood and blood products before 1985, before the advent of routine screening for the AIDS virus in blood donors.
- Accidental exposure to contaminated blood in the health care setting.

Because a small number of health care workers have contracted the AIDS virus through occupational exposure, the Centers for Disease Control and Prevention (CDC) recommends that universal blood and body fluid precautions be used for all patients within the health care setting.

The Occupational Safety and Health Administration (OSHA) has also mandated that personal protective garb, including latex gloves, face masks, eye shields, and water-proof gowns, must be made available to all health care workers when necessary.

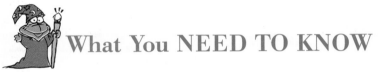

What You NEED TO KNOW

Clinical Manifestations

AIDS is not a single isolated disease process; rather, it is a syndrome with a wide variety of symptoms. During the period of initial infection, some patients experience flulike symptoms from 2 to 8 weeks after the initial exposure. These symptoms include fever, chills, headache, arthralgia, vomiting, diarrhea, sore throat, and rash. During this period, an accelerated rate of viral replication occurs, which may temporarily lower the CD4 count. Within several weeks, the body's immune system is able to suppress viral replication.

This initial infection begins a period of latency that may last 7 to 10 years before other symptoms occur. In some cases, patients experience persistent generalized swelling of the lymph nodes (lymphadenopathy). Two or more sets of lymph nodes in different locations in the body may remain chronically swollen and painful for 3 months or more. During the period of latency, the CD4 cells gradually decrease. Eventually, the individual becomes susceptible to opportunistic infections and malignancies, most of which are rare in the healthy individual.

With progressive impairment in the immune system, the typical adult patient presents with malnutrition, weight loss, diarrhea, and gastroenteritis. Infections that attack the mucosal lining of the gastrointestinal system impair the functioning of the gastrointestinal tract, causing profuse, watery diarrhea that can lead to a fluid loss of several liters per day. The herpes simplex virus and cytomegalovirus can cause ulcerations beginning in the mouth and extend all the way to the anus. These viral infections cause severe pain and interfere with normal digestive processes. Candida infections of the mouth and esophagus can cause difficulty eating and swallowing, leading to further weight loss and malnutrition.

Other symptoms can involve the respiratory tract. Early complaints include a persistent dry cough and progressive shortness of breath during exertion.

Pneumocystis carinii is a common organism found both in soil and in living spaces that does not cause illness in people with a normal immune system. In people with suppressed immune systems, this organism multiplies rapidly and causes pneumonia.

Central nervous system (CNS) abnormalities are present in many AIDS patients. These symptoms can be the consequence of secondary infections from organisms such as *Toxoplasma gondii*, or may be a result of the effects of the retrovirus on the CNS. Progressive multifocal leukoencephalopathy is a condition found in people with AIDS that causes a loss of the myelin covering of the nerves in the CNS. Lesions in the brain can cause dementia, blindness, and paralysis. Few people with this condition survive more than 1 year.

AIDS dementia complex has been identified as a neurologic syndrome associated with HIV. Symptoms of this disorder include a gradual decrease in cognitive function, changes in behavior, impaired concentration and memory, and social withdrawal.

People with AIDS also tend to have a higher incidence of certain malignant tumors, some of which are considered to be indicator diseases for the diagnosis of AIDS. Malignancies that are frequently present in the AIDS population include Kaposi's sarcoma, rapidly progressive cervical carcinoma, non-Hodgkin's lymphoma, and primary CNS lymphoma.

Prognosis

Although a small percentage of individuals who are HIV positive have been identified as having nonprogressive forms of the disease, AIDS is nonetheless considered to be a terminal disease. Recent advances in the field of antiretroviral therapy have allowed many people with AIDS to experience a complete regression of symptoms and live normal lives, although they continue to harbor the virus and can transmit it to others.

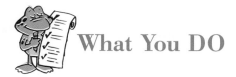

What You DO

Treatment

Currently, the goal of therapy for HIV disease is to decrease replication of the virus. Several different antiretroviral agents combine to accomplish this task. Properly taken, these drugs can suppress the virus to clinically nondetectable levels. The therapy itself can pose many problems for HIV patients.

Combination drug therapy can be extremely costly and is frequently difficult for patients to obtain. Paying the cost of medical care is a significant concern for AIDS patients, because they are frequently unable to work because of their illness and, consequently, may have no health insurance benefits. Additionally, combination drug therapy has many side effects that cause some patients to be noncompliant with their medication regimen. The other goal of treatment is to provide prompt aggressive therapy for secondary diseases and complications associated with HIV.

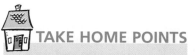

TAKE HOME POINTS

- The person with immunocompromise from AIDS is susceptible to unusual diseases and infections, including toxoplasmosis, systemic histoplasmosis, rare malignancies, and neurologic deterioration.
- AIDS is a terminal disease that is transmitted by the exchange of body fluids.
- The average life expectancy of the person with AIDS is 7 to 10 years.

Without treatment, the chances are 35% that the child of a mother infected with HIV disease will develop AIDS by age 5. Children with HIV disease respond well to highly active antiretroviral therapy and may have a better response to therapy than do adults. Complications associated with pediatric HIV include cognitive dysfunction and cardiac abnormalities.

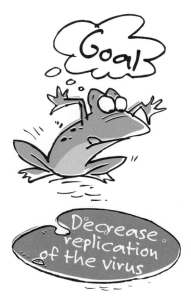

See Chapter 1B in
RWNSG: *Pharmacology*

⚠ **Antiretroviral agents must be taken correctly and on a tightly fixed schedule to obtain maximal therapeutic benefit.**

⚠ **Immunocompromise renders patients with AIDS extremely vulnerable, and they experience a high rate of mortality, particularly when timely treatment for complications of AIDS is not implemented promptly.**

Nursing Responsibilities

The nurse's role in caring for the patient with HIV is two-fold. The nurse must:

- Prevent the spread of HIV to uninfected people.
- Help patients with HIV achieve and maintain an optimal level of health for as long as possible

In view of the pandemic proportions of HIV infection, the general public must be educated in detail about measures to prevent the spread of the virus, but without inspiring fear to the extent that HIV-positive individuals are shunned, stigmatized, or isolated from the rest of society.

When caring for people with HIV, the nurse must design and implement a series of interventions that are tailored to meet the specific needs of the individual throughout the course of the illness. Extensive education forms a core component of care for the patient with HIV. Most patients experience a state of shock and despair after they have been informed of their HIV-positive status. These individuals will require extensive emotional support, guidance, and counseling from the entire health care team.

Information about the implications of their illness must be carefully provided when the individuals indicate they are ready to receive it. Even then, the nurse must be prepared to reinforce information with multiple repetitions and written literature. Severe emotional distress can impair the ability of the individual to recall and use vital information. Patient education must include the following:

 Measures to prevent spreading the disease:
- Avoid sharing needles.
- Use barrier precautions to prevent the exchange of body secretions during intercourse.
- Refrain from donating blood in the presence of high-risk behaviors or possible exposure to HIV.

 Provide detailed information on treatment regimens, such as how to self-administer medications appropriately.

 Reduce co-factors that may contribute to immune compromise:
- Protein-calorie malnutrition
- Pregnancy
- Stress
- Alcohol
- Intravenous and recreational drug use

 Manage side effects associated with treatments and medications.

 Teach self-care measures to minimize disease-related symptoms, such as wasting and malnutrition.

 Prevent opportunistic infection:
- Avoid contact with organisms found in soil, water, and human and animal feces.
- Adhere to food safety precautions.
- Encourage careful washing of produce.
- Avoid raw or undercooked eggs.

- Avoid nonpasteurized dairy products.
- Avoid raw meats or seafood.
- Teach hand-washing precautions.
- Provide chemoprophylaxis against *P. carinii*, cytomegalovirus, *T. gondii*
- Provide skills to cope with body image changes.
- Provide information where to obtain counseling, legal advice, and psychosocial support.
- Teach signs and symptoms that indicate the need to seek medical intervention.

Careful monitoring and evaluation for AIDS-associated complications must be carried out with each patient contact. Fever, cough, shortness of breath, weight loss, changes in mental status are all potential indications of secondary diseases that must be addressed promptly to maximize the patient's chances for survival.

Nurses caring for patients with HIV and AIDS must also be prepared to cope with the emotional and social implications. For many people, this disease carries a great deal of shame and stigma. Patients may have been rejected by friends and family because of their sexual orientation, or they may have hidden their sexual orientation and now suffer severe depression and isolation because they are separated from a partner during their illness. Extensive and compassionate emotional support must be provided for this population.

Do You UNDERSTAND?

DIRECTIONS: **Choose the correct answer to each of the following questions, and write the corresponding letter in the spaces provided.**

_____ 1. Which one of the following are stimulated by CD4 cells to produce antibodies?
    a. Monocyte
    b. Neutrophil
    c. T lymphocyte
    d. B lymphocyte

_____ 2. Which one of the following is a sign and symptom of AIDS dementia?
    a. Cognitive impairment
    b. Loss of short-term memory only
    c. Hyperactivity
    d. Gait disturbances

_____ 3. A patient with AIDS has shown sudden changes in his physical status and behavior, including declining ability to perform simple tasks, such as cooking a meal or personal hygiene and grooming. Other symptoms include poor coordination and lethargy. Which one of the following is a possible cause of these changes?
    a. CNS infection
    b. CNS lymphoma
    c. Multifocal leukoencephalopathy
    d. All of the above

HIV/AIDS Treatment Information Service (ATIS)
Provides information in English and Spanish about federally approved treatment guidelines for HIV and AIDS
http://www.hivatis.org
AIDSmeds.com
Contains complete and easy-to-read information on the treatment of HIV and AIDS
http://www.aidsmeds.com
Journal of the American Medical Association (JAMA)
HIV/AIDS Information Center
http://www.ama-assn.org/special/hiv/
National AIDS Treatment Advocacy Project
Dedicated to informing the HIV-positive population about the latest HIV treatment and advocating on the treatment and policy issues for people with HIV
http://www.natap.org/

Answers: 1. d; 2. a; 3. d.

_____ 4. The AIDS virus is more likely to be transmitted in the presence of which of the following?
a. Dry, chapped skin
b. Genital ulcerations
c. Preexisting illness
d. Other infections

_____ 5. The period of latency for HIV infection usually ends within which timeframe?
a. 2 to 5 years
b. 5 to 7 years
c. 7 to 10 years
d. None of the above

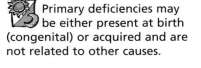 Primary deficiencies may be either present at birth (congenital) or acquired and are not related to other causes.

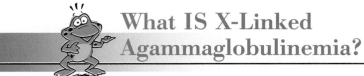

What IS X-Linked Agammaglobulinemia?

X-linked agammaglobulinemia is a recessive genetic disorder that affects primarily men. This condition is passed on from a mother who is a carrier of the gene to her son. Few or no B cells in the blood or lymphoid tissue is a characteristic of this disorder. Lymph nodes are extremely small and tonsils never develop. Because B lymphocytes are needed to produce antibodies, the blood of these people usually contains no IgA, IgM, IgD, or IgE, and extremely small amounts of IgG.

Pathogenesis

Symptoms do not typically appear until after 6 to 12 months of age because of initial protection conveyed by maternal antibodies. After that time, these individuals are vulnerable to a wide range of bacterial infections, particularly of the upper respiratory tract, ears, conjunctiva, CNS, and skin.

At-Risk Populations

Any individual with a family history of immune deficiency disorders has a potential for inheriting this disorder.

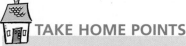 **TAKE HOME POINTS**

This disorder is present predominantly in young men because it is an x-linked recessive trait that is transmitted on the X chromosome. Females do not inherit the recessive traits of the maternal X chromosome unless the paternal Y chromosome contains the same recessive trait; this is highly unusual.

Any infant or young child suffering from persistent infections should be evaluated for possible immunodeficiency disorders, particularly in the presence of a positive family history.

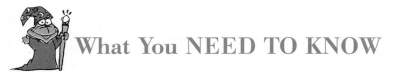

What You NEED TO KNOW

Clinical Manifestations

Signs and symptoms of this disorder include a pattern of recurrent, severe bacterial infections, particularly of the ears, lungs, CNS, conjunctiva, and skin. Patients tend to respond poorly to antibiotics and require prolonged extensive therapy.

Prognosis

Without treatment, these individuals die at an early age of overwhelming infection. Even with treatment, survival beyond adolescence or early adulthood is rare. If children with X-linked agammaglobulinemia survive to adulthood, tissue damage and inflammation from repeated infections can leave them with arthritis in the large joints.

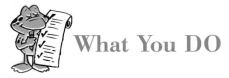

What You DO

Treatment

To date, no cure is available, and treatment is directed toward prevention of infection and aggressive therapy with antimicrobials when infection occurs.

Treatment includes giving intravenous gamma globulin to convey short-term passive immunity, prophylactic antibiotic therapy, chest physical therapy to maintain respiratory function, and periodic x-rays of the chest and sinuses to detect infection while in the early stages.

Nursing Responsibilities

Similar to caring for any immunocompromised patient, thorough, comprehensive physical assessments must be carried out on a routine basis to detect infection in the early stages when it is most readily treated.

- Inspect the conjunctiva for redness and drainage, and be prepared to send any drainage to the laboratory for a culture and sensitivity, particularly when it is purulent or dark colored.
- Examine for evidence of otitis media. Very young children may pull at their ears and be inconsolable when suffering pain from otitis media.
- Check for a runny nose and cough, which can be evidence of a sinus infection.
- Evaluate for increased respiratory rate or decreased or abnormal breath sounds, which may be observed in the patient with respiratory involvement.
- Inspect the skin and nails carefully for rashes or lesions. Remember to use a comb to part the patient's hair to help assess the scalp.

Many children with X-linked agammaglobulinemia die of infection before their sixth birthday.

TAKE HOME POINTS

- A deficiency of B cells characterizes X-linked agammaglobulinemia, which leads to a deficiency or lack of antibodies.
- Transmission occurs from a mother to her son.
- Signs and symptoms of this disorder include recurrent severe bacterial infections that are frequently slow to respond to treatment.
- Treatment includes prevention of infection and prompt aggressive treatment of infection when it occurs.

Children with this disorder are prone to many complications, including chronic sinus and pulmonary disease, autoimmune disease, leukemia, and lymphoma.

Evaluate the infant or child for changes in behavior, eating patterns, irritability, and decreases in activity.

Monitor vital signs for changes indicative of infection, particularly temperatures of 100.5° F or more. Infection requires immediate aggressive treatment. Never wait to report fever or symptoms of infection in an immunocompromised individual.

For the older child, teach good hand-washing practices after using the bathroom.

- Design a plan of care to minimize the risk of infection. For these patients, a private room is medically necessary whenever they are hospitalized. In an in-patient setting:
  - Post signs on the patient's room reminding staff and visitors with contagious illnesses, such as colds or influenza to avoid direct contact.
  - Observe strict medical asepsis and good hand washing with each patient contact.
  - Administer antibiotics and antimicrobials on time as ordered.
- Teach the patient's caregiver the precautions to prevent infection and minimize sources of infection in the home environment.
- Protect the patient from injury to the skin whenever possible; direct contact with people with contagious illnesses in the home environment must be avoided.
- Inform patients and caregiver that pets might have to be removed from the home to decrease exposure to pathogens.
- Remind the parents of an affected child to maintain safe food handling and storage practices to decrease the risk of food-borne illnesses.
- Provide caregivers with written and verbal information on signs and symptoms of infection that indicate the need to seek medical attention. Help the parents and child develop positive coping mechanisms that will bolster the integrity of the family and improve their ability to cope with a potentially life-threatening condition.

Do You UNDERSTAND?

DIRECTIONS: Choose the correct answer to each of the following questions, and write the corresponding letter in the spaces provided.

_____ 1. Patients with X-lined agammaglobulinemia are susceptible to which one of the following?
   a. Viral infections
   b. Bacterial infections
   c. Fungal infections
   d. Protozoan infections

_____ 2. Intravenous gamma globulin may be given for which one of the following?
   a. Provide short-term passive immunity
   b. Treat active infection
   c. Prevent the development of infection
   d. a and c only

_____ 3. Signs and symptoms of infection in the infant include which one of the following?
   a. Changes in behavior
   b. Changes in eating and sleeping patterns
   c. Crying and fussiness
   d. All of the above

Answers: 1. b; 2. d; 3. d.

_____ 4. Which one of the following nursing interventions decrease the risk of infection?
  a. Maintaining meticulous hand-washing precautions
  b. Maintaining medical asepsis
  c. Prohibiting contact with people carrying contagious illnesses
  d. All of the above

What IS DiGeorge Syndrome?

DiGeorge syndrome (congenital thymic hypoplasia) is an autosomal-dominant genetic condition. The term syndrome indicates a pattern of features that tend to occur together. Depending on the amount of thymic tissue that is present, these patients can have varying degrees of T-cell dysfunction.

Pathogenesis

DiGeorge syndrome is the consequence of an error in development of the thymus in utero. T-cell deficiency varies depending on the extent to which the thymus is adversely affected.

Because the parathyroid glands and the structures of the face are derived from the same site in utero, problems with hypocalcemia and facial deformities may develop, including a cleft palate.

This disorder is the result of deletion of a genetic segment on the long arm of chromosome 22 and may now be detected by genetic testing.

At-Risk Populations

Because this disorder can arise spontaneously and is present at birth, identifying those who are at risk for this disorder is nearly impossible. Potential parents who are aware of a family history of genetic disorders, particularly disorders involving the immune system, should be referred to a geneticist for testing and evaluation.

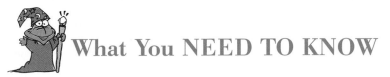

What You NEED TO KNOW

Clinical Manifestations

In some cases, malformations of the heart may be observed, including Tetralogy of Fallot, ventricular septal defect, and malformations of the aortic arch. Hypoparathyroidism may be present, which leads to low levels of the parathyroid hormone and subsequent hypocalcemia and hyperphosphatemia.

Varying degrees of T-cell deficiency may be present, resulting in persistent infections. As these children grow, they may experience developmental delay with a small stature and have both learning difficulties and emotional and behavioral problems.

DiGeorge syndrome
http://www3.ncbi.nlm.nih.gov/htbin-post/Omim/dispmim?188400

Children with severe T-cell dysfunction are susceptible to bacterial, viral, and fungal infections. Infants with an extremely small but functional thymus may initially have problems with T-cell function but usually have normal function by the age of 5 years.

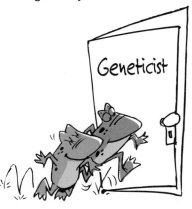

Velo-cardio Facial Syndrome Educational Foundation
http://vx4.cs.hscsyr.edu/~vcfsef/home.html

Answer: 4. d.

Children with this disorder tend to have characteristic facial features, including widely set eyes, low-set ears, and a shortened upper lip. Particularly during infancy, these children may have extremely small heads (microcephaly).

TAKE HOME POINTS

- DiGeorge syndrome is the consequence of an error in development of the thymus in utero.
- Patients with DiGeorge syndrome may have varying degrees of immune dysfunction, as well as abnormalities in facial appearance and cardiac malformations.
- Patients with DiGeorge syndrome may have short stature, delayed physical development, and learning disabilities.
- Hypoparathyroidism may result in hypocalcemia.

See Chapter 11 in
RWNSG: *Pharmacology*

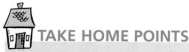
TAKE HOME POINTS

- Patients with T-cell dysfunction are at risk for graft-versus-host disease.
- When T cells in grafted tissue (e.g., transfused blood) are mature, they may attack and destroy the host's tissues.

Prognosis

Depending on the severity of the physical problems associated with this syndrome and access to appropriate medical care, patients with DiGeorge syndrome can live to adulthood. Metabolic abnormalities such as hypocalcemia require correction. Cardiac anomalies may require surgical intervention. Immunodeficiency states will require prompt aggressive treatment of infection, as discussed in the section on X-linked agammaglobulinemia.

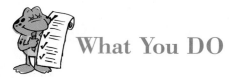 # What You DO

Treatment

Calcium supplementation must be implemented promptly to prevent tetany and seizures. All patients who have other clinical features suggestive of this disorder should be screened for cardiac defects. When present, depending on the nature of these defects, on-going medical care or surgical intervention may be required. Investigations of transplantation of thymus tissue in young infants with severely depleted T-cell function have been carried out. Preliminary research indicates that early transplantation of the thymus before infections arise can provide immune reconstitution for some patients with this syndrome.

Nursing Responsibilities

For the patient with an immunodeficient state, primary emphasis is placed on prevention and early detection of infections. Remember that defective T-cell function can lead to inadequate function of B cells, because properly functioning T cells are required to initiate certain aspects of B-cell activity.

Because this disorder can potentially affect many aspects of health, the nurse must:
- Coordinate and organize care provided by many different disciplines, such as cardiology, infectious disease specialists, and speech pathologists.
- Design a plan of care to meet the unique needs of that patient in the most efficient and timely possible manner.
- Provide parents of the child who are dealing with a new diagnosis of a genetic disease the opportunity to grieve for the loss of the hoped-for "perfect child" and a quiet private environment in which they may express their concerns and fears. Parents of a child with this disorder can feel overwhelmed by guilt and blame themselves because the syndrome arises from a genetic defect. Parents must deal with their loss and disappointment to be effective caregivers, particularly when the child has multiple medical problems.

One of the nurse's most important roles is to support the child's parents' ability to be competent parents. Topics to address for patient and family education include:
- Prevention of infection
- Signs and symptoms of infection

- Growth and developmental milestones
- Need for early assessment for learning disabilities
- Need for ongoing medical care and evaluation

Parents may also obtain important information and emotional support from networking with other parents of children with similar health problems.

Do You UNDERSTAND?

DIRECTIONS: **Complete the sentences using words from the list below. Not all words will be used.**

1. DiGeorge syndrome is caused by errors in development of the _____ gland.
2. Physical characteristics commonly present with DiGeorge syndrome include _____, short _____, and short upper lip.
3. _____ supplementation should be implemented promptly to prevent tetany and seizures.

calcium	pituitary	thymus
microcephaly	stature	vitamin

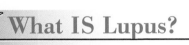

SECTION C
AUTOIMMUNE DISORDERS

Disturbances in the immune system can result in a variety of complications, including the development of autoimmune diseases. Generally, a disease is considered to be autoimmune when the body creates autoantibodies and T-cell activity against the host tissue. This section provides an overview of systemic lupus erythematosus (SLE), one of the more commonly occurring autoimmune diseases. Two other diseases are also discussed—scleroderma and Sjögren's syndrome. These conditions can occur in conjunction with lupus or appear separately.

What IS Lupus?

SLE (lupus) is a chronic, progressive inflammatory disease that is characterized by periods of exacerbation and remission of symptoms. Discoid lupus erythematosus tends to involve only the skin and generally does not affect the internal organs. SLE can eventually affect not only the skin, but also internal organs, including the kidneys, joints, lungs, heart, CNS, and gastrointestinal tract.

SLE occurs most common-ly in women between the ages of 20 and 40, although it has been diagnosed in both young children and older individuals.

African-American women have three times the inci-dence of lupus than do Caucasian women. In this population, the disease tends to develop at a younger age and have a higher rate of serious complications and mortality than it does in other ethnic groups.

Pathogenesis

Lupus develops because the body forms antibodies to its own normal healthy tissue (autoantibodies), including erythrocytes, coagulation proteins, lymphocytes, and platelets. These antibodies react with the patient's tissues and lead to the formation of immune complexes. Immune complexes are accumulations of antigens and their corresponding antibodies. These immune complexes leave the circulation and may be deposited in capillaries, joints, skin, and internal organs in which they initiate an immune response. The severity of the disease is thought to be a reflection of the degree of immune response initiated by the immune complexes.

The cause of this disease is unknown. Research suggests that the development of autoantibodies may be a result of many different factors, including genetic traits, hormonal influences, and immunologic and environmental factors. Environmental influences include exposure to chemicals, ultraviolet light, certain foods, and infectious agents. The tendency of certain drugs to invoke a lupuslike reaction in susceptible individuals is well documented. Drug-induced lupus is most commonly observed with procainamide, isoniazid, hydralazine, and D-penicillamine. Contrary to the primary form of the disease, drug-induced lupus usually goes into complete remission when the causative agents are eliminated.

At-Risk Populations

SLE occurs most commonly in women between the ages of 20 and 40, although it has been diagnosed in both young children and elderly individuals.

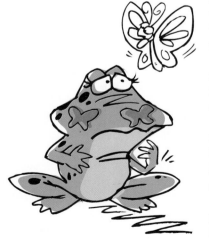

What You NEED TO KNOW

Clinical Manifestations

Lupus has been called "the great pretender" because of the ability to mimic many other diseases and is consequently frequently misdiagnosed. One of the few "classic" symptoms of lupus is a red, butterfly-shaped rash that covers the nose and cheeks.

Less commonly observed symptoms involving the skin include mottled redness on the sides of the palms and the fingers, redness and swelling around the fingernails, and bruises (purpura). Approximately 40% of patients with lupus are sensitive to the sun.

The majority of lupus patients experience joint pain and arthritislike symptoms at some time over the course of the disease. The arthritis associated with lupus rarely causes joint destruction, but complications such as osteonecrosis, local heat and swelling, stiffness, joint pain, and ulnar deviation of the fingers are frequently present.

Other symptoms include persistent fevers and malaise (in the absence of proven infections), vascular headaches, seizures, and psychoses. Symptoms involving connective tissue can include arthritis-like joint pain that is occasionally present for years before other evidence of the disease appears. Renal compromise can appear at any time over the course of the disease, even when other symptoms of lupus are absent.

Over one half of patients with lupus experience skin changes that may potentially cause pain, itching, and scarring. The facial butterfly rash characteristic of lupus can range from faint redness to severe eruptions and scaling. Ulcerations may also develop in the mucosa, and scalp hair loss occurs in up to one half of lupus patients. Severe itching can occur with lupus skin lesions.

Pericarditis, myocarditis, and vasculitis are frequently part of the disease process. Vascular abnormalities cause the patient to have an increased risk of venous and arterial blood clots (arteria thromboses) in the extremities. Complaints of chest pain that worsens with deep inspirations (pleuritic chest pain) are believed to be a result of inflammation of the pleural lining. These abnormalities can result in decreased cardiac function, impaired gas exchange, and poor tissue perfusion.

Most lupus patients have asymptomatic renal damage as a consequence of their disease. Less than one half of lupus patients have clinically detectable renal disease. Potential warning signs include nausea and vomiting, pruritus, anorexia, facial swelling, weight gain, edema of the lower extremities, breathlessness, cough, proteinuria, nocturia, and urinary frequency.

Neurologic changes secondary to lupus are common and can vary in severity. Cerebrovascular accidents occur in approximately 15% of patients, and up to 20% of patients develop seizure disorders. Cranial and peripheral neuropathies can limit self-care ability and have a significant effect on quality of life. Cognitive impairment can also occur.

Prognosis

The outcome of lupus is highly variable and depends on the severity of the disease, the degree of organ damage, and the presence of drug-induced complications. Patients who require long-term immunosuppressive drug therapy to control lupus are at an increased risk for malignancies and complications associated with infection. Chronic long-term use of corticosteroids can lead to coronary artery disease, diabetes, osteoporosis, and aseptic necrosis of the bones. When the initial acute phase of the disease is adequately controlled and the patient has access to health care, the long-term prognosis is usually good, with greater than 95% surviving 10 years after diagnosis.

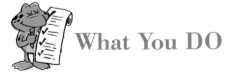 What You DO

Treatment

Mild or sporadic flares of lupus may require little or no treatment. Body aches can be controlled with nonsteroidal antiinflammatory drugs (NSAIDS), and judicious use of aspirin can be helpful. Antimalarial drugs such as Plaquenil can be given to decrease the inflammatory response.

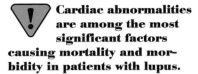 **Cardiac abnormalities are among the most significant factors causing mortality and morbidity in patients with lupus.**

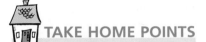 Myocardial infarctions secondary to atherosclerosis has been observed in patients under 35 years of age.

TAKE HOME POINTS

- SLE is a chronic autoimmune disease that affects connective tissue and is characterized by periods of exacerbation and remission.
- Lupus is thought to develop as a consequence of antibodies that the body creates against its own healthy tissue.
- The development of lupus has been linked to genetic influences, estrogen, environmental factors, and exposure to drugs.
- Lupus can affect the skin, serous membranes, lungs, heart, joints, muscles, kidneys, and blood-forming system.

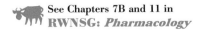 See Chapters 7B and 11 in RWNSG: *Pharmacology*

Corticosteroid therapy is indicated for severe disease to preserve organ function. Generally, combinations of prednisone and immunosuppressive therapy such as azathioprine and cyclophosphamide are used. For patients with coagulopathies, heparin and maintenance therapy with warfarin may be required.

Because of complications associated with long-term corticosteroid and immunosuppressive therapy, medical management is directed toward using the minimal possible dose of either drug required to control symptoms of the disease. After control of symptoms is achieved, corticosteroid doses are gradually decreased by 10% at intervals, the goal being to eliminate steroids completely.

Nursing Responsibilities

Nursing management of the patient with lupus is directed toward controlling adverse symptoms, optimizing overall health, and promoting the patient's ability to cope with the disease. Because the disease has such a wide spectrum of symptoms that may change over time, and because the disease often has periods of exacerbation and remission, the nurse must frequently reassess the patient's status and adjust nursing care and interventions accordingly.

- Conduct and document a baseline neurologic assessment at the time of diagnosis.
- After diagnosis, regularly monitor the patient throughout the course of the disease for evidence of neurologic changes, including abnormalities of the cranial nerves, changes in mental status, depression, and cognitive decline. Symptoms of cognitive decline include confusion, difficulty in understanding abstract concepts, organizing, and solving problems.

Nursing Care of Skin Manifestations
- Conduct a baseline assessment of the skin to evaluate the appearance, severity, and duration of skin lesions.
- Educate the patient regarding skin care measures and avoidance of exposure to ultraviolet (UV) rays from the sun, as well as fluorescent and halogen lights. Warn the patient that glass does not provide complete protection from UV rays. Instruct the patient to use a sunscreen with a sun-protection factor (SPF) of at least 15 or more every time they are exposed to the sun, and advise them to wear protective clothing, such as broad-brimmed hats, long-sleeved shirts, and pants made of fabric capable of blocking UV rays. Hair dyes and over-the-counter creams and lotions can increase photosensitivity, as do certain drugs.

Nursing Care of Musculoskeletal Manifestations
Nursing care is directed toward helping the patient maintain joint function and increasing muscle strength.
- Inform the patient that an inflamed or swollen joint should not bear weight; however, gentle range-of-motion exercises can be helpful to maintain flexibility. A regular exercise plan should be maintained during periods of remission to promote muscle tone and overall fitness.

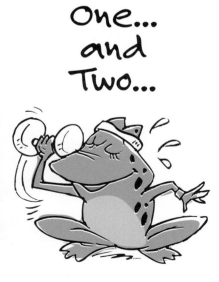

National Institute of Arthritis and Musculoskeletal and Skin Diseases
http://www.nih.gov/niams/
Lupus: A Patient Care Guide for Nurses and Other Health Professionals
http://www.nih.gov/niams/healthinfo/lupusguide/ordrfrm.htm

One...
and
Two...

- Treat pain cautiously with analgesics but only under direct medical supervision.
- Remind the patient not to self-medicate with over-the-counter drugs without obtaining their health care provider's approval.

Nursing Care Associated with Cardiac Involvement

- Conduct a careful physical assessment.
- Monitor for evidence of cardiovascular complications and thrombus formation.
- Teach patients the measures to maintain cardiovascular health, including frequent monitoring of blood pressure, regular aerobic exercise (when not otherwise contraindicated), avoidance of smoking, and the importance of following a diet low in fat and sodium.
- Instruct the patient on the signs and symptoms of cardiac and pulmonary compromise that warrant medical intervention.

Nursing Care Associated with Renal Involvement

- Regularly assess renal function.
- Monitor diagnostic laboratory studies.
- Conduct a periodic evaluation for signs and symptoms of renal compromise.
- Decrease fluid retention and edema.
- Maintain electrolyte balance.
- Institute measures to decrease the risk of infection.
- Instruct the patient with dietary and fluid restrictions on the importance of daily weighing for evidence of fluid retention and on the correct way to measure blood pressure.
- Teach the patient about the signs and symptoms of fluid overload and the point at which to seek medical assistance.

TAKE HOME POINTS

Warm baths or heating pads after arising can help to loosen stiff joints and improve comfort.

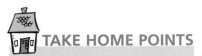

TAKE HOME POINTS

Corticosteroid and immunosuppressive therapy can leave the patient at risk for infections. Teach the patient about the signs and symptoms of urinary tract infection, including frequent urination, urgency, cloudy urine, and incomplete emptying of the bladder. Advise the patient to avoid contact with people having contagious illnesses, such as upper respiratory infections and influenza.

Do You UNDERSTAND?

DIRECTIONS: Choose the correct answer to each of the following questions, and write the corresponding letter in the spaces provided.

_____ 1. When is a disease considered to be autoimmune?
a. B-cell activity against host tissue is present.
b. T-cell activity against host tissue is present.
c. Persistent inflammatory response is present.
d. Macrophage activity is accelerated.

_____ 2. When deposited in tissue, immune complexes tend to do what to an immune response?
a. Initiate
b. Delay
c. Suppress
d. Maintain

_____ 3. The most important aspect of skin care for the patient with lupus involves which of the following?
   a. Keeping the skin moist and lubricated with a protective cream
   b. Using mild soaps
   c. Avoiding over-the-counter skin care preparations
   d. Avoiding exposure to ultraviolet rays

_____ 4. Patients whose lupus is currently in remission should be advised to do which of the following?
   a. Maintain a regular exercise program to improve muscle strength.
   b. Avoid contact with people with contagious illnesses.
   c. Gradually taper doses of corticosteroids.
   d. Avoid stress.

_____ 5. A patient with previously well-controlled lupus notes facial and pedal edema, along with dyspnea on exertion over the last few days. The patient should do which of the following?
   a. Decrease salt and fluid intake.
   b. Elevate the feet.
   c. Take a diuretic.
   d. Notify the physician.

What IS Systemic Sclerosis?

Systemic sclerosis is a term used to describe a disorder that can affect not only the skin, but also most of the internal organs. Previously called scleroderma, this term is now most commonly used when the disorder affects only the skin. Systemic sclerosis is a relatively rare chronic autoimmune condition that is characterized by large deposits of collagen that lead to thickening and fibrosis of the skin, particularly on the hands and face. In some patients, the disease is limited to the skin, but the more severe form can also adversely affect vascular, organ, and immunologic function.

Pathogenesis

Currently, the cause of the abnormal autoimmune process leading to systemic sclerosis is unknown. The exact mechanisms of this disease are also poorly understood. The current consensus is such that systemic sclerosis is the consequence of abnormal inflammatory mechanisms, similar in nature to those that cause lupus. Autoantibodies and abnormal accumulations of T cells cause damage to arterioles. These damaged vessels then leak plasma into the surrounding tissue. Chemical factors are released that lead to the excess production of collagen, a tissue protein. This collagen accumulates and leads to hardness and tightening of the skin. Similar to lupus, this disorder has many different manifestations. Inflammation, fibrosis, and sclerosing of not only the skin, but also the vital organs are all characteristics of progressive systemic sclerosis.

Answers: 3. d; 4. a; 5. d.

At-Risk Populations

No genetic link has been identified, although connective tissue disorders tend to occur more commonly in some families. Some studies suggest that scleroderma may be linked to chemical exposure. Recent research from the Institute of Allergy and Infectious Disease suggests that persistent fetal cells in a woman's circulation may lead to abnormalities in immune regulation.

 Sclerosis is most prevalent among women between the ages of 35 and 54.

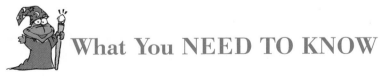

What You NEED TO KNOW

Clinical Manifestations

Presenting symptoms vary from patient to patient and also depend on the stage and type of sclerosis encountered. Typically, patients will have painless edema in both hands and fingers, which can extend to the upper and lower extremities and the face. The skin is taut and shiny. As the disease progresses, the edematous areas become tight, hard, and thickened. Because of decreased elasticity, patients can loose range of motion in joints and develop contractures, occasionally to the extent that they are unable to perform activities of daily living (ADLs) independently. Calcium deposits in the subcutaneous tissue cause small white lumps under the skin that may leak and drain.

When the sclerosis is progressive, this process of hardening and fibrosis can adversely affect internal organs and structures. Disruption of the gastrointestinal tract is common and is manifested by complaints of persistent indigestion, reflux, bloating, and early satiety with meals. Fibrotic changes in the esophagus lead to dysmotility, along with dysphagia and reflux disease. Peristalsis is decreased, which can cause symptoms similar to a small bowel obstruction.

Fibrotic changes in the myocardium may lead to electrocardiogram changes, abnormal heartbeats, chest pain, and heart failure. Most patients experience some degree of compromise in arterial circulation to the hands and feet, causing severe pain and even loss of fingers and toes. When exposed to emotional stress or cold, arterioles in the fingers and toes constrict, causing the digits to become blue, cold, and painful. In severe cases, the tips of the fingers and toes become necrotic. Renal involvement can lead to malignant hypertension and death. Changes in blood pressure may be the first indication of renal compromise.

Symptoms of pulmonary involvement include shortness of breath and a nonproductive cough. Fibrosis of the lung tissue is present in nearly all patients with progressive disease, although many individuals are asymptomatic.

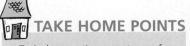 **TAKE HOME POINTS**

- Typical presenting symptoms of sclerosis are painless edema in the hands and fingers and Raynaud's phenomenon.
- Loss of skin elasticity can lead to impaired range of motion in joints and contractures, occasionally to the extent that patients are unable to perform ADLs.

Prognosis

The prognosis for sclerosis is variable, depending on the type of disease and the presence of other co-morbid factors. Most patients with involvement limited to their skin have a good prognosis. However, approximately 10% will gradually develop severe respiratory compromise over a period of approximately 10 to 20 years. Patients with rapidly progressing skin involvement or organ involvement tend to have a poorer prognosis. Currently, slightly more than one half of these patients survive for 10 years or longer.

Involvement of internal organs can lead to severe hypertension, congestive heart failure, and respiratory and renal failure.

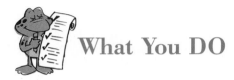

What You DO

Treatment

Unfortunately, no effective therapy for sclerosis is available. Medical care is directed toward control of symptoms and support of organ function. Some alleviation of symptoms has been obtained with drug therapy, specifically immunosuppressive agents, antiinflammatory agents, and some drugs with vasodilation effects. Gastrointestinal agents such as Prevacid, Pepcid, or Prilosec can be used to support and maintain gastrointestinal function.

During the early stages of the disease, patients can benefit from occupational and physical therapy to prevent contractures of the fingers and arms. Rapidly progressive tightening of the skin can cause pressure, pain, and inflammation of underlying muscles and tendons, leading to a painful inflammation of the muscles (myositis). This condition may be improved by the administration of low dose oral steroids.

Nursing Responsibilities

The nurse should:
- Assess all skin surfaces carefully for evidence of circulatory compromise or vasculitic lesions. Treat ulcers and breaks in skin integrity promptly, because poor peripheral circulation will make healing problematic.
- Teach the patient ways to protect their skin in areas with poor circulation. Mild soap, lubricating lotions, and protective gloves and socks should be worn if the patient is able to tolerate the contact against the skin. For cases of severe skin involvement, a bed cradle and/or footboard can be helpful in removing bed linens from sensitive areas.
- Instruct the patient to avoid cold temperatures whenever possible because of the increased risk of vasospasm.
- Advise the patient to avoid tobacco and caffeine because of their vasoconstrictive effects.
- Offer the patient with esophageal dysfunction small and frequent meals that are soft and bland.
- Advise patients to avoid foods that are spicy and high in fat and alcohol because these ingredients stimulate the production of gastric acid.
- Teach the patient to keep the head elevated for at least 2 hours after eating. Histamine antagonists can be beneficial for some patients to decrease production of gastric acid.
- Monitor the patient on an ongoing basis for signs and symptoms of organ involvement. Changes in blood pressure, cardiovascular, pulmonary, and renal status should be reported to the health care provider immediately.

See Chapters 1C, 7B, 8A, and 11 in
RWNSG: *Pharmacology*

Because of the toxic effects of many drugs used to treat sclerosis, careful medical monitoring and frequent diagnostic testing is indicated to detect adverse effects before damage is severe or irreversible.

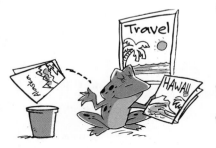

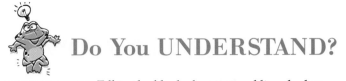

Do You UNDERSTAND?

DIRECTIONS: **Fill in the blanks by unscrambling the letters.**

1. The most common symptom of sclerosis is _____ of the skin. (*chengtinik*)
2. Sclerosis is thought to be the result of damage to _____. (*triolesare*)
3. A patient with sclerosis complains of new difficulties with dysphagia, bloating, and indigestion after eating. This patient is most likely experiencing _____. (*tarestalingsotin*)
4. Precautions to maintain _____ is one of the most important education topics for patients with sclerosis. (*inks triginety*)

What IS Sjögren's Syndrome?

Sjögren's syndrome (SS) is a progressive, incurable autoimmune disorder that is characterized by dry eyes and dry mouth (keratoconjunctivitis sicca [KCS] and xerostomia). SS can occur as an isolated disorder, or it can be present in association with other autoimmune diseases, such as rheumatoid arthritis or lupus. This disease affects primarily the tear glands and salivary glands, although it may occasionally affect other exocrine glands, including those lining the vagina or the respiratory and gastrointestinal tract. SS is the result of abnormal infiltration of the lacrimal and salivary glands with T lymphocytes. The exact cause of this disease is unknown. Some research indicates that viruses may be potential causative agents of this disorder.

Pathogenesis

During the early stages of SS, molecules that attract lymphocytes are released from the venules. T lymphocytes adhere to the venules and migrate into the gland in which they are activated and release interleukin-2 and tumor necrosis factors. Activated B cells in the gland produce antibodies. With progressive infiltration and inflammation of the glandular tissue, glandular function decreases and the patient experiences the characteristic dryness of the mouth, eyes, and vagina that are the chief complaints associated with the disease.

At-Risk Populations

Approximately 90% of people with this disease are women. Most women are diagnosed after menopause, although this disorder can appear in younger women. Approximately 50% of cases occur in conjunction with another autoimmune or connective tissue disorder.

Children of women with this disease have an increased risk of serious cardiac defects.

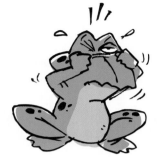

What You NEED TO KNOW

Clinical Manifestations

Patients with SS usually complain of painful, burning dry eyes. Many people will complain of a foreign body sensation when they blink. These symptoms are a result of a decreased volume of flow of tears. For some patients, the corneal dryness is severe to the extent that they have corneal ulcerations.

An additional symptom is a severe dry mouth. The patient may require water to swallow food and may be forced to carry water at all times. Diminished production of saliva can lead to a sore, inflamed tongue; painful, irritated oral mucosa; oral *Candida albicans* infections; and severe dental caries.

This disease can adversely affect any organ in the body. Signs and symptoms of musculoskeletal involvement include arthralgias and myalgias. Other potential sites of organ involvement include the lungs, liver, kidneys, and hematopoietic system. Diagnoses commonly observed with organ involvement include inflammation of the lungs (pneumonitis), biliary cirrhosis, interstitial nephritis, leukopenia, thrombocytopenia, and anemia.

Fatigue is commonly present in conjunction with SS and can be severe and debilitating. In the presence of active immune disease, the fatigue is thought to be a result of the action of cytokines such as IL-1 or tumor necrosis factor (TNF) on the CNS.

Prognosis

In the absence of other diseases or organ involvement, the rate of long-term survival for patients with SS is good. Importantly, however, these patients may suffer multiple complications such as dental and ophthalmic diseases, as well as poor quality of life and persistent prolonged discomfort.

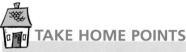
TAKE HOME POINTS

- SS is a progressive, chronic autoimmune disorder that is characterized by dry eyes and dry mouth.
- This disease results from abnormal infiltration of exocrine glands by T lymphocytes.
- Complications of SS include damage to the eyes, periodontal disease, and oral infections.

 Patients with persistent swelling of the parotid or submandibular glands should be carefully evaluated for malignancies. Patients with SS have a greatly increased risk of developing non-Hodgkin's lymphoma, particularly in the lymph nodes of the neck.

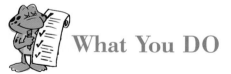
What You DO

Treatment

Management of this disorder is directed primarily toward palliation of distressing symptoms and prevention of complications. Oral dryness may be alleviated with saliva substitutes and oral moisturizers. A variety of solutions are available and have been used with varying degrees of success in different patients. Sialogogues (drugs that stimulate the production of saliva) can also offer some benefit to patients who have some remaining functional salivary glands. Pilocarpine hydrochloride (Salagen) has been shown to be safe and effective for long-term use and has been approved by the U.S. Food and Drug Administration for this purpose.

Nursing Responsibilities

The nurse should:

- Advise patients suffering from dry mouth to drink liquids throughout their waking hours, but avoid caffeinated beverages, such as tea and coffee. Sugarless candy and gum can help stimulate the flow of saliva.
- Warn patients to avoid alcohol and tobacco because these substances can damage delicate oral mucosa.
- Teach the patient to maintain meticulous oral hygiene, avoid acidic foods, and see a dentist at frequent intervals to avoid the high risk of cavities and periodontal disease.
- Recommend using artificial tears to help the treatment of dry eyes. Because of the decreased volume of natural tears, some agents with preservatives can cause increased pain and irritation for the patient with SS. Preservative-free liquid tears are available in single-dose units, which decreases the risk of pathogens growing in the solution. Ocular lubricants can also be helpful at night, but are usually unsuitable for use during waking hours because of their tendency to cloud the vision. A minor surgical procedure that occludes tear drainage, which then allows tears to accumulate and moisten the eyes, can help relieve severe dryness of the eye.

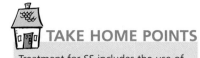

TAKE HOME POINTS

Treatment for SS includes the use of oral and ophthalmic lubricants.

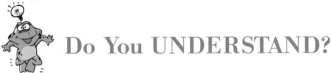

Do You UNDERSTAND?

DIRECTIONS: **Choose the correct answer to each of the following questions, and write the corresponding letter in the spaces provided.**

_____ 1. SS is characterized by which one of the following?
    a. Dry mucous membranes
    b. Weight loss
    c. Fluid retention
    d. Anorexia

_____ 2. Preventive screening measures for all patients with SS include which one of the following?
    a. Testing of stool for occult blood
    b. Evaluation of pulmonary function
    c. Annual colonoscopy
    d. Frequent evaluation for head and neck cancers

_____ 3. A patient with SS has persistent swelling in the left parotid gland. The nurse should do which one of the following?
    a. Apply an ice pack to the area.
    b. Apply a heating pad to the area.
    c. Suggest that the patient take over-the-counter NSAIDS.
    d. Inform the patient's health care provider.

Answers: 1. a; 2. d; 3. d.

_____ 4. Which nursing intervention would not be appropriate for a patient with SS?

    a. Offer the patient saliva substitutes and oral moisturizers.

    b. Advise the patient to use an alcohol-based mouthwash to maintain oral hygiene.

    c. Suggest the patient use gum and hard sugarless candy to stimulate flow of saliva.

    d. Instruct the patient to use liquid tears in single-dose units.

_____ 5. Which foods or beverages should be avoided?

    a. Coffee

    b. Red meats

    c. Milk

    d. Caffeine-free sodas

Answers: 4. b; 5. a.

Neurologic and Neurovascular Systems

CEREBROVASCULAR DISEASE

The nervous system allows humans to interact with and respond to the world around them. Regardless of the cause, dysfunctions in the nervous system can adversely affect the ability to think, reason, predict, or carry out simple activities of daily living.

The central nervous system (CNS) may be considered as the master control system of the body; it allows us to interpret, use and act on the input from our senses, and it helps protect and maintain the integrity and normal function of the body. The nervous system has central and peripheral components. The brain and spinal cord are the major components of the CNS.

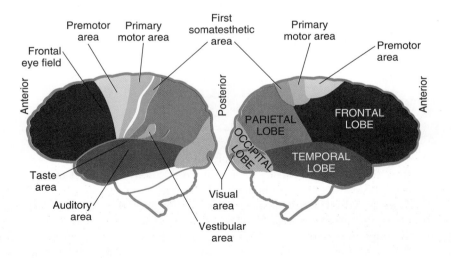

The autonomic nervous system (ANS) is responsible for maintaining and regulating the function of glands and smooth muscles within the body and promoting the coordinated functioning of the visceral organs. The ANS has two subdivisions: the sympathetic and the parasympathetic systems. The sympathetic nervous system is responsible for initiating the protective "fight-or-flight" response when the body is exposed to stress.

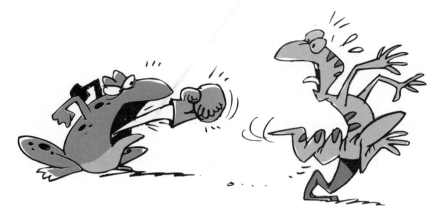

The parasympathetic system transmits impulses to the visceral organs and is responsible for "vegetative" functions of the body that are not under conscious control.

Nerve cells have a limited ability to recover from damage, which is an important consideration when considering the effect of disease and trauma to the CNS. The brain is a delicate organ and requires a constant supply of glucose and oxygen. At any given time, the brain receives 15% of cardiac output (blood ejected by the heart) and consumes 20% of the body's total oxygen requirements. Any event or process that decreases the brain's supply of oxygen and nutrients is a serious threat to the normal integrity and function of the brain and CNS.

What IS a Cerebrovascular Accident?

National Stroke Association
http://www.stroke.org/intro.html
National Institute of Neurologic Disorders and Stroke
http://www.ninds.nih.gov/

Cerebrovascular accidents (CVA) are also called strokes or brain attacks. A stroke occurs when a sudden interruption of blood flow to a part of the brain occurs. A stroke should not be confused with a transient ischemic attack (TIA). A stroke is defined as a neurologic deficit lasting over 24 hours that occurs as a result of interrupted arterial blood flow to a part of the brain. With a stroke, the interruption of oxygen and nutrients to brain cells can cause permanent brain damage and impaired functioning. A TIA is a neurologic deficit that lasts for less than 24 hours. Most TIAs resolve within a few hours, and the patient regains full neurologic functioning.

Pathogenesis

CVAs or brain attacks are the result of disturbance in blood flow to the brain. Various factors can deprive the brain of oxygen and nutrients, causing the brain tissue to become ischemic. Most cerebrovascular damage to the brain is the indirect result of either atherosclerosis or hypertension. Strokes are generally occlusive, embolic, or hemorrhagic in origin.

Occlusive. Atherosclerosis of the vessels in the brain can lead to the gradual narrowing or stenosis of the cerebral arteries, with complete blockage (occlusion) as the ultimate result. Alternatively, fatty plaques can break off into the circulation and form a thrombus in distal cerebral vessels, ultimately causing a blockage.

Hemorrhagic. Hypertension can lead to damage to cerebral vessels and subsequent intracerebral hemorrhage. Bleeding can occur into the ventricular, subdural, or subarachnoid spaces. Other vascular conditions that lead to cerebral hemorrhage include ruptured cerebral aneurysms and arteriovenous malformations (AVM). An aneurysm is an abnormally dilated area or blister on the arterial wall. When subjected to increased pressure from hypertension, the arterial wall becomes progressively thinner, more fragile, and eventually ruptures, allowing blood to leak into the cerebral tissues.

An arteriovenous malformation is a tangle of twisted, abnormally shaped blood vessels that are frequently described as resembling a "nest of worms." These vessels can become abnormally dilated and fragile and frequently leak blood, which can cause a stroke.

Embolic. Cardiovascular conditions such as atrial arrhythmias and recent myocardial infarction can cause clots (emboli) to be released into the systemic circulation in which they eventually lodge in a cerebral vessel and block blood flow. Certain blood disorders and hyperviscosity syndromes can increase an individual's risk for stroke. The abnormal hemoglobin associated with sickle cell disease causes abnormally shaped, rigid red blood cells to form, resulting in increased viscosity and microvascular sludging. Myeloproliferative disorders such as polycythemia vera can cause increased blood viscosity and impaired blood flow to vital organs.

Whatever the cause may be, the result of impaired arterial blood flow to the brain is ischemia and hypoxia of cerebral tissues. The brain's oxygen supply is exhausted within 10 seconds after cessation of blood flow. Irreversible tissue damage occurs within 2 to 4 minutes after the stroke unless the blood supply is reestablished. These tissues then begin to undergo anaerobic glycolysis. Lactic acid accumulates and ionic gradients are altered, allowing sodium, calcium, chloride, and water to enter the cells. Excess intracellular calcium leads to further damage of the cells, causing prostaglandins, cytokines, and leukotrienes to be released, resulting in further cell damage. Synaptic transmission is decreased as a result of inadequate adenine triphosphate (ATP). When blood flow is restored promptly, the damage may be reversed. Otherwise, intracellular homeostasis is permanently disrupted, with subsequent cellular swelling and the death of neurons.

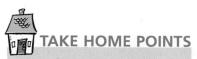

TAKE HOME POINTS

- Any event that decreases or compromises the supply of blood and oxygen to cerebral tissue can cause a stroke and impose permanent neurologic damage.
- A blockage in blood flow to the brain by fatty deposits or a blood clot or bleeding into the cerebral tissue usually causes strokes.

Women over the age of 35 who take oral contraceptives have an increased risk of stroke. The risk is even higher when the individual smokes.

African-American men have a higher incidence of stroke than do Caucasian men, and they appear to experience increased mortality and morbidity from stroke. One possible cause for this phenomenon is an increased incidence of hypertension at an early age. Other contributing factors include inadequate access to preventive health care and financial constraints that limit their ability to adhere to a prescribed medical regimen.

Regardless of race or ethnicity, strokes are increasingly likely to occur in people over the age of 60.

In the case of hemorrhagic strokes, damage to delicate brain tissue is compounded by the presence of blood within the tissue, which tends to cause increased intracranial pressure and subsequent extension of brain damage.

At-Risk Populations

Any individual with disease that compromises normal blood flow is at risk for a stroke. These diseases include prolonged uncontrolled hypertension, diabetes mellitus, heart disease, atherosclerosis, and blood disorders, such as sickle cell anemia and polycythemia vera.

To some extent, the tendency toward cardiovascular disease appears to be an inherited trait. Patients with a strong family history of cardiovascular disease, including myocardial infarction or hypertension, particularly in people under the age of 50, are at risk.

Behaviors that are strongly correlated with an increased risk for stroke include use of alcohol, tobacco, and cocaine.

Age, gender, and race are nonmodifiable risk factors that are not under patient control. Modifiable risk factors involve individual decisions, and are frequently, but not always, subject to the patient's control. Lifestyle modification and elimination of high-risk behaviors such as smoking and consuming a diet low in fat and sodium can accomplish a great deal in decreasing the risk of stroke and cardiovascular disease.

Preventive measures should include careful management and, when possible, elimination of risk factors. People who are physically active, maintain ideal body weight, consume a diet low in animal and saturated fats, and abstain from smoking have a significantly decreased risk for coronary and vascular disease. Patients who have problems with hypertension, hyperlipidemia, or those with a family history of stroke or cardiovascular disease require careful monitoring and care by a qualified health care provider.

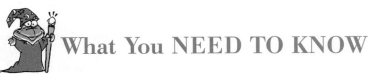

What You NEED TO KNOW

Clinical Manifestations

Signs and symptoms of a stroke will vary according to the area of the brain that has been damaged. Symptoms can be gradual in onset or sudden and acute. Strokes from cerebral thrombosis exhibit fluctuating symptoms characterized by periods of regression and improvement. Progression of the blockage is indicated through a pattern of increasing neurologic deficits. This process is referred to as a "stroke in evolution." Early symptoms of a thrombotic stroke include confusion, aphasia, vertigo, and headache.

Hemorrhagic strokes tend to occur during activity. Of the three main types of strokes, hemorrhagic strokes tend to have the highest rate of mortality. Intracerebral bleeding occurs abruptly, and the symptoms evolve quickly. Early warning signs of a cerebral hemorrhage include severe headache and nausea.

Embolic stroke tends to cause symptoms that are sudden and acute in onset. In contrast to hemorrhagic strokes, embolic strokes tend to occur during sleep. Symptoms of embolic stroke include weakness or numbness on one side of the body, visual changes or blindness, paralysis, and difficulty speaking or understanding speech. Speech difficulties experienced by the stroke patient can be particularly distressing because they deprive a patient of the ability to communicate. Strokes can also cause cognitive impairment and decreased self-care ability.

Strokes that involve the right portion of the brain tend to adversely affect visual and spatial awareness and orientation, but these stokes can leave the patient unaware of any deficits. These patients tend to be impulsive in their behaviors, exhibiting poor judgment. The left hemisphere of the brain is, for most people, the center for language, math, and analytic skills. A stroke in this area can result in varying degrees of aphasia, as well as problems with reading and writing. Patients with this type of injury tend to be slower and more cautious in their behavior, and they are often anxious, depressed, and tend to have labile emotions.

Motor deficits associated with CVAs tend to affect the opposite side of the body from the cerebral hemisphere in which the stroke occurred. Depending on the nature and extent of the injury, muscle tone can be flaccid or spastic. Neurologic damage can also result in a spastic bladder and problems with bowel function.

Sensory deficits can cause significant impairment, leaving the patient unable to read, write, or carry out purposeful activities, such as shaving or grooming. Neglect syndrome is a result of this sensory deficit, rendering the patient unaware of their paralyzed side. This problem tends to be more severe in patients with a right hemispheric stroke. Patients with this syndrome may leave the affected leg dragging underneath a wheelchair or neglect to comb one side of their hair or shave one side of their face.

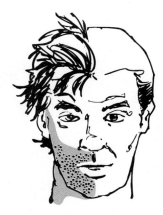

Prognosis

The chance for recovery from a stroke is highly variable and depends on the extent and severity of cerebral tissue damage. Hemorrhagic stroke has a mortality rate of up to 70%, particularly when intracerebral bleeding is extensive. Overall, approximately 10% to 15% of patients with an ischemic stroke fail to survive. Approximately 20% of individuals who manage to survive require long-term institutionalization, and up to one half of those remaining experience varying degrees of disability.

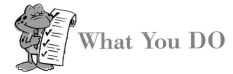

What You DO

Treatment

To determine a course of treatment, the exact cause of the stroke must be identified as soon as possible. Computerized tomography (CT) or magnetic resonance imaging (MRI) is used to evaluate the brain and identify the presence of a hemorrhage or aneurysm. Cerebral angiograms may be performed to evaluate the vasculature of the brain and detect clots and areas of vasospasm or rupture.

Depending on the extent of the damage involved, most stroke patients are kept in a fasting state immediately after their attack. Many stroke patients experience difficulty with the mechanics of speech and swallowing and are consequently at risk for aspiration. Indications of potential problems with eating include slurred speech and an absent or diminished gag reflex.

Medical management of a patient with a stroke is directed toward minimizing damage resulting from the stroke, maintaining adequate cerebral perfusion, and decreasing the risk of extension of the stroke and a subsequent recurrence. A tissue plasminogen activator (tPA) can reverse the effects of the stroke when given within 3 hours after the onset of symptoms. Patients with an embolic or thrombotic stroke are usually anticoagulated with heparin and will likely require long-term anticoagulant therapy after leaving the hospital. Alternative management involves the administration of platelet aggregation inhibiters that are given to decrease the risk of clot formation.

Coexisting medical conditions that may have contributed to the stroke, such as diabetes mellitus or hypertension, are also evaluated and treated in an attempt to decrease the patient's future risk of another stroke. As soon as the patient is medically stable and does not appear at risk for extension of the stroke, rehabilitation therapy can begin to help minimize the effect of neurologic deficits.

During the acute phase, care is focused on timely implementation of therapeutic measures and on careful monitoring for evidence of extension of the stroke. Optimal care of the patient with a stroke involves collaboration among many different disciplines. The nurse is frequently responsible for ensuring that care is coordinated among the various disciplines and that the care is implemented in an effective, timely manner.

After a hemorrhagic stroke has been ruled out with diagnostic studies, patients with an ischemic or thrombotic stroke can benefit from the administration of thrombolytic therapy, particularly when treated within 3 hours of the initial occurrence of symptoms. The patient who has had a previous stroke within the last 2 months has active internal bleeding or has a history of aneurysms is not a candidate for thrombolytic therapy.

Nursing Responsibilities

Care is directed toward maintaining adequate cerebral tissue perfusion and decreasing the risk for increased intracranial pressure with careful positioning. A

TAKE HOME POINTS

Do not offer food to patients who have had a stroke without a prescribing health care provider's order or without the evaluation of his or her swallowing ability by a speech pathologist.

See Chapters 1, 3A, and 11 in
RWNSG: *Pharmacology*

precise history of the symptoms can help identify the area of the brain that has been damaged and can also help identify possible causes of the stroke. For a patient with a new onset of stroke:

- Gather information on the nature of the symptoms, the length of time that they have been present, and whether the symptoms have resolved, are improving, or appear to be worsening.
- Obtain the patient's medical history, particularly risk factors such as diabetes, cardiovascular disease, and hyperlipidemia.
- Assess neurologic function, including level of consciousness; motor and sensory deficits; cognitive, memory, or intellectual impairments; and difficulties with speech, hearing, or vision. Because of the possibility of cognitive and memory deficits, obtain a description of baseline status before the stroke from a friend or family member.
- Evaluate the patient for evidence of further neurologic deterioration or increased intracranial pressure throughout the hospital stay. A comprehensive neurologic assessment should be performed at least every 2 to 4 hours. Complete vital signs must be obtained at least every 4 hours.
- The head of the bed should not be lower than 30 degrees, and the head and neck should be in a neutral position. Extreme hip and neck flexion should be avoided. Procedures that increase intracranial pressure, such as bathing or suctioning, should be widely spaced to allow rest periods. Evaluate oxygen saturation levels frequently, keeping oxygen levels above 95% when possible. Elevated carbon dioxide (CO_2) levels tend to increase intracranial pressure.

Care is also directed toward minimizing and preventing complications associated with a stroke:

- Place patients with hemiplegia or hemiparesis in proper body alignment at all times, and begin passive and active range-of-motion exercises when feasible. Supportive devices such as hand and wrist splints, slings, and footboards may be needed to keep the patient in normal anatomic alignment and prevent contractures.
- Reposition immobile patients every 2 hours, and assess every 8 hours for skin breakdown, particularly over bony prominences.

Care must be planned to accommodate for possible sensory deficits. Communication can be difficult, particularly when the patient has aphasia. The nurse should perform the following:

- Avoid the temptation to finish the patient's sentences, and be prepared to devise alternate methods of communication. For example, a patient with expressive aphasia may have difficulty saying, "I'm thirsty," but may be able to point to a picture of a glass of water. Approach the patient from the unaffected side, and place frequently used items within the patient's visual field.
- When the patient has neglect syndrome, touch the affected side frequently and protect these areas from injury.
- Collaborate with physical and occupational therapy to help identify a treatment plan that will either help the patient regain function or compensate for deficits. Helping a stroke patient relearn old skills or relearn new ways of doing old tasks takes a great deal of time, repetition, and patience.

Any deterioration in neurologic status must be reported to the health care provider immediately.

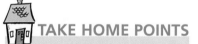
TAKE HOME POINTS

Be careful to support joints and extremities when performing passive range-of-motion activities. Patients with flaccid muscle tone are at risk for dislocations and joint damage.

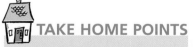
TAKE HOME POINTS

The rehabilitative phase of stroke care is directed toward helping the patient regain lost function or learn new ways of carrying out activities of daily living.

TAKE HOME POINTS

Patients with poor impulse control should be placed directly across from the nurses' station and may require passive restraint to keep them safely seated in a wheelchair. Electronic alarms may also be used to alert staff to a patient who is attempting to get out of bed or out of a chair unsupervised. These alarms are also safer when compared with a restraint device.

- Make the patient's family and caregivers a part of the rehabilitation process, and keep them informed about the goals of care so they can promote and encourage independence whenever possible.
Safety measures include:
- Protecting the patient from falls and potential sources of injury
- Answering the patient's calls for assistance promptly and offering the chance for toileting every 2 hours while awake to decrease episodes of incontinence
Emotional and personality changes and intellectual deficits are frequently the most devastating of all the complications experienced by a stroke patient. Because of cognitive changes, break down complex instructions into short, simple, concrete steps, and be prepared to repeat instructions frequently. Distractions in the environment must be minimized, and expectations must be realistic and achievable.

The patient who is emotionally labile requires a safe, supportive, predictable environment with routine and structure. Nurses and caregivers must learn to disregard emotional outbreaks and be respectful of the patient's dignity at all times. Family and friends must be advised that behavior and personality changes are a consequence of the illness and may be irreversible.

Because of their potentially devastating, even lethal outcomes, strokes should be prevented whenever possible. Nurses have a duty to educate the public on cardiovascular health, including the role of exercise, weight management, abstinence from smoking, and prompt aggressive control of hypertension and diabetes. Meticulous nursing care and collaboration with other health care disciplines, including dietitians, physical therapists, occupational therapists, and social workers, can help minimize the damage associated with stroke and facilitate the patient's recovery.

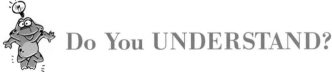

Do You UNDERSTAND?

DIRECTIONS: Fill in the blanks to complete the following statements.

1. The _____ lobe of the brain is responsible for vision.
2. The _____ lobe of the brain is responsible for judgment.
3. A stroke patient tends to be impulsive and falls frequently. This patient's stroke likely occurred in the _____ side of the brain.
4. The _____ type of stroke is usually treated with heparin.

DIRECTIONS: Circle the correct answers.

5. Which diseases and disorders increase a patient's risk for stroke?

diabetes mellitus   asthma   sickle cell anemia

hypertension   hemolytic anemia

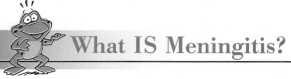

SECTION B
CNS INFLAMMATION AND INFECTION

Despite the physical and innate protection that the body affords to the brain and CNS, infectious and inflammatory agents can disrupt normal functioning of the CNS. This section describes and discusses infectious and inflammatory processes affecting the CNS that cause meningitis.

What IS Meningitis?

Infections and inflammatory processes of the CNS are identified based on the portion or portions of the CNS that are infected. The term meningitis is used to describe the infectious process that is limited to the subarachnoid space and meninges. Meningitis tends to spread rapidly because the infection is readily disseminated throughout the CNS by cerebrospinal fluid (CSF).

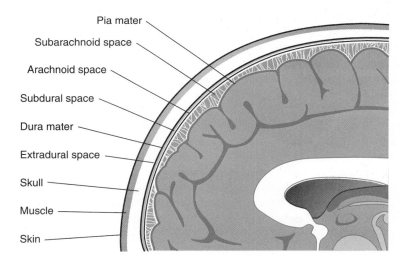

Pia mater
Subarachnoid space
Arachnoid space
Subdural space
Dura mater
Extradural space
Skull
Muscle
Skin

Pathogenesis

In most cases, either bacteria or enteroviruses cause meningitis. Common bacteria include *Haemophilus influenzae*, *Neisseria meningitidis*, *Streptococcus pneumoniae*, and *Escherichia coli*. Bacterial meningitis can occur when an infection elsewhere in the body spreads into the CNS via the bloodstream. Enteroviruses grow and replicate in the intestinal tract from which they are ultimately transmitted to the brain and nervous system. Fungal organisms can also infect the CNS, particularly when the patient is immunocompromised.

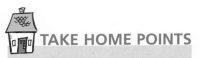

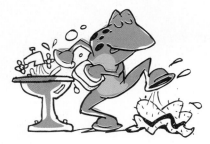

Bacterial meningitis is common in children under 5 years of age. Pneumococcal meningitis is a major threat for the extremely young and the extremely old, particularly when these individuals are compromised by coexisting illnesses.

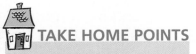

Many different types of viruses, including Epstein-Barr, mumps, Coxsackie, and the human immunodeficiency viruses can cause viral meningitis. Viruses can enter the body through many different routes, including the nose and mouth, animal or mosquito bites, and by passing across the placenta to the fetus.

Occasionally, patients who have cancer develop meningitis because of infiltration of the meninges by tumor cells. The result is increased intracranial pressure, fibrosis, and further inflammation of brain tissue.

Common sources of infectious organisms include the respiratory tract, the sinuses, the mastoid sinuses, and middle ear. Infectious organisms enter the CNS by one of three routes: the blood, either via the arterial route or through connections between facial veins and the cerebral circulation; traumatic insertion of an organism, such as during a medical procedure; or by local extension from an established infection.

Problems associated with a CNS infection are the result of organisms or bacterial toxins that cause either direct or indirect damage to tissue. The presence of endotoxins and cell wall fragments is thought to activate the immune response, with subsequent tissue damage resulting from the inflammatory response. Research suggests that inflammatory mediators disrupt the blood-brain barrier, allowing pathogens, neutrophils, and protein into the CSF.

At-Risk Populations

Risk factors include living in cramped, crowded quarters, such as military barracks or college dormitories, or the presence of a basilar skull fracture, otitis media, sinusitis or mastoiditis, neurosurgery, dermal sinus tracts, certain types of immunocompromise, and systemic sepsis.

By no means are all CNS infections preventable, although prudent health care measures can help decrease the incidence and severity of infection. With the availability of effective oral antibiotics, the incidence of serious otitis media has decreased significantly in the last few decades, thereby decreasing what was once a major risk factor for meningitis. Early detection and prompt treatment of infection, particularly when involving the head, neck, and respiratory system, can also decrease the risk for meningitis and encephalitis. Careful hand washing with bacteriocidal agents can also help decrease the transmission of disease causing organisms.

Vaccination against childhood illnesses, particularly mumps, measles, rubella, and varicella, conveys a high degree of protection against these diseases and is also an important measure to decrease the risk for meningitis. Vaccination is available against certain organisms such as *Neisseria meningitidis* and *Streptococcal pneumoniae* and should be offered to high-risk groups.

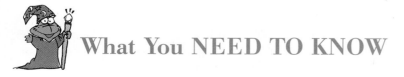

What You NEED TO KNOW

Clinical Manifestations

Symptoms associated with meningitis vary depending on the causative agent, as well as the extent and location of the infection. A headache, fever, myalgia, malaise, photophobia, pain in the eyes and neck, stiffness in the neck and back, and a positive Kernig's sign are all characteristic of meningitis.

Meningococcal meningitis usually causes a petechial rash, in addition to the previously mentioned symptoms. Patients may develop tremors and convulsions. A decreased level of consciousness is usually present, with progressive confusion and drowsiness that will eventually progress to a coma and death if prompt aggressive treatment is not initiated.

Microscopic examination and cultures of the CSF are important in differentiating between bacterial and viral meningitis. In bacterial meningitis, the CSF is cloudy, with elevated neutrophil and protein levels and a low glucose level. In contrast, with viral meningitis, examination of the CSF typically reveals elevated leukocyte count, a mild to moderate elevation in protein, and a normal glucose level.

Prognosis

Most patients with viral meningitis achieve a complete recovery within 10 to 14 days after the onset of symptoms, although some patients complain of persistent fatigue and weakness for months afterward. In a host who is otherwise healthy, viral meningitis is usually self-limiting, and the patient responds well to symptomatic and supportive care.

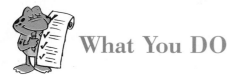

What You DO

Treatment

Infections of the CNS are emergencies and require immediate medical intervention. Because the signs and symptoms of viral and bacterial meningitis can be similar, obtaining a thorough health history and diagnostic evaluation is important to aid in determining the possible cause and source of infection, particularly in the absence of a positive culture.

Medical treatment for bacterial meningitis emphasizes prompt initiation of antibiotic therapy because of the high risk for mortality. Meningococcal meningitis is usually susceptible to penicillin, which represents first line therapy. Alternate drugs include ceftriaxone and cefotaxime.

Because meningococcal infections are contagious, people who have had close contact with patients with meningococcal meningitis should be given prophylactic antibiotic therapy to decrease their risk for developing the infection.

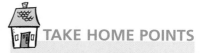
TAKE HOME POINTS

To test for Kernig's sign, instruct the patient to lay on the back with one leg bent at the knee. Raise the knee toward the chest. Pain with this maneuver is considered to be a positive Kernig's sign, which is a result of meningeal irritation.

The extremely young and the extremely old as a group tend to experience the highest rates of mortality from meningitis.

Bacterial meningitis tends to have high rates of mortality and morbidity and is likely to be fatal if prompt treatment is not quickly initiated. One third of survivors have neurologic sequelae, including deafness, hydrocephalus, and mental retardation.

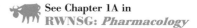
See Chapter 1A in RWNSG: *Pharmacology*

Chemoprophylaxis can be accomplished with Rifampin, ciprofloxacin, or a single dose of ceftriaxone. In cases caused by other bacteria such as *Haemophilus influenzae*, corticosteroids can be helpful as an adjunct therapy to reduce the incidence of disease related complications (e.g., hearing loss) and to decrease the chance of other neurologic deficits.

Medical treatment of acute viral infections of the CNS is directed toward supportive care, prevention and treatment of complications, and alleviation of distressing symptoms. Even patients with severe cases involving coma and seizures are likely to make a full recovery but may require management in an intensive care unit in which respiratory and nutritional support can be provided.

Nursing Responsibilities

The nurse should:

- Administer scheduled antibiotics and antiinfectives carefully, accurately, and on time.
- Monitor serologic studies, particularly electrolyte, renal, and liver function tests routinely, to detect potential drug induced toxicities.
- Assess the patient for evidence of drug-induced adverse reactions, such as gastrointestinal distress, rashes, and allergic reactions.
- Perform a comprehensive physical and neurologic assessment at least every 4 hours during the acute phases of the infection.
- Report changes in vital signs and deterioration in neurologic status promptly to the health care provider.
- Leave low-grade fevers untreated unless they are causing the patient discomfort. Low-grade fevers are thought to enhance the body's natural immune defenses. Temperatures of 40° C (104° F) or higher usually require vigorous treatment with antipyretics and possibly a cooling blanket.
- Routinely assess all four extremities for normal pulses and adequate perfusion. Severe bacterial infections carry an increased risk of septic emboli, with subsequent obstruction of microcirculation in the hands and feet.
- Assess carefully for evidence of abnormal bleeding, such as unexplained bruises and resumption of bleeding from old venipuncture sites. Septic emboli can also trigger the clotting cascade and cause disseminated intravascular coagulation (DIC).
- Establish seizure precautions for all patients. Keep the side rails up at all times, and have a portable suction device plugged in and ready for immediate use at the bedside in the event of aspiration. An oral airway is kept at the seizure-prone patient's bedside.
- Maintain adequate nutrition and hydration, particularly in the febrile patient with decreased levels of consciousness.
- Monitor intake and output, and collaborate with the health care provider to make certain that adequate fluids and nutrition are provided.
- The head of the patient's bed should be kept elevated 30 to 45 degrees at all times to decrease intracranial pressure, unless otherwise contraindicated. Activities that can increase intracranial pressure, such as deep endotracheal suction, should be carried out only when necessary and with extreme caution.

For the immobilized, obtunded, or comatose patient, routine nursing measures should be carried out to prevent the complications associated with immobility (e.g., decubitus ulcers, renal calculi). Discharge planning should include the need for possible physical therapy and rehabilitation to help the patient regain prior levels of functioning.

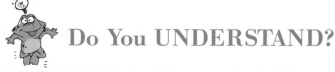

Do You UNDERSTAND?

DIRECTIONS: Fill in the blanks to complete the following statements.

1. The covering of the brain closest to the skull is called the

   _____.

2. At least three measures that help prevent the development of CNS infection include _____,

   _____, and _____.

3. Meningococcal meningitis usually causes a _____, in addition to other neurologic symptoms.

4. _____ meningitis tends to have a high rate of mortality and morbidity.

SECTION C
HEAD INJURY

Head injury is a common problem and is one of the most frequently observed diagnoses in children and adults seeking emergency care. Approximately 500,000 people each year need hospitalization for treatment of head trauma. Individuals who survive a head injury can be left with severe neurologic deficits. This section addresses various types of injury, including concussions, coup and contrecoup, hematomas, and skull fractures.

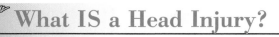

What IS a Head Injury?

Head injury involves physical damage to brain tissue that is caused by external physical force. Depending on the severity of the insult and the location of the brain injury, the changes in brain tissue and function can be temporary or permanent. Head injuries are categorized according to the type of damage that occurs or the nature of the mechanism that caused the injury.

Pathogenesis

Closed Head Injury. A closed head injury means that after a blow, the skull is left intact and no obvious external damage has occurred. This type of injury is usually the result of sudden acceleration-deceleration accidents. Because the brain is suspended in a hard container (the skull) and is surrounded by a layer of CSF, the process of rapid acceleration-deceleration can result in injury at the site of impact. After the initial blow, the brain "bounces" back in the other direction within its container, striking the hard, rough inner surface of the skull. Another name for this type of injury is "coup, contre-coup."

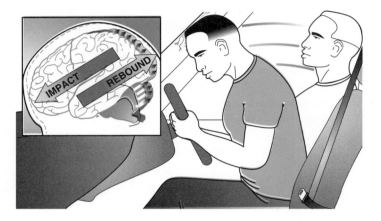

Open Head Injury. An open head injury occurs when penetration of the scalp, skull, meninges, or brain has occurred. Open head injuries are typically associated with skull fractures and carry a high risk of infection. Depressed or broken fragments of the skull can penetrate brain tissue and cause further damage.

After a blow to the head, both primary and secondary injuries can occur. Primary injuries are those that occur as a direct consequence of the physical trauma and are further categorized as focal or diffuse. Examples of focal primary injuries include contusion, laceration, and hemorrhage. Diffuse injuries include concussion, contusion, diffuse axonal injury, and hypoxic brain injury. Diffuse axonal injuries are commonly associated with strong acceleration-deceleration forces that cause damage to axons and neuronal pathways. Severe diffuse axonal injury can cause coma and autonomic dysfunction. The damage results in microscopic hemorrhages throughout the brain.

Concussions. Concussions are the least severe form of axonal injury. Sudden movement of the brain within the cranial vault that leads to diffuse but reversible injury is characteristic of concussions.

Skull Fractures. Fractures of the skull are a relatively common head injury, but they do not, in and of themselves, cause neurologic damage. An open skull fracture means that the dura mater is torn. This type of injury requires surgery. With closed skull fracture, the dura mater is intact. Blows to the face and nose can fracture the bones of the floor of the skull, creating an abnormal opening

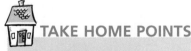

TAKE HOME POINTS

Head injuries are categorized according to the type of damage that occurs. A closed head injury means that the skull is left intact. An open head injury means that the skull, scalp, meninges, or brain has been penetrated.

between the sinuses and the brain through which infectious organisms can enter the CNS.

Secondary brain injury occurs as a consequence of the original insult. The initial injury generates an inflammatory response that becomes maladaptive because the reaction is taking place within the tight confines of the skull. The inflammatory response leads to cerebral edema and increased intracranial pressure (ICP). Because increased pressure damages cells, the inflammatory response worsens. Cerebral edema compromises blood flow to cerebral tissue. Subsequent hypoxia causes anaerobic glycolysis and failure of the sodium and potassium pump, leading to an excess accumulation of sodium in the cell. Water moves into the cell, causing further swelling and a decrease in cerebral perfusion. Scarring and fibrosis of brain tissue occurs as a consequence of this process.

Hematomas. Hematomas are an indirect consequence of head trauma. A hematoma is an accumulation or a collection of blood that escapes from a damaged vessel. Ordinarily, a hematoma would be no great cause for concern because the body eventually reabsorbs the blood. However, when the accumulation of blood pools within the confines of the cranial vault, cerebral perfusion can be jeopardized. The patient experiences increased ICP, tissue damage, and activation of the inflammatory response.

Hematomas are described based on the location where they occur. Epidural hematomas are usually the result of arterial bleeding from a skull fracture. Because arteries are under high pressure, a rapid accumulation of blood in the epidural space usually occurs.

Subdural hematomas have a wide range of symptoms and can be acute, subacute, or chronic in nature. These hematomas are typically associated with torn cerebral veins but can occasionally occur from arterial sources. Acute subdural hematomas tend to appear rapidly and are characterized by a sudden decline in neurologic status. This type of intracranial bleeding is an emergency that requires immediate surgical intervention.

Subacute subdural hematomas are of venous origins, in which blood tends to accumulate more slowly. Symptoms can appear anywhere from 4 to 21 days after the injury and typically involve neurologic deficits, changes in mental status, and complaints of severe headache.

Chronic subdural hematoma does not typically develop until several weeks after the initial injury. This type of injury can result from seemingly insignificant head trauma. Symptoms are vague, nonspecific, and are often mistakenly diagnosed as dementia or stroke.

Subarachnoid hemorrhage occurs as a result of head trauma that damages vascular structures in the subarachnoid space or a rupture of cerebral aneurysms within intracerebral arteries. This type of injury can cause vasospasm of cerebral blood vessels, which then leads to hypoxia and ischemia of brain tissue, leaving the patient at risk for further brain damage.

Chronic subdural hematoma is commonly observed in older patients or in younger adults with a history of alcohol abuse.

At-Risk Populations

Head injuries can happen to anyone in the course of normal daily activities. One half of all brain injuries occur in motor-vehicle, pedestrian, bicycle, or pedestri-

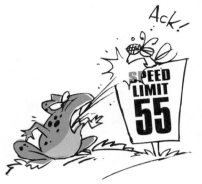

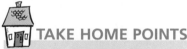 The highest incidence for traumatic brain injury is for people 15 to 24 years and aged 75 and older. Falls among elderly adults and young children are the second most frequent cause of brain trauma.

TAKE HOME POINTS

Safety precautions such as the use of safety belts, helmets, air bags, and child and infant seats can help prevent head injuries.

an-vehicle accidents. Males are more than twice as likely as are females to sustain a brain injury. A second, less drastic peak occurs in children age 5 and under. Alcohol is thought to be a factor in one half of all traumatic head injuries. However, changes in speed limits and highway design have helped to decrease the incidence of head trauma.

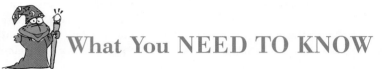 # What You NEED TO KNOW

Clinical Manifestations

Signs and symptoms of head injury vary according to the location and extent of the damage to cerebral tissue.

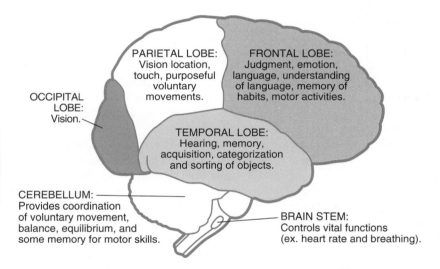

PARIETAL LOBE: Vision location, touch, purposeful voluntary movements.

FRONTAL LOBE: Judgment, emotion, language, understanding of language, memory of habits, motor activities.

OCCIPITAL LOBE: Vision.

TEMPORAL LOBE: Hearing, memory, acquisition, categorization and sorting of objects.

CEREBELLUM: Provides coordination of voluntary movement, balance, equilibrium, and some memory for motor skills.

BRAIN STEM: Controls vital functions (ex. heart rate and breathing).

After the initial trauma, patients may experience a brief or prolonged loss of consciousness, decreased level of consciousness, somnolence, confusion, and disorientation, as well as psychologic, cognitive, and motor deficits. A decline in level of consciousness is frequently the first sign of increasing ICP. Other signs and symptoms include headache, nausea, restlessness, increasing systolic blood pressure, decreasing pulse rate, and changes in pupillary reaction.

A localized injury can cause specific symptoms, whereas a more diffuse injury involving shifting of cerebral tissue can result in a different pattern of injury, including changes in level of consciousness, contralateral muscle weakness, and coma. Injury can also produce changes in physical, cognitive, mental, and emotional functioning. Patients with a severe diffuse axonal injury may be deeply comatose, with decerebrate or decorticate posturing and disruption of vital organ function and temperature regulation.

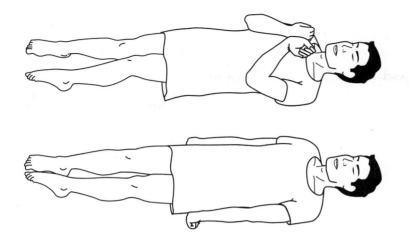

A brief loss of consciousness is characteristic of a concussion. Most patients recover fully without any neurologic deficit, although research suggests that a postconcussion syndrome involving headache, irritability, insomnia, and poor concentration may occur. These symptoms can persist for several months after the initial injury.

Even after the individual is recovered and medically stable, a variety of neurologic and psychomotor deficits can exist. Although they may appear physically normal, many survivors of traumatic brain injury have many functional problems that make it difficult for them to fulfill their previous role. These problems include difficulties in attention, concentration, language use, and visual perception. Learning ability may be altered, and previously acquired complex knowledge and skills may be lost. Behavioral alterations include verbal and physical aggression, agitation, impulsivity, and social disinhibition. Changes in personality, labile emotions, depression, and anxiety are also common findings.

Depending on the degree and location of damage, brain injury can impair motor function and cause hemiparesis or hemiplegia. Although some patients may retain voluntary control over movement, they may have problems with spasticity and abnormal posturing. Decorticate posturing is present in the patient with lesions in the corticospinal pathways. Decerebrate posturing is typically observed in patients with damage in the brainstem.

Depending on the extent, location, and severity of injury, deficits can be permanent, show partial improvement, or resolve completely. However, even patients with mild traumatic brain injury can experience permanent damage.

Brain Injuries and Associated Symptoms

LOCATION OF INJURY	ASSOCIATED SYMPTOMS
Right hemisphere	Left-sided paralysis
Left hemisphere	Right-sided paralysis
Broca's area	Expressive aphasia
Wernicke's area	Poor auditory comprehension, fluent speech but with phrasing error and/or meaningless jargon
Cerebellum	Impaired movement and balance; loss of fine motor function
Frontal lobe	Impairments in fine motor movements, speech, and the ability to use and manipulate tools
Temporal lobe	Hearing disturbances, long-term memory loss
Occipital lobe	Decreased ability to interpret the meaning of visual images

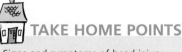

TAKE HOME POINTS

Signs and symptoms of head injury vary according to the location and extent of damage to cerebral tissue. Possible signs and symptoms include changes in level of consciousness, headache, nausea, restlessness, increasing systolic blood pressure, decreasing pulse rate, and changes in pupillary reaction.

Patients with an open skull fracture, particularly of the basilar area, may experience a CSF leak and are at increased risk for CNS infections. Signs and symptoms of CSF leaks include clear drainage from the nose or ears.

Prognosis

The chances of recovery from brain injury depend on the location and severity of the injury and the extent of damage. Even minor injuries such as a concussion can leave a patient with residual neurologic deficits, such as problems with memory. Patients with more severe injuries have improved outcomes when appropriate medical treatment is initiated within the first hour after the injury. Patients with severe injuries can have mortality rates of 35% or more. Survivors of this type of injury frequently experience profound personality changes, as well as neurologic and psychologic deficits.

Patients who are experiencing elevated ICP that does not respond adequately to therapy tend to have a poor outcome. After the acute phase of injury is resolved, rehabilitative care significantly influences the degree of recovery of neurologic function. Individuals with severe damage to the extent that they are unable to benefit from rehabilitative care usually require placement in a long-term care facility.

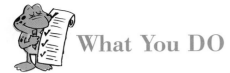

What You DO

Treatment

For optimal outcomes, treatment must begin as soon as possible after the injury. Initial interventions involve radiologic assessment of the brain for lesions, such as a hematoma or a depressed skull fracture, that require surgical intervention.

Generally, the goal of medical care is to restore and maintain normal ICP, oxygen and CO_2 levels, and blood supply to cerebral tissue. Because of the high risk for CNS infections, patients with open head injuries are typically treated with prophylactic antibiotics. ICP monitoring may be required to evaluate the status of the patient and facilitate prompt treatment of elevations in pressure.

A variety of pharmacologic approaches may be needed to decrease ICP. Restlessness and agitation, frequently present with head injury, can increase ICP and can be successfully treated with narcotics and benzodiazepines. When no benefit is obtained from sedation and the patient has rising ICP, has increased muscle tone, or is resisting the ventilator, paralyzing agents such as pancuronium or vecuronium may be used. Mannitol may be given to decrease ICP by osmotic diuresis. High-dose glucocorticoids are given to decrease cerebral edema. As a last step to control rising ICP, large doses of barbiturates may be used to induce coma. Patients with expanding brain injury, such as from a growing intracerebral hematoma, may require surgical intervention to remove the hematoma and preserve the integrity of cerebral tissue.

Nursing Responsibilities

Safety belts, helmets, air bags, and child and infant seats have accomplished a great deal in decreasing the incidence of brain trauma. Nurses must be actively involved in educating the public about the ways that these measures help decrease the incidence of head injury. Appropriate assessment of safety and fall risks can lead to interventions that will decrease the risk of injury. These interventions may include the use of assistive devices such as walkers and handrails and early screening and treatment of osteoporosis.

The goals of nursing care for the patient with a head injury are to decrease ICP, promote the delivery of oxygen and nutrients to the brain, and minimize complications and adverse effects associated with the brain injury. Immediately after the injury, patients with major head trauma require supportive measures in an intensive care setting to maintain all vital functions.

Begin with a comprehensive assessment to establish a baseline, and document findings in the patient's record.

- Assess the patient carefully for evidence of seizure activity. In many cases, seizure activity is limited to one part of the body, such as an eyelid, corner of the mouth, or fingers, hand, or arm (i.e., focal seizures). Any focal seizure can progress to generalized seizures. Seizures are cause for concern because they can lead to cerebral hypoxia.

TAKE HOME POINTS

Medical care for the patient with a head injury is directed toward restoring and maintaining normal ICP, oxygen and CO_2 levels, and blood supply to cerebral tissue.

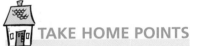 **See Chapters 1A, 2C, 2F, 7B, and 14 in RWNSG: *Pharmacology***

TAKE HOME POINTS

- A lumbar puncture is contraindicated in the presence of known or suspected head injury.
- Patients with head injury are likely to have a cervical spine injury as well. Radiologic evaluation as a part of the initial diagnostic evaluation after the injury should rule out this possibility.

Increasing ICP is an emergency and must be treated. Without prompt intervention, the patient can suffer permanent brain damage or death.

> ⚠ **Any suspected seizure activity must be reported immediately thus drug therapy can be initiated.**

> ⚠ **Subtle changes such as drowsiness may be indicative of further intracranial bleeding. Any subsequent deterioration in baseline neurologic examination must be reported immediately.**

- After the initial baseline has been established, comprehensive examinations may need to be carried out as often as every hour. Temperature regulation can be a problem for patients with head injury, particularly when they have suffered damage to the hypothalamus. A correlation frequently exists between elevated temperature and poor outcomes in this population. Moderate hypothermia causes a reduction in cerebral blood flow thus decreasing ICP.

- Pay special attention to oxygenation levels and blood pressure. Hypotension has been shown to reduce cerebral perfusion pressure and oxygenation. A blood pressure that is too low can compromise cerebral blood flow and increase damage to cerebral tissue. Uncontrolled hypotension has been associated with twice the mortality rates in head injury patients. Autoregulation of vital signs is often adversely affected by brain injury. Blood pressure must be carefully controlled. Elevated blood pressure can increase cerebral blood volume and indirectly cause more cerebral ischemia. Mechanical ventilation may be required to maintain adequate control of oxygen and CO_2. Keeping CO_2 levels within normal ranges is important. Excess levels of CO_2 causes increased cerebral blood flow and ICP, ultimately leading to cerebral ischemia. Decreased levels of CO_2 can cause constriction of cerebral arteries.

- Report any findings that are suggestive of skull fracture, including blood behind the eardrum, "raccoon's eyes" (periorbital ecchymosis), or bruising over the mastoid bone (Battle's sign) to the health care provider immediately. Clear, thin fluid coming from the nose or ears is suggestive of a CSF leak. When the drainage is CSF, it will test positive for glucose and form a halo when applied to tissue paper. Patients with a CSF leak may also complain of a persistent salty or sweet taste. For patients with a confirmed CSF leak, avoid placing anything in the patient's nose or ears because of the increased risk for CNS infection.

- 🍎 Teach the patient with a skull fracture to avoid blowing the nose and apply a mustache dressing over the upper lip to absorb drainage.

- Elevate the head of the patient's bed 15 to 30 degrees, unless contraindicated.

- Avoid flexing the patient's neck or knees or turning the patient's head to either side. Abnormal muscle tone, spasticity, posturing, and disrupted motor reflexes make positioning a brain-injured patient in normal anatomic alignment difficult. Special care must be taken in positioning to compensate for abnormal reflexes and muscle tone. These patients may require supportive devices such as pillows, foam wedges, and rolls to maintain good body alignment. Unless other medical contraindications exist, such as increased ICP, these patients should have routine passive and active range-of-motion exercises within the levels of their ability and should also be inspected daily for evidence of skin breakdown. Keep in mind that abnormal movement and spasticity can cause skin breakdown in unusual locations.

- Minimize extraneous stimulation such as loud noise, conversations, and lights, all of which have been shown to increase ICP. Suctioning, painful procedures, baths, and emotionally charged conversations within the patient's hearing can also increase ICP.

Sedatives and analgesics may be required to decrease fear, anxiety, and pain. These drugs can also help decrease combativeness and agitation and facilitate mechanical ventilation. Because these drugs can make evaluating mental and neurologic status difficult, they may need to be withheld periodically to obtain an accurate assessment. Sedation can mask symptoms of neurologic deterioration and should not be used without ICP monitoring.

After the patient is medically stable, a referral should be made to a brain injury rehabilitation team. Recovery from head injury is frequently prolonged and difficult not only for the patient, but also for the patient's significant others.

 In contrast to other types of head injuries, the patient with a basilar skull fracture should be placed nearly flat to prevent pressure on the brain stem, unless other contraindications exist.

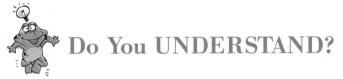

Do You UNDERSTAND?

DIRECTIONS: Provide answers to the following questions.

1. What type of head injury carries the greatest risk for infection?

   _____

2. A patient with a recent head injury complains of a persistent sweet taste. This is likely a result of what?

   _____

3. What position is safest for the patient with a basilar skull fracture? Why?

   _____

4. Why should hypotension be avoided when treating a patient with a head injury?

   _____

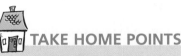 **TAKE HOME POINTS**

Nursing responsibilities include frequent comprehensive neurologic and physical assessments. General nursing care measures emphasize the prevention of increased ICP, maintaining adequate cerebral tissue perfusion, and minimizing complications and adverse effects associated with brain injury.

 SECTION D
MOVEMENT DISORDERS

This section provides an overview of neurologic diseases that alter motor and sensory function, also known as movement disorders.

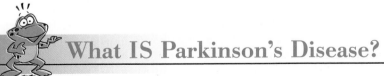 What IS Parkinson's Disease?

Pathogenesis

Parkinson's disease is a progressive neurologic disorder that results from degeneration of dopaminergic neurons of the substantia nigra in the midbrain. The loss of neurons causes a decline in the amount of the neurotransmitter dopamine. Dopamine is responsible for controlling movement. Damage to this area causes the rigidity, abnormal movement, and muscle tone that are characteristic of this disorder.

Answers: 1. open; 2. CSF leak; 3. flat, prevents pressure on the brain stem; 4. hypotension leads to decreased cerebral perfusion pressure and oxygenation.

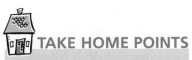

TAKE HOME POINTS

Parkinson's disease is a degenerative neurologic disorder characterized by resting tremor, rigidity, and bradykinesia.

The primary form of Parkinson's is most common in men over the age of 60. Older women are more likely to develop drug-induced Parkinson's than are men. On rare occasions, Parkinson's disease develops in children and adolescents.

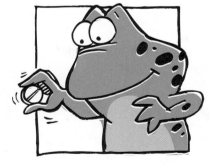

Parkinson's disease is classified as either primary (of unknown cause) or secondary. This disorder is slightly more common in men than it is in women. Some research suggests a genetic component to primary Parkinson's disease. Secondary Parkinson's is the result of conditions that interfere with the activity of dopamine. These conditions include the ingestion of certain drugs, such as haloperidol (Haldol) and reserpine, as well as hydrocephalus, cerebrovascular disease, and lesions in the midbrain.

At-Risk Populations

In rare cases, Parkinson's disease is an autosomal dominant condition. People with cerebrovascular disease or those who take certain drugs are also at risk for secondary Parkinson's. In patients with a drug-induced version of the disease, the symptoms may or may not resolve after the drugs are discontinued.

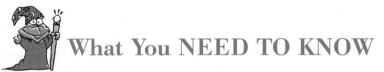

What You NEED TO KNOW

Clinical Manifestations

In the early stages, patients may notice a decrease in the speed of their movement and their ability to carry out certain tasks. Generalized stiffness and poorly localized muscle pain may also be present. Friends and family members may remark that the patient has a masklike facial expression (masked facies) and that the voice is softer and more monotonous in tone.

Tremors typically occur when the patient is at rest or when the arms are raised. The tremor is frequently described as a "pill-rolling" because the hands move from supination to pronation as the fingers are flexing and extending. The tremor usually decreases with voluntary movement. In many patients, the legs are also affected, causing a shuffling gait and problems with posture and balance.

As the disease progresses, the patient's automatic movements gradually decrease. Patients frequently have difficulty rising from a sitting position and may have problems with balance, resulting in falls. Eye blinking, smiling, crossing the legs, and swinging the arms while walking are typically affected. The term bradykinesia is used to describe the slowing of voluntary and involuntary movement. The length of the patient's stride becomes progressively smaller, causing the patient to take small, shuffling steps (festinating gait). Patients with this disease tend to have stiff muscle tone (cogwheel rigidity). The stiff muscle tone produces a ratchetlike resistance when performing range-of-motion activities.

Prognosis

The prognosis for Parkinson's disease varies, depending on the severity of symptoms, the presence of dementia at the time of diagnosis, and the patient's responsiveness to medical therapy. In the later stages of the disease, patients may require 24-hour care. Many patients die of complications of the illness, such as aspiration pneumonia and falls. Patients with milder forms of the disease can continue to work for as long as 10 years after diagnosis. Individuals with more severe, rapidly progressive forms of the illness may survive only 5 to 7 years after diagnosis.

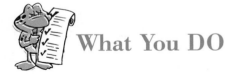

What You DO

Treatment
Drugs are the mainstay of therapy for Parkinson's disease. Levodopa is the most helpful agent for this illness, although the drug has to be given at frequent intervals because of the short duration of action. Other drugs shown to be beneficial include dopamine agonists, MAO inhibitors, and COMT inhibitors. Because some patients ultimately become resistant to drug therapy, neurosurgical interventions can be helpful in some cases. Thalamotomy, thalamic stimulation, and pallidotomy have been shown to decrease and, in some cases, eliminate tremors.

See Chapter 2D in **RWNSG:** *Pharmacology*

Nursing Responsibilities
Nursing care is directed toward helping the patient maintain the activities of daily living while minimizing symptoms and complications. The nurse should:

- Teach the patient and family about drugs the patient is taking, including side effects and drug-drug interactions.
- Focus on minimizing complications of the disease itself and maximizing existing system functioning. Physical therapy can help patients improve gait, postural stability, joint flexibility, and range of motion.
- Be certain that the patient is upright when eating or drinking to prevent aspiration. A suction device should be placed at the bedside. Loss of spontaneous automatic movements such as swallowing can decrease a patient's food intake and place them at risk for aspiration.
- Encourage the use of dietary supplements as needed to supplement nutritional intake. The texture and consistency of the patient's diet may require modification according to the patient's swallowing ability.
- In the hospital setting, place the call bell within the patient's reach at all times. Encourage the use of safety devices such as hand rails and elevated toilet seats in the home. Because of impaired gait and postural instability, patients are at significant risk for falls.
- Allow the patient sufficient time to communicate because speech is frequently difficult in later stages of the disease.

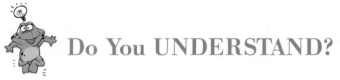

Do You UNDERSTAND?

DIRECTIONS: Fill in the blanks to complete the following statements.
1. Parkinson's disease is caused by the loss of _____, a neurotransmitter.
2. The most disabling symptom of Parkinson's disease is problems with initiation of _____.
3. The most common causes of secondary Parkinson's include _____ and _____.

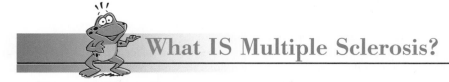

What IS Multiple Sclerosis?

Pathogenesis

Multiple sclerosis (MS) is a disease of the CNS that is characterized by recurrent inflammations of neural tissue. MS is also characterized by the random formation of plaque in the CNS, along with destruction of the myelin sheath. Damage to the myelin sheath disrupts transmission of nerve impulses. Although this process can occur at any location within the CNS, commonly affected areas include the optic nerves, cervical spinal cord, and the region between the thoracic and lumbar spine.

The origin of the abnormal inflammatory process has yet to be identified. Research is ongoing regarding the possible role of viral and bacterial infections, trauma, autoimmunity, and heredity.

At-Risk Populations

MS is most common in cold climates. Because MS is more likely to occur in people who have a first-degree relative with the disorder, a genetic component to the development of this disease may exist.

MS is most frequently observed in people ages 20 to 40 and is more frequent in women than it is in men.

People of European origin are more likely to develop MS than are those of Asian, African, or Native-American descent.

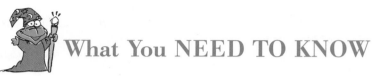

What You NEED TO KNOW

Clinical Manifestations

The signs and symptoms of MS depend on the area of the CNS that is affected. Common presenting symptoms include blurred vision, double vision, weakness in the arms and legs, a history of falls, and difficulty walking. Early symptoms can be transient, and the patient may experience a period of remission before symptoms occur again.

Answers: 1. dopamine; 2. movement; 3. cerebrovascular disease, drugs.

As the disease advances, periods of remission no longer occur. Nerve cells are destroyed and new symptoms appear, leading to gradually increasing disability. Late symptoms of the disease typically include involuntary movement of the eyes (nystagmus), intention tremors, difficulty speaking, paraplegia, and emotional lability.

 Women and people under 40 years of age at the time of diagnosis appear to have a more favorable prognosis.

Prognosis

MS is a chronic, incurable disease that has a variable clinical course. Many people with MS are able to walk and maintain gainful employment decades after their diagnosis. Most MS patients live nearly as long as do people without the disease.

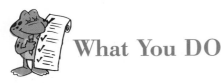 # What You DO

Treatment

Treatment is directed toward control of symptoms, prevention of complications, and maintenance and promotion of normal function. Commonly used drugs include biologic response modifiers such as interferon β-1b and interferon β-1a, glucocorticosteroids, and immunosuppressant agents, such as azathioprine and methotrexate.

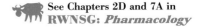 **See Chapters 2D and 7A in RWNSG: *Pharmacology***

Nursing Responsibilities

Successful management of MS requires a multidisciplinary approach involving the collaborative efforts of many disciplines, including the primary care provider, physical therapy, occupational therapy, and psychologic counseling. Coordinating the various levels of care is frequently the responsibility of the nurse and includes the following:

- Teach the patient about the proper ways to administer medications safely and to follow and adhere to an exercise regimen, as well as the need for adequate rest, stress reduction, skin care, and prevention of infection.
- Teach patients to avoid people with contagious respiratory illnesses and to avoid prolonged inactivity whenever possible. Remind the patient to receive the vaccination for pneumococcal pneumonia and yearly influenza vaccinations is also included.
- Provide active and passive range-of-motion exercises and inspect the patient's skin daily for evidence of breakdown, paying special attention to pressure points, which helps minimize complications, including decubitus ulcers and contracted extremities.
- Place grab bars and handrails in strategic places in the patient's home to help decrease the risk of injury from falls. Assistive devices such as walkers, canes, and wheelchairs can help the patient maintain independence and mobility.

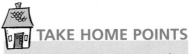 **TAKE HOME POINTS**

Infection is a major complication of MS, usually occurring in the lungs or urinary tract. Infection can also trigger an exacerbation of the disease.

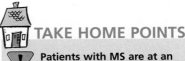 **TAKE HOME POINTS**

Patients with MS are at an increased risk of falling. Monitor ambulatory patients and provide assistive devices whenever possible.

Do You UNDERSTAND?

DIRECTIONS: Indicate in the space provided whether each statement is
true or *false*. If false, then correct the statement in the
margin space to the left to make it true.

_____ 1. MS is more likely to affect men compared with women.

_____ 2. MS typically occurs in women over the age of 50.

_____ 3. Symptoms associated with MS are the result of the disruption of the
transmission of nerve impulses.

_____ 4. Biologic response modifying drugs can be helpful in slowing the progression of the disease.

What IS Myasthenia Gravis?

Pathogenesis

Myasthenia gravis (MG) is a chronic neurologic disease resulting from an abnormality of the neuromuscular junction. Decreased receptor sites for acetylcholine—a neurotransmitter—cause decreased muscle function. The abnormality results in rapid fatigue of voluntary muscles.

MG is thought to be the result of an autoimmune response. Antibodies to
acetylcholine receptors can be found in the blood of patients with MG. These
antibodies are thought to cause damage to the receptors located on surface of
muscle fibers at the neuromuscular junction. Without receptors, acetylcholine
cannot stimulate muscle activity.

At-Risk Populations

MG occurs most frequently in people between the ages of 20 and 30 and is three
times more common in women than it is in men.

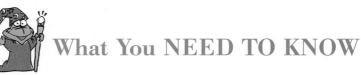

In approximately 10% of
cases, pregnant women
who have MG pass the disease
to their infants. In these infants,
the disorder disappears within a
few weeks after birth.

What You NEED TO KNOW

Clinical Manifestations

The course of MG is highly variable. The earliest symptom is weakness of eye
muscles. Patients can experience drooping of the eyelids and double vision.
With progressive disease, the patient experiences weakness of the head, neck,
and facial muscles, leading to difficulty chewing, speaking, smiling, and swallowing. Other problems include weakness of the limbs, leading to difficulty with
walking and lifting objects.

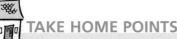

TAKE HOME POINTS

Weakened respiratory mus-
cles can place a patient in
respiratory compromise and can
be life threatening.

Answers: 1. false, MS is more likely to affect
women; 2. false, MS typically occurs in
women ages 20 to 40; 3. true; 4. true.

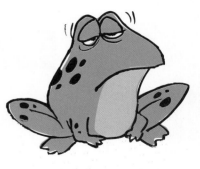

Prognosis

MG is typically characterized by a series of disease-free intervals alternating with relapses. Without appropriate treatment, a patient's symptoms can progress to respiratory failure and eventual respiratory arrest. Patients whose disease is limited to eye muscles (ocular myasthenia) typically have an excellent prognosis with minimal disease-related complications.

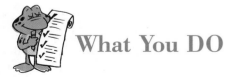

What You DO

Treatment

Treatment of MG involves the use of anticholinesterase drugs, biologic response-modifying drugs, and glucocorticosteroids. For patients with severe disease, plasmapheresis can be a lifesaving procedure. Patients with MG who have a tumor of the thymus gland (thymoma) may require removal of the thymus (thymectomy) to obtain a remission of symptoms.

See Chapters 2D and 7B in RWNSG: *Pharmacology*

Nursing Responsibilities

Nursing responsibilities focus on minimizing the complications and disability associated with MG and include the following:

- Administer medications consistently and on time to maintain therapeutic blood levels and improve muscle strength.
- Provide assistance with activities of daily living as needed and schedule activities that require exertion early in the day to minimize fatigue.
- Maintain good aseptic techniques and teach the patient to avoid potential sources of infection.
- Monitor the patient closely for sudden increase in weakness and difficulty with oral secretions, swallowing, or breathing. These symptoms can be indicative of either a myasthenic crisis or a cholinergic crisis.

⚠ **Patients with sudden increases in weakness and difficulty with oral secretions, swallowing, or breathing may be in myasthenic or cholinergic crisis. Without appropriate treatment and supportive care, the patient can die quickly of respiratory failure.**

Do You UNDERSTAND?

DIRECTIONS: **Provide answers to the following questions.**

1. What is the deficiency that causes the symptoms associated with MG?

   _____

2. What is the most common initial symptom associated with MG?

   _____

3. What can be done to maximize the effectiveness of MG drug therapy?

   _____

Answers: 1. Acetylcholine; 2. Droopy eyelids (ptosis of the eyelids); 3. Administer anticholinesterase medications consistently and on time.

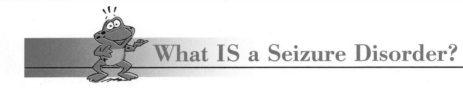

What IS a Seizure Disorder?

Pathogenesis

A seizure is an abnormal discharge of electrical impulses within the brain. Abnormal impulses result in changes in awareness, sensory alterations, and involuntary muscle movement. Seizures can be a symptom of an underlying condition or illness and may resolve spontaneously when the problem is treated. Three or more recurring seizures are usually a result of a disease called epilepsy.

Isolated seizures occur from a variety of conditions and disorders, including electrolyte imbalance, renal and liver failure, hypertensive encephalopathy, and acute head trauma. In patients with epilepsy, a lesion or injury to the brain may be identified. In many cases, the structural lesion causing the disease is never identified. Approximately 40% of epilepsy in adults and children is inherited.

At-Risk Populations

Patients with seizure disorders have more than one risk factor in their medical history. Patients who have experienced a single, isolated seizure have a 25% risk of developing epilepsy.

What You NEED TO KNOW

Clinical Manifestations

Seizure activity varies, depending on the area of the brain involved. Simple partial seizures do not involve loss of consciousness and can begin with involuntary twitching of an extremity, loss of ability to speak, or strange vocalizations. The patient may also express fear or a sense of impending doom.

Complex partial seizures involve impaired levels of consciousness, with automatic movements noted such as chewing, swallowing, or picking at clothes. Partial seizures can evolve into tonic-clonic seizures (previously known as grand mal seizures).

Absence seizures are characterized by loss of awareness and loss of muscle tone, typically lasting from 10 to 15 seconds. Patients with uncontrolled absence seizures can have one hundred or more episodes per day.

Myoclonic seizures are characterized by jerking of one or more muscle groups, with a tendency to occur early in the morning. Tonic-clonic seizures begin on both sides of the body. During the initial tonic phase, the muscles are rigid, and the patient may stop breathing for a brief period. The clonic phase involves a rhythmic jerking of muscles, with deep breathing at the end of the seizure. The patient may bite the tongue and become incontinent of urine and feces. After returning to consciousness, the patient may be confused, complain of headache,

Seizures can occur in infants and young children because of birth injury, hypoxia, or high fever. In the older adult, seizures can occur after a stroke.

Newborns with birth trauma, hypoxia, or those with a family history of seizures or neurologic diseases are at risk for seizures.

Epilepsy frequently causes depression and a sense of social isolation, particularly in children and adolescents.

Children with undiagnosed absence seizures are frequently accused of inattentiveness and inappropriate behavior, particularly in the classroom setting. Any child with a sudden change in behavior requires physical evaluation by a qualified health care provider.

and be sleepy. Some patients with epilepsy experience an aura—an abnormal sensation or sensory perception that is a warning of an impending seizure.

Prognosis

Approximately 80% of patients with epilepsy respond to drug therapy, have good quality of life, and live a normal life span. Most other cases can be cured by surgery. A few patients who are unable to or unwilling to comply with drug therapy can succumb to complications of status epilepticus, usually a stroke or heart failure.

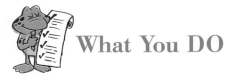

What You DO

Treatment

Patients who have a single seizure, have no risk factors for epilepsy, and a normal electroencephalogram (EEG) and neurologic examination require no antiepileptic treatment.

After ruling out underlying causes of seizures, such as metabolic disorders or structural defects within the brain, patients may be started on antiepileptic medication. Approximately 40% to 60% of patients obtain complete control of seizure activity with drugs, such as phenytoin (Dilantin), carbamazepine (Tegretol), primidone (Mysoline). The remainder of patients may require more than one drug to control their seizures satisfactorily.

A small percentage of patients have refractory seizures that fail to respond to medications. These patients can be helped by neurosurgery that involves destroying or ablating the epileptic focus within the brain or sectioning the corpus callosum between the hemispheres to decrease the transmission of abnormal impulses.

Nursing Responsibilities

Care of the patient with a seizure disorder is complex and involves intensive education and emotional support. The nurse should:

- Teach the patient to avoid factors that can precipitate a seizure, including stress, excessive heat, alcohol, sleep deprivation, and certain drugs.
- Teach the family about the ways to intervene when a seizure occurs, the importance of adherence to drug therapy, and the ways to manage side effects.
- Advise patients who have a history of poorly controlled or recurrent seizures to avoid driving a car or engaging in activities in which they can be at risk for injury. Children or adults may require helmets or other protective devices to decrease the risk for injury.
- Encourage patients with epilepsy to express their concerns and referring them to a support group available in their area.

⚠ **Status epilepticus, a condition involving persistent, prolonged tonic-clonic seizures is life threatening and requires immediate emergency medical intervention.**

⚠ **Individuals with recurrent seizures must begin drug therapy immediately to avoid further damage to brain tissue.**

See Chapter 2D in RWNSG: *Pharmacology*

☀ Pregnancy lowers the seizure threshold. Patients of childbearing age should be cautioned about possible adverse effects of antiseizure medications on a developing fetus.

⚠ **Patients on antiseizure drugs must be instructed to avoid discontinuing the drugs without medical assistance and supervision because of the danger of recurrent seizures, including status epilepticus.**

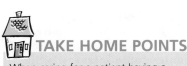
Do You UNDERSTAND?

DIRECTIONS: **Indicate in the space provided whether each statement is *true* or *false*. If false, then correct the statement in the margin space under the "TAKE HOME POINTS" to make it true.**

_____ 1. Seizure disorders can be inherited.

_____ 2. Adults can experience febrile seizures.

_____ 3. To be diagnosed with epilepsy, a person must have three or more seizures.

_____ 4. Pregnancy can lower the seizure threshold.

SECTION E

DEGENERATIVE NEUROLOGIC DISORDERS

Degenerative neurologic diseases frequently deprive the individual of independence. The nature of the disease reflects a process of loss, which is usually both cognitive and physical. The functional rate of decline will vary depending on the particular disease process and the individual patient. Additionally, adjustments and ability to cope will depend on the patient's perception of the loss of function. This section provides information on commonly observed neurodegenerative diseases. An understanding of these disorders will assist the nurse in developing strategies that will help patients cope with loss and set realistic goals.

What IS Alzheimer's Disease?

National Alzheimer's Association
www.alz.org
National Institute of Health Alzheimer's Disease Page
www.ninds.nih.gov

Alzheimer's disease (AD) is a chronic, progressive, degenerative disorder involving the brain that is characterized by profound impairment of cognitive function.

Pathogenesis

The cognitive impairment commonly observed in AD is thought to be a result of abnormalities in cholinergic neurotransmitters, which cause a decrease in acetylcholine synthesis. Confirmation of the diagnosis can be made only at autopsy, during which cerebral atrophy and cellular degeneration are documented. The cellular degenerative changes occur primarily in the temporoparietal and anterior frontal areas and include neurofibrillary tangles and amyloidal plaque deposits.

Answers: 1. true; 2. false, children most often experience febrile seizures; 3. true; 4. true.

The exact cause of AD is unknown. However, deficits in the neurotransmitter acetylcholine, which is necessary for memory, are thought to be responsible for symptoms. Approximately 10% of cases have been linked to a gene located on chromosome 21. This gene is closely linked to the genes for apo-protein and for beta amyloid, which are present in increased concentrations in patients with AD.

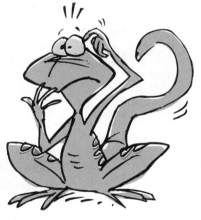

TAKE HOME POINTS

Positive family history and presence of Down syndrome are the only established risk factors for AD.

At-Risk Populations

A positive family history of AD and the presence of Down syndrome appear to be the only two risk factors. Other proposed risk factors include previous head trauma, a family history of Down syndrome, thyroid disease, hearing loss, maternal age, and exposure to aluminum. The evidence, however, is conflicting and insufficient.

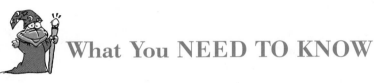

What You NEED TO KNOW

Clinical Manifestations

Progressive deterioration of short- and long-term memory is responsible for the clinical manifestations of AD. In many instances, depression is one of the first symptoms. Although the stages vary between patients, a few time approximations and characteristic behaviors have been identified.

STAGE 1: EARLY (2-4 YEARS)

- Exhibits forgetfulness; usually subtle
- May attempt to cover up using lists and notes
- Demonstrates declining interest in environment, people, and affairs
- Demonstrates uncertainty and hesitancy in initiating tasks
- Performs poorly at work, may be terminated from job

STAGE 2: MIDDLE (2-12 YEARS)

- Exhibits progressive memory loss
- Hesitates when questioned; shows signs of aphasia
- Displays difficulty following simple instructions or completing simple calculations
- Exhibits bouts of irritability
- Becomes anxious, evasive, and physically active
- Becomes more active at night rather than sleeping
- Wanders, particularly at night

Continued

STAGE 3: END-STAGE

- Becomes apraxic for basic activities
- Loses important papers
- Loses way in familiar surroundings or inside own home
- Forgets to pay bills; neglects household chores; becomes noncompliant with medication administration
- Loses possessions, then claims someone stole them; exhibits paranoid delusions
- Neglects personal hygiene
- Loses social graces; embarrasses family and friends
- Refuses to eat and drink fluids in adequate amounts
- Exhibits dysphagia
- Is unable to communicate verbally or in writing
- Fails to recognize family
- Is incontinent of urine and feces
- Is predisposed to major seizures
- Loses ability to stand and walk
- Death usually results from sepsis (i.e., aspiration pneumonia)

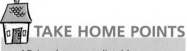

TAKE HOME POINTS

- AD involves a predictable progressive decline in cognitive and physical function.
- Continuous activity places client at risk for safety, agitated delirium, and dehydration.
- In the final stage, families are faced with making end-of-life decisions regarding initiation of tube feeding, nursing home placement, and hospice.

Prognosis

Progressive decline generally reaches the final stage in 10 to 12 years. Death generally occurs within 6 to 9 months after reaching the final stage.

What IS Multiinfarct Dementia?

Multiinfarct dementia (MID) (vascular dementia) is a nondegenerative type of dementia.

Pathogenesis

Multiple cortical embolic infarcts are responsible for neurologic symptoms. In individuals with subcortical white matter or lacunar infarctions, progressive deterioration in cognition without focal deficits may be present. Carotid and cardiac emboli, cerebral arterial and venous thrombosis, and vasculitis all contribute to MID. Infarcts on CT or MRI scans are necessary to establish a diagnosis. Many subjects diagnosed with MID are found to have a mixture of MID and AD on autopsy.

At-Risk Populations

Hypertension, heart disease, positive family history, hypercholesterolemia, cocaine abuse, and smoking place patients at an increased risk for MID.

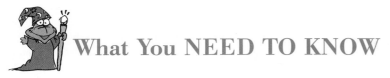

What You NEED TO KNOW

Clinical Manifestations

Hallmark findings of MID include mental slowing, dysphagia, shuffling gait, urinary incontinence, and bilateral motor abnormalities. Fewer behavioral problems associated with MID exist as compared with other types of dementia. When other symptoms commonly associated with AD are present, such as wandering, mixed dementia should be included in the differential diagnosis.

Prognosis

Because MID is a nondegenerative disease, prevention of additional cerebral infarcts preserves cognitive function and positively affects the prognosis.

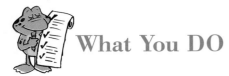

What You DO

AD Treatment

Currently, no cure for AD is available. Treatment is limited to palliation. Behavioral and pharmacologic interventions focus on improving both cognitive and physical levels of function. Newer drugs, which increase brain acetylcholine levels, called cholinesterase inhibitors (donepezil and rivastigmine), can improve cognitive function when initiated in the early stages of AD. Antipsychotic medications are frequently used to manage hallucinations and delusions.

MID Treatment

The goal of treatment is to optimize the patient's functional level of independence. Treatment strategies include:
- Encouraging physical and cognitive activities that promote the highest level of functional ability
- Therapies directed at correcting underlying medical conditions
- Medications such as aspirin or potent antiplatelet agents (ticlopidine or clopidogrel) to prevent recurrent stroke
- Minimizing environmental stressors
- Avoiding medications with CNS effects
- Managing behavioral problems

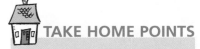

TAKE HOME POINTS
- MID is a nondegenerative type of dementia.
- MID occurs as a result of cerebral infarction.
- Mental slowing, dysphagia, shuffling gait, and urinary incontinence are classic symptoms of MID.

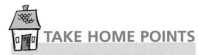

TAKE HOME POINTS

Prevention of cerebral infarcts positively affects prognosis.

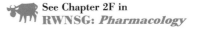

See Chapter 2F in RWNSG: *Pharmacology*

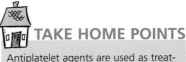

TAKE HOME POINTS

Antiplatelet agents are used as treatment for MID.

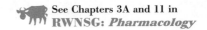

See Chapters 3A and 11 in RWNSG: *Pharmacology*

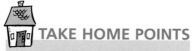

TAKE HOME POINTS

Nursing responsibilities for MID include stressing the importance of compliance with treatment of the underlying cause of MID as an essential element in preserving cerebral function. Although fewer behavioral problems associated with MID are present compared with other types of dementia, many of the same forms of interventions are beneficial.

TAKE HOME POINTS

- Treatment of AD is limited to palliation.
- Cholinesterase inhibitors and antipsychotics are frequently used to improve cognitive function and manage psychotic behavior in AD and MID.

Nursing Responsibilities

Nursing responsibilities for both AD and MID focus on optimizing the patient's level of cognitive and physical function. When diagnosis is established early, patients are usually mentally competent and capable of making decisions regarding end-of-life care. In these situations, the health care provider is in a strategic position to facilitate dialog among the patient, family, and health care professional regarding issues of tube feeding, nursing home placement, and resuscitative efforts, which generally need addressing during the final stage.

Consistency, stability, and active participation are essential in enhancing cognitive function. The following programs have been identified as helpful adjuncts:

- *Social skills therapy:* Reinforce behaviors used when interacting with others positively.
- *Communication therapy:* Improve speech patterns; minimize sensory deprivation.
- *Memory retaining therapy:* Provide reality orientation.
- Reminiscence therapy: using story telling and memory recall of past experiences.
- *Stress management:* Identify factors that minimize stress and methods of effective management.
- *Behavioral therapy:* Maintain consistency and structure to identify behavioral expectations; use written directions and schedules to assist with activities; provide day care programs.
- *Pharmacologic therapy:* Use medications to improve cognitive function and manage behaviors.
  The nurse should:
- Administer cholinesterase inhibitors (donepezil and rivastigmine) as ordered. These drugs can improve cognitive function when initiated in the early stages.
- Administer antipsychotic medications as ordered. Antipsychotics are frequently required to manage behavioral problems.
- Minimize stressors to optimize cognitive function as a result of associated decreases in acetylcholine levels from catecholamine surges.
- Regularly assess patient medications used to treat other health problems, paying particular attention to effects on baseline mental status. For instance, medications with anticholinergic properties also negatively affect acetylcholine levels and can significantly affect cognitive function.
- Educate caregivers regarding meeting nutritional and physical needs. Caregiver stress tends to increase with progressive decline in independence, particularly in patients who exhibit wandering behaviors. Ongoing assessment of caregiver burden and referral to support groups becomes important because of the effect on the patient's care.

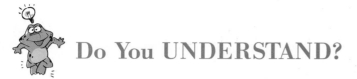

Do You UNDERSTAND?

DIRECTIONS: **Indicate in the spaces provided whether the listed activity is likely to increase (I) or decrease (D) the functional level of independence for the patient with AD.**

_____ 1. Being home alone

_____ 2. Watching old movies

_____ 3. Taking a 25 mg Phenergan suppository

_____ 4. 1500 calorie diet in the middle-stage patient

_____ 5. Day care program

_____ 6. Benadryl 25 mg PO for sleep

_____ 7. Trips to the zoo

_____ 8. Scheduled toileting every 3 hours while awake

DIRECTIONS: **Indicate in the spaces provided whether the following statements are *true* or *false*.**

_____ 9. MID is not preventable.

_____ 10. Day care programs are not as effective in patients with MID as it is in patients with AD.

_____ 11. Platelet aggregation inhibitors play an essential role in treatment of MID.

_____ 12. Patient with MID are at an increased risk for falls.

What IS Huntington's Disease?

Huntington's disease (HD) is a hereditary degenerative brain disease characterized by dementia and involuntary movements (chorea).

Pathogenesis

HD results from genetically programmed degeneration of neurons in certain areas of the brain. Neurons of the basal ganglia are specifically affected, causing uncoordinated movement. Within the basal ganglia, HD targets the striatum, particularly neurons in the caudate nuclei and pallidum. The cerebral cortex is also affected and responsible for symptoms associated with psychiatric disorders and dementia.

HD is a result of an inherited autosomal dominant disorder. The genetic defect responsible for HD is a small sequence of DNA on chromosome 4 in which an unstable trinucleotide.

A small number of cases are sporadic in that they occur although no family history exists. A new genetic mutation is thought to be the cause of these cases that occurs during sperm development and brings the number of CAG repeats into the range that causes HD.

National Institute of Stroke and Neurologic Diseases
www.ninds.nih.gov

At-Risk Populations

Each child of a parent with HD has a 50% chance of inheriting the HD gene. A person who inherits the HD gene and survives long enough will eventually develop the disease.

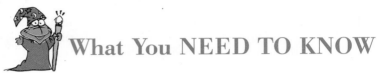

What You NEED TO KNOW

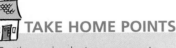

Clinical Manifestations

Early manifestations of the disease vary. Adult-onset HD with its disabling chorea frequently begins in middle age. However, other variations of HD are distinguished not simply by age at onset, but rather by the clinical picture.

Initially symptoms may be overlooked as mood swings or uncharacteristic irritability progresses to depression, hostile outbursts, and dementia. In some patients, symptoms begin with mild clumsiness, balance problems, or continuous uncontrollable movement in the fingers, feet, face, or trunk. These movements frequently intensify with anxiety. Because chorea causes problems with walking, increased falls result. As neurodegeneration progresses, speech becomes slurred and associated functions, such as swallowing, eating, and speaking, continue to decline.

Prognosis

The duration of the illness ranges from 10 to 30 years. Generally, the earlier the symptoms appear, the more rapidly the disease progresses. The most common causes of death are sepsis and injuries related to a fall.

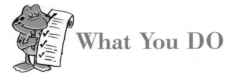

What You DO

Treatment

Treatment is limited to palliative management of the emotional and movement problems associated with HD. Benzodiazepines and antipsychotic agents can help alleviate choreic movements, as well as control hallucinations, delusions, and violent outbursts. Antidepressants can be helpful during the early stages of HD.

Nursing Responsibilities

**See Chapter 2F in
RWNSG: *Pharmacology***

Nursing responsibilities focus on optimizing the patient's level of cognitive and physical function. Because of the genetic predisposition to the disease, patients may receive explicit directions regarding the aggressive nature of their care and end-of-life issues. Choreic movements can necessitate the use of muscle relaxants. Antipsychotic agents can also be used to control psychiatric disorders and dementia.

The nurse should:
- Explain the indications and side effects of all prescribed drugs to patients, their families, and their caregivers.
- Instruct caregivers on preventing skin problems and preventing aspirations. Choreic movements frequently cause limited mobility and difficulties with swallowing.
- Educate families regarding the importance of genetic counseling.

Do You UNDERSTAND?

DIRECTIONS: **Indicate in the space provided whether each statement is** *true* **or** *false.* **If false, correct the statement to make it true in the space provided.**

_____ 1. Lorazepam is frequently used to treat the choreic movements associated with HD.

_____ 2. Aspiration is not a common occurrence in the patient with HD.

_____ 3. Patients with HD frequently die from complications associated with fractures.

_____ 4. Families with a positive history for HD should be referred for genetic counseling.

3 Hematologic System

DISTURBANCES IN COAGULATION

In this section, diseases and disorders affecting coagulation of the blood are examined. Coagulation is an essential, protective part of the controlling and stopping of bleeding (hemostasis) to prevent blood loss when a vessel is damaged. Coagulation is the ability of blood to change from a fluid to a semisolid mass. This mechanism of clot initiation and formation involves a series of sequential cascadelike reactions that employ several factors in the blood and injured tissue. Control of bleeding is accomplished through the following sequence:

1. Immediately after the wall of a vessel is injured, contraction of the vessel decreases the flow of blood into and out of the vessel. This constriction is a protective mechanism because it helps limit blood loss.

2. Damage to the blood vessel causes platelet plugs to form. With disruption of the endothelial lining of the vessel, the underlying collagen is exposed.

3. When platelets are exposed to collagen or other foreign surfaces, such as antigen-antibody complexes, thrombin, proteolytic enzymes, endotoxins, or viruses, they undergo a change. The platelets begin to swell and form irregular shapes with processes protruding from their surfaces. Eventually, these platelets become sticky and adhere to the collagen and basement membrane of the vessel.

4. The platelets release adenosine diphosphate (ADP), which attracts other platelets and aids in platelet adhesion and aggregation. ADP is also released from disrupted red blood cells and damaged tissue.

5. Enzymes released from the platelet cause the formation of thromboxane A in the plasma.

6. Both ADP and thromboxane A activate platelets that adhere to the original platelets. The platelet plug results, causing the damaged endothelial vessel wall to adhere to the collagen fibers. When the tear is small, the plug arrests the circulation.

7. Later, fibrin threads that result from the process of coagulation form a tight plug. Usually the plugging mechanism seals the tear in the vessel.

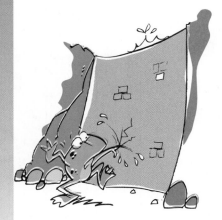

Coagulation is achieved through three basic reactions, which constitute the sequential pathway for blood coagulation. The intrinsic or extrinsic pathway in response to tissue or endothelial damage forms prothrombin activator. Prothrombin activator catalyzes the conversion of prothrombin to thrombin. Thrombin catalyzes the conversion of soluble fibrinogen to solid fibrin polymer threads. These fibrin threads form the meshwork on which plasma, blood cells, and platelets aggregate to make the clot.

Clot formation must occur before coagulation can be achieved. Clotting factors are a series of plasma proteins that are generally inactive forms of proteolytic enzymes. The enzymatic proteolytic actions cause successive reactions of the clotting process in a cascadelike sequence. One factor is important for the activation of the next factor.

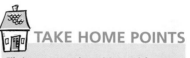

TAKE HOME POINTS

Fibrinogen, prothrombin, and factors VII, IX, and X are essential procoagulation factors that are synthesized in the liver according to the body's requirements.

 Pregnancy and oral contraceptives can adversely affect the coagulation process.

 ## What IS Idiopathic Thrombocytopenia Purpura?

Idiopathic thrombocytopenia purpura (ITP) is a bleeding disorder characterized by a marked increase of platelet destruction, resulting in multiple bruises and hemorrhage into the tissue.

Pathogenesis

Low platelet count (thrombocytopenia) results from immunologic platelet destruction. ITP resulting from auto antibodies directed against certain platelet antigens is the most common type of immune thrombocytopenia.

At-Risk Populations

The reported prevalence of ITP in adults and children is 1 to 13 per 100,000 persons. In children, both sexes are affected; in adults, the disease is predominant in women.

 Platelet Disorder Support Association
http://www.itppeople.com/
Platelets On The Internet
http://moon.ouhsc.edu/jgeorge/

 Acute ITP is usually more common in children. Fewer than 40% of all patients with ITP are younger than 10 years of age. Pregnant women may also be affected with ITP.

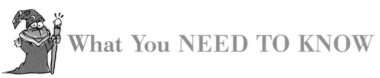 ## What You NEED TO KNOW

Immunization is important. Patients are encouraged to receive Haemophilus influenza type B conjugated vaccine, polyvalent pneumococcal vaccine, and quadrivalent meningococcal polysaccharide vaccine at least 2 weeks before elective splenectomy.

Clinical Manifestations

The physical examination is usually normal except for purpura. A platelet count of less than 20,000/mm^3 and a prolonged bleeding time are indicative of ITP. Platelet size and appearance may be abnormal, and anemia may be present when extensive bleeding has occurred. Bone marrow studies reveal an abundance of megakaryocytes. Platelet survival time is decreased from 3 to 7 days to only several hours.

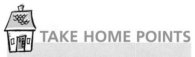

TAKE HOME POINTS

- Patients with the human immunodeficiency virus (HIV) may also have associated ITP.
- ITP has the same stigmas associated with a chronic disease, for example, time lost from work or school.
- Weight gain and mood swings, observed with steroid treatment, is also a concern of some patients.

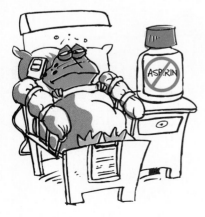

Older patients have hemorrhagic complications more often than do younger patients with the same platelet counts.

Chronic acute idiopathic or autoimmune thrombocytopenia purpura (AITP) occurs most frequently in adults.

See Chapters 1C and 7C in RWNSG: *Pharmacology*

Treatment of children with acute ITP continues to be debated. Usually, AITP resolves spontaneously within 6 months. Children are usually treated with a short course of tapering steroids. Unless an emergency exists, platelet transfusions are not administered.

The Jehovah's Witness population does not permit transfusion of blood products. Their religious beliefs may preclude the use of IVIG, primarily because it is derived from blood.

Avoid all aspirin in any form and other drugs that can impair coagulation.

Prognosis

Spontaneous remission occurs in children 83% of the time compared with 2% in adults. Rare intracranial hemorrhage is the most common cause of death, affecting only 3% to 4% of patients.

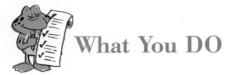

What You DO

Treatment

Treatment is generally designed to prevent life-threatening complications, such as intracranial hemorrhage. The treatment for ITP ranges from a simple steroid treatment to a splenectomy with long-term follow-up.

ITP can be present for many years and is characterized by periodic flare-ups or exacerbations. Supportive care and the institution of bleeding precautions are advised.

Adults with ITP are given corticosteroids as the initial treatment to promote capillary integrity. Intravenous immunoglobulin (IVIG) may also be administered on a weekly basis. Other treatments include intravenous azathioprine, danazol, immunosuppressive therapy, plasmapheresis, and splenectomy. Splenectomy is not performed as initial therapy in patients who have bleeding symptoms or minor purpura.

Nursing Responsibilities

When caring for a hospitalized patient with clotting problems, the nurse should take every precaution against bleeding and should:

- Protect the patient from trauma, keeping the side rails up and padded when possible.
- Promote the use of an electric razor and soft toothbrush.
- Avoid invasive procedures, such as venipuncture or urinary catheterization when possible.
- Monitor platelets at least daily.
- Test stool for guaiac, dipstick urine, and emesis for blood.
- Watch for symptoms of bleeding, such as petechiae, ecchymosis, surgical or gastrointestinal bleeding, and menorrhagia.
- Advise the patient to avoid constipation, straining during bowel movements, and coughing, which can lead to increased intracranial pressure.
- During periods of active bleeding, enforce strict bed rest.
- When administering platelet transfusions, remember that platelets are fragile, thus infuse quickly with the proper administration set.

Do You UNDERSTAND?

DIRECTIONS: **In the space provided, write the letter that corresponds to the correct answer for each of the following questions.**

_____ 1. A patient diagnosed with ITP will have which of the following?
   a. High platelet count and hemoglobin.
   b. High platelet count and low hemoglobin.
   c. Low platelet count.
   d. High hemoglobin.

_____ 2. Nursing management of the patient diagnosed with ITP should include what?
   a. Monitoring of bleeding.
   b. Heme testing of stools and emesis.
   c. Padding bed rails when bed rest is necessary.
   d. Instructions for the patient to avoid taking over-the-counter medications, particularly aspirin products.
   e. All of the above.
   f. a, b, and d.

What IS Thrombotic Thrombocytopenia Purpura?

Thrombotic thrombocytopenia purpura (TTP) is a syndrome characterized by intravascular thrombosis with extreme thrombocytopenia, extreme elevation of lactate dehydrogenase (LDH), neurologic symptoms, fever, and renal dysfunction.

Pathogenesis

TTP is a syndrome with diverse etiologic aspects and many possible precipitating causes. More than 90% of cases of TTP develop without an apparent cause or underlying disease process. Medications that have been implicated in TTP development include oral contraceptives, antineoplastic agents, immunosuppressive drugs, antibiotics, iodine, and ticlopidine hydrochloride.

Infectious agents have also been associated with TTP. Disseminated thrombotic occlusions of the microcirculation and end-organ injury facilitate the symptoms. Evidence suggests that platelet or endothelial cell injury may be the initial pathologic event. A number of factors in the patient's plasma, including immunoglobulins, can mediate cellular injury.

See Chapters 10A, 1D, 1C, and 1A in **RWNSG:** *Pharmacology*

At-Risk Population

Patients with lymphoma, acute myelogenous leukemia, some adenocarcinomas, and bone marrow transplant patients are at risk. Patients who have *Escherichia coli*, Coxsackie B virus, mycoplasma pneumonia, HIV, or a nonspecific upper respiratory infection can develop the disease.

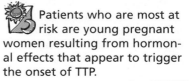 Patients who are most at risk are young pregnant women resulting from hormonal effects that appear to trigger the onset of TTP.

Answers: 1. c; 2. e.

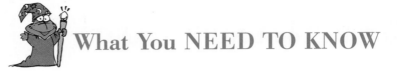

What You NEED TO KNOW

Clinical Manifestations

Profound thrombocytopenia, intravascular hemolysis with erythrocyte fragmentation (schistocytosis), extreme elevations in serum LDH, and mental status changes can occur with TTP. The blood supply to the brain is compromised in approximately 50% to 75% of TTP episodes. Neurologic symptoms may be intermittent and fluctuate but are usually the most common presenting symptom. Headaches of unknown origin, confusion, stupor, coma and paresis, and cranial nerve palsies are common.

Hemorrhagic complications are the second most common presenting symptom. Approximately 40% of patients present with bleeding complications and 80% to 90% of patients develop bleeding complications. A patient may experience overwhelming hemorrhage as characterized by petechiae, purpura, and bruises, (ecchymoses), and hemorrhage from the gastrointestinal or urinary tracts.

Fever is an uncommon presenting symptom but eventually occurs in 60% to 100% of patients and may be as high as 102° to 105° F. Usually, no source of infection is found. Fever may also be the result of tissue necrosis, release of the products of hemolysis, or the release of endogenous pyrogenic substances from leukocytes damaged by the antigen-antibody reaction.

Renal dysfunction is common. Approximately 80% to 90% of patients present with hematuria. Proteinuria is observed in 50% of patients.

Prognosis

Without treatment, 90% of patients will die of their disease and 30% of patients die in spite of therapy.

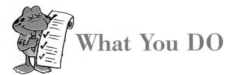

What You DO

See Chapters 1C, 7C, and 11 in RWNSG: *Pharmacology*

Patients who are unwilling to accept transfusion with blood products or plasma because of cultural issues or religious beliefs can die from uncontrolled hemorrhage.

Treatment

Treatment includes steroid therapy, dipyridamole, daily aspirin, and fresh frozen plasma (FFP) at the rate of 1 unit per hour until plasmapheresis can be arranged. Plasma exchange or infusion is the single most important intervention for improved outcomes. Patients must receive plasma exchange daily or twice per day, depending on their LDH levels, platelet levels, and symptoms. Other treatments include immunosuppressive agents, such as cyclophosphamide, azathioprine, and intravenous gamma globulins.

Splenectomy has an 87% response rate when performed in conjunction with steroids and Dextran.

Nursing Responsibilities

Nurses should institute bleeding precautions as was discussed for ITP. Meticulous hand washing before contact with the patient and between patients to prevent spread of infection is important. Intravenous lines must be swabbed with alcohol before entry. Central venous catheters must have dressings changed per institutional guidelines and monitored for infection. Renal function should improve with plasma pheresis. The nurse should:

- Protect the patient from harm by padding side rails and having the patient use an electric razor.
- Test stool for guaiac, dipstick urine, and emesis for blood.
- Instruct the patient to avoid all aspirin products.
- Administer stool softeners, when necessary, to help patients avoid straining with bowel movements.
- Advise the patient not to engage in sexual intercourse of any kind while platelet counts are below institutional guidelines.

 No intramuscular injections or suppositories should be used in patients with TTP.

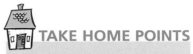 **Monitoring for the symptoms of serious bleeding complications is imperative in patients with TTP.**

 # Do You UNDERSTAND?

DIRECTIONS: In the space provided, write the letter that corresponds to the correct answer for each of the following questions.

_____ 1. TTP is associated with which of the following?
  a. Renal dysfunction
  b. Neurologic manifestation
  c. Thrombocytopenia and bleeding
  d. All of the above

_____ 2. Plasmapheresis is which of the following:
  a. Blood transfusion
  b. Plasma exchange
  c. IVIG
  d. Platelet exchange

_____ 3. Patients diagnosed with TTP usually have what?
  a. Elevated LDH 5 to 10 times greater than is the normal limit.
  b. Elevated blood urea nitrogen (BUN) and creatinine levels.
  c. High platelet counts.
  d. Elevated bilirubin.
  e. a, b, and d.

TAKE HOME POINTS

- TTP is a syndrome characterized by microvascular thrombosis with thrombocytopenia, neurologic symptoms, fever, and renal dysfunction.
- Plasma exchange or infusion is the single most important therapeutic intervention.

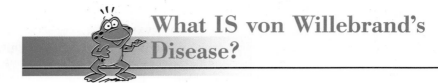

What IS von Willebrand's Disease?

Characterized by a prolonged bleeding time, moderate deficiency of clotting factor VIII (antihemophilic factor), and impaired platelet function, von Willebrand's disease (VWD) is the most common hereditary bleeding disorder. The hallmark feature is impaired platelet plug formation and thrombus formation, both of which cause increased risk for bleeding problems.

Pathogenesis

A glycoprotein that is synthesized in the megakaryocytes and endothelial cells is the von Willebrand's factor (VWF). The primary hemostatic property is the binding of VWF to the subendothelium and platelet glycoproteins. This binding forms a bridge between platelets and subendothelium. VWF promotes platelet-to-platelet binding. VWF's additional hemostatic effect is its binding with factor VIII to form a stable complex and protect it from rapid removal from circulation.

At-Risk Populations

VWD is predominately inherited as an autosomal dominant trait and occurs equally in men and women. Although determining the prevalence is difficult, because mild cases often go undetected, the worldwide prevalence of the disorder is estimated to be as high as 1%.

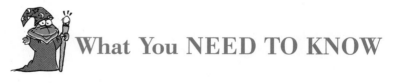

What You NEED TO KNOW

Clinical Manifestations

VWD can be distinguished from classic hemophilia because (1) both sexes are equally affected because of the autosomal mode of inheritance, (2) the bleeding time is prolonged, and (3) mucosal bleeding manifestations are typical, although deep tissue hemorrhage is rare.

The clinical symptoms include bleeding episodes involving the skin and mucous membranes, nosebleed (epistaxis), easy bruising, gingival bleeding, and menorrhagia. Epistaxis is the most common manifestation and is frequently the first indication of the bleeding disorder. Severe forms of this disease can cause hemorrhage after laceration or surgery, menorrhagia, and gastrointestinal bleeding.

Also, the blood group O has been associated with low levels of VWF.

Typical laboratory test results include a prolonged bleeding time (more than 6 minutes), slightly prolonged partial thromboplastin time (more than 45 seconds), absent or reduced levels of factor VIII related antigens, low factor VIII

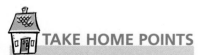

TAKE HOME POINTS

The most frequent laboratory finding in VWF is a prolonged bleeding time in the presence of a normal platelet count.

activity level, defective in vitro platelet aggregation, and normal platelet count with normal clot retraction. The same patient will have varying levels of VWF at different episodes. No single laboratory test to define VWD is available.

Prognosis

Patients with VWD usually respond well to treatment. Fatal hemorrhage is rare.

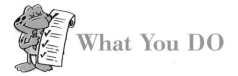

What You DO

Treatment

Therapy is aimed at shortening the bleeding time by local measures and replacement of factor VIII by infusion of cryoprecipitate or blood fractions that are rich in factor VIII. Before surgery, intravenous infusion of cryoprecipitate or FFP generally shortens bleeding time. Factor VIII should be 50% of normal before invasive procedures begin. Superficial bleeding can be managed with topical hemostatic agents, pressure dressings, and sutures. Women treated with the exogenous administration of estrogen are reported to have increased levels of VWF and factor VIII. The administration of DDAVP (desmopressin) is widely used for mild cases of VWF to regain hemostasis in bleeding episodes. DDAVP may be given intravenously, subcutaneously, and intranasally.

Nursing Responsibilities

The nurse should:

- Teach patients local measures to control bleeding during bleeding episodes; immediately elevate the injured part and apply cold compresses and gentle pressure to the site.
- Instruct patients on ways to prevent bleeding, unnecessary trauma, and complications.
- Warn patients to inform health care providers and other medical personnel that they have a bleeding disorder before undergoing invasive procedures.

Do You UNDERSTAND?

DIRECTIONS: Fill in the blanks to complete the following statements.

1. VWD is the most common _____
   _____ _____.
2. The treatment for VWD is _____
   of _____.
3. von Willebrand's disease is _____
   and _____.

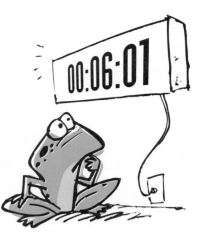

See Chapters 7B and 10A in
RWNSG: *Pharmacology*

VWF concentration can also be altered by pregnancy, oral contraceptive administration, liver disease, advanced age, and stress, in which increased levels are observed.

Warn patients to avoid nonsteroidal antiinflammatory agents and drugs containing aspirin products; these can further inhibit platelet activity. Contact sports should also be avoided.

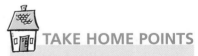

TAKE HOME POINTS

Therapy attempts to shorten the bleeding time by local measures and replacement of factor VIII by infusion of cryoprecipitate or blood fractions that are rich in factor VIII.

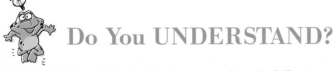

Answers: 1. inherited bleeding disorder; 2. transfusion, cryoprecipitate; 3. acquired, inherited.

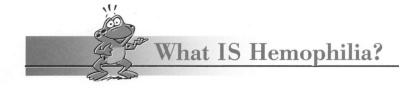

What IS Hemophilia?

Pathogenesis

Hemophilia is a group of inherited blood coagulation disorders. A deficiency exists of one of the factors necessary for blood coagulation, which leads to hemorrhage or excessive bleeding, even from minor injuries. The two most common forms are hemophilia A (classic) and hemophilia B (Christmas disease). Approximately 80% of persons with the disease have classic hemophilia, which is the result of a deficiency or absence of antihemophilic factor VIII. Hemophilia is usually inherited in males as an X-linked recessive trait. In hemophilia B, factor IX is missing, which causes a deficiency of plasma thromboplastin compound.

World Federation of Hemophilia
http://www.wfh.org/
National Hemophilia Foundation
http://www.hemophilia.org/splash.htm

At-Risk Population

The sons of a hemophiliac female carrier have a 50% chance of inheriting the gene. Hemophilia is estimated to occur in 25 per 100,000 males.

What You NEED TO KNOW

Clinical Manifestations

The plasma levels of factor VIII or IX procoagulation activity affect the severity of the illness and bleeding manifestations. Patients with levels less than 1% have an increased chance of spontaneous and severe bleeding complications.

Hematuria, mucous membrane bleeding, and intracranial hemorrhage can also occur. Moderately affected patients (with factor VIII:C or factor IX:C levels below 5% or normal) bleed after trauma or surgery. These patients can also develop spontaneous bleeding. Hematuria and gastrointestinal bleeding is also common, especially when the patient has a local lesion (e.g., ulcer, polyp, inflammatory process).

Hemophilia is frequently first noted as a result of circumcision. During the toddler years, children may develop repeated blood within the joints (hemarthroses), which can lead to chronic synovitis or the destruction of bone and cartilage.

Prognosis

With appropriate treatment and precautions, the life expectancy of the hemophiliac patient is comparable to that of the unaffected male population.

All patients with hemophilia develop excessive bleeding after dental extraction. Any surgery or trauma should be considered life threatening.

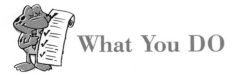

What You DO

Treatment

Treatment consists of replacement with factor VIII or factor IX concentrates. This replacement may be administered to treat bleeding episodes or as a prophylactic in patients with severe disease. Replacement factors are also administered before surgery or dental extraction. DDAVP or antifibrinolytic agents or both may be administered as a prophylactic measure. Social and psychologic support is especially important. Patients and their significant others should be encouraged to join a support group of specialized health care providers.

See Chapters 3B and 7B in RWNSG: *Pharmacology*

Nursing Responsibilities

The patient who is diagnosed with hemophilia can be faced with exposure to viral infection and HIV exposure from replacement factors derived from human blood. The use of recombinant factors VIII and IX have made exposure less of an issue in recent times. This chronic disease places a stress on the family, socially, psychologically and financially. Guilt on the part of the mother who may have not known she was a carrier may also be present. The nurse should:

- Counsel parents about the importance of avoiding injury in children with hemophilia.
- Encourage regular check-ups with the dentist.
- Teach parents of young children with hemophilia and adult patients about the administration of factor VIII and IX concentrates. The goal of therapy is to minimize the development of chronic synovitis or progressive arthropathy. Treatment of acute hemarthrosis must begin immediately, with intensive therapy and pain control, physical therapy, wedging casts, night splints, or traction in conjunction with regular infusions of factor concentrates.

Patients and their families need to be educated early about complications and the need for immediate therapy.

Do You UNDERSTAND?

DIRECTIONS: Unscramble the italicized words to complete the statements.

1. Hemophilia is inherited as an X-linked defect from the
_____. (*thremo*)
2. Hemophiliac patients develop excessive bleeding after

_____ _____.

(*nadtle tronixctea*)

TAKE HOME POINTS

- Therapy should begin promptly for the patient who is diagnosed with hemophilia to prevent further complications. If the bleeding cannot be controlled immediately, then the patient should be advised as to the ways to contact their health care provider for possible plasma pheresis and further treatment.
- The patient and family should receive counseling and guidance at diagnosis. Many social and psychologic problems affect the patient and their significant others.
- A high incidence of drug addictions is present with hemophiliac patients because of the frequent need for pain medication.

SECTION B

DISORDERS OF ERYTHROPOIESIS AND ERYTHROCYTE FUNCTION

This section discusses diseases and disorders affecting red blood cells (erythrocytes). The erythrocyte cell is a component of blood that the body uses to transport oxygen to the tissues. Under the microscope, these cells appear flat and concave. The red blood cell is sturdy and flexible, which allows it to travel through small capillaries and vessels without being trapped or destroyed. Hemoglobin is an important component of the red cell because of its ability to bind with oxygen and carbon dioxide. The hemoglobin contained in red blood cells releases oxygen to the tissues and organs through gas exchange in the capillaries.

The average life span of the red blood cell is approximately 4 months, after which time it is removed from the circulation by macrophages in the spleen and liver. Bone marrow must rapidly create new cells. The body must have adequate amounts of iron to create hemoglobin. Vitamin B_{12} and folic acid are required for the synthesis of erythrocyte precursors needed for the formation of properly functioning cells.

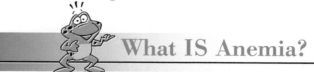

What IS Anemia?

Anemia is a decrease in hemoglobin concentration, circulating red blood cells (RBCs), or hematocrit (packed RBC volume). Anemias are classified according to their cause and the appearance of the RBCs when viewed under a microscope. The size of the RBCs may be larger (macrocytic) or smaller (microcytic) than is normal, and the hemoglobin concentration will be pale (hypochromic) or more highly colored (hyperchromic) than is usual.

See Chapter 12 in
RWNSG: *Pharmacology*

Pathogenesis

Three possible causes for anemia include blood loss, destruction or hemolysis of RBCs because of disease or drugs, and ineffective production of RBCs as a result of disease or nutritional deficits.

At-Risk Populations

Individuals who are particularly at risk include children, pregnant women, and older adults.

Anemia can occur in nearly any age group and be the consequence of a wide variety of physical disorders. Any person with poor nutrition can develop anemia.

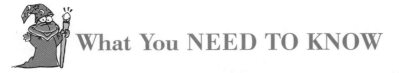

What You NEED TO KNOW

Clinical Manifestations

Because RBCs are responsible for carrying oxygen throughout the body, the symptoms of anemia are usually reflective of the degree of oxygen deficiency (hypoxemia). Some patients are asymptomatic if their anemia developed gradually. Blood tests during a routine examination can first detect the problem. Initially, some general fatigue and weakness may be present. As hypoxemia progresses, patients can experience headaches, tinnitus, roaring in the ears, light-headedness, and near syncope.

As the body tries to compensate for the decrease in available oxygen, patients may progress from dyspnea on exertion (DOE) to shortness of breath at rest with accompanying tachycardia or cardiac arrhythmia. Patients with cardiovascular disease are particularly at risk for anemia-related problems, including congestive heart failure and angina. Other symptoms can be associated with specific causes of the anemia.

Caucasian patients with anemia may be pale or have pallor. In the dark-skinned individual, pallor may be noted in the conjunctiva, oral mucosa, the palms of the hands, and the plantar surfaces of the feet.

Prognosis

Most patients recover completely from anemia when the underlying cause is treated.

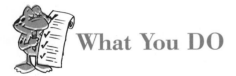

What You DO

Treatment

Treatment of anemia includes not only correcting the imbalance, but also finding and treating the underlying cause or causes of the condition. Supplementation with oral or parenteral iron, folic acid, and vitamin B_{12} may be indicated. Transfusions with packed red blood cells are indicated in severe anemias associated with acute blood loss or in patients with coexisting cardiopulmonary disease. Whole blood may be required for patients who are anemic and hypovolemic.

 Blood Net
www.bloodnet.org

Nursing Responsibilities

Diagnostic evaluation of anemia is targeted toward identifying the source of the problem. The nurse should:
- Help patients understand the cause of and treatment for their anemia.
- Counsel the patient to conserve energy during treatment. Nurses can help patients explore ways to avoid fatigue and over-exertion.
- Conduct laboratory studies that include a complete blood count with hemoglobin, hematocrit, RBC count, white blood cell (WBC) count, indices, and differential. Additional blood tests may include a reticulocyte count,

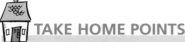

TAKE HOME POINTS

Oxygen therapy helps decrease dyspnea and treat compensatory tachycardia.

Jehovah's Witnesses may decline treatment with blood products because of their religious beliefs.

folate level, vitamin B_{12} level, serum iron level, total iron binding capacity (TIBC), and transferrin saturation. When hemolysis is suspected, the haptoglobin and direct and indirect Coombs' tests may be ordered.
- Examine the upper and lower gastrointestinal tract for occult blood loss in the gut, when necessary.
- Conduct bone marrow biopsies, when necessary, to rule out potential problems with hematopoiesis.
- Administer transfusions, when ordered.
- Teach patients about the risks associated with transfusions.
- Monitor for transfusion reactions.

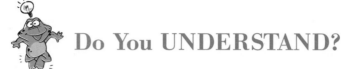

Do You UNDERSTAND?

DIRECTIONS: **Unscramble the italicized letters to form a key point about anemia.**
1. Three _____: (*ussace*)
2. _____ loss (*odlob*)
3. _____ of RBCs (*trudetonics*)
4. Ineffective _____ of RBCs (*dropnutcoi*)

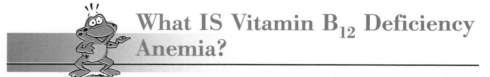

What IS Vitamin B_{12} Deficiency Anemia?

Vitamin B_{12} deficiency anemia (**pernicious anemia**) is a megaloblastic anemia in which the RBCs appear larger than normal on examination under the microscope. This condition is reflected in laboratory studies indicating an elevated mean corpuscular volume (MCV), which estimates the size of RBCs. The RBCs are large and immature, which leaves them unable to function normally, resulting in premature removal of the cells from circulation. Hypersegmented neutrophils can be noted on the blood smear during microscopic examination. The diagnosis is confirmed with a serum B_{12} level and a Schilling test. The Schilling test involves the administration of radiolabeled cyanocobalamin (vitamin B_{12}) and a 24-hour urine collection to determine malabsorption of B_{12}.

Pathogenesis

Vitamin B_{12} is needed for the formation of DNA, which is essential for the growth of mature, properly functioning RBCs. Vitamin B_{12} deficiency anemia is nearly always the result of an inadequate absorption of this nutrient in the ileum from a lack of intrinsic factor. Intrinsic factor is normally secreted by the gastric mucosa to promote the absorption of vitamin B_{12}.

Patients are usually older, and an autoimmune component to this anemia may be present.

Answers: 1. causes; 2. blood; 3. destruction; 4. production.

At-Risk Populations

Other patients at risk for vitamin B_{12} deficiency anemia are those who have undergone gastrectomy, ileal resection, or those with inflammatory bowel syndromes. Individuals with poor dietary habits or alcoholism are also at risk for this disorder.

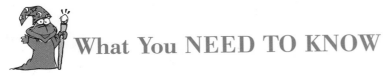

What You NEED TO KNOW

Clinical Manifestations

Vitamin B_{12} deficiency anemia usually develops slowly, over years, primarily because the body can have a 3-year store of vitamin B_{12}. The body compensates for the gradual loss of RBCs and the symptoms of anemia as listed may not become apparent until late in the development of the anemia. Because vitamin B_{12} is also essential for myelin integrity in the nervous system, symptoms can include neurologic manifestations. Gradually worsening soreness and burning of the tongue can occur. Patients might complain of symmetric numbness or tingling in the extremities, and ataxia or a loss of vibratory sense may be noted. Patients may exhibit changes in mental status, or they may develop memory loss, dementia, and depression. Indigestion, constipation, or diarrhea can also be present.

Prognosis

Without treatment, pernicious anemia will result in irreversible neurologic damage and cause life-threatening complications, particularly for the weak or vulnerable patient who is already compromised from preexisting conditions or age.

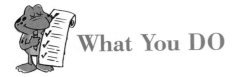

What You DO

Treatment

Treatment can begin with daily vitamin B_{12} injections while the patient is hospitalized, after which the injections can then become monthly.

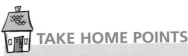
See Chapter 12 in RWNSG: *Pharmacology*

Nursing Responsibilities

The nurse should:
- Help patients understand that treatment must continue for their life span, except in cases in which the underlying cause of the condition is reversible.
- Provide assistance with ambulation, and take appropriate safety precautions in patients with neurologic deficits from vitamin B_{12} deficiency, when needed.
- Teach the patient or caregiver the proper way to administer B_{12} injections at home.

  Neurologic deficits do not always resolve with treatment. Patients may need physical or occupational therapy directed toward helping them maintain independent activities of daily living.

TAKE HOME POINTS

- Individuals at risk include older adults and those who have undergone gastrectomy or ileal resection, or those with an inflammatory bowel disease, poor dietary habits, or alcoholism.
- Treatment involves daily vitamin B_{12} injections.

Do You UNDERSTAND?

DIRECTIONS: **Fill in the numbers to complete each statement.**

1. The body can store vitamin B _____ for _____ years.
2. The Schilling test involves collecting urine for _____ hours.

What IS Folate Deficiency Anemia?

Folic acid is required for the synthesis of DNA and the development of red cells in the bone marrow. A deficiency of folic acid will cause a megaloblastic anemia with large RBCs and an elevated MCV. Additionally, decreased folate levels in the serum are present.

Pathogenesis

Chronic alcohol abuse is the classic cause of folate deficiency anemia. Alcoholics frequently have an inadequate diet and tend to have decreased absorption of nutrients in the gut. This deficiency can also be the result of mal-nutrition or an increased need for folate as in pregnancy, hemolysis, or malab-sorption syndromes in the bowel. Common drugs that interfere with folate absorption are phenytoin, methotrexate, trimethoprim, and triamterene.

At-Risk Populations

Individuals with an inadequate diet as a result of either environmental factors or biologic factors are at risk for folate deficiency anemia. Groups that tend to have an inadequate diet are those from low socioeconomic classes, alcoholics, drug abusers, those with nutritional disorders (e.g., bulimia, anorexia), and pregnant women.

 During pregnancy, low folate levels in the mother can lead to an increased risk of neural tube defects in the newborn. For this reason, pregnant women or those who are attempting to conceive should have daily supplements of oral folic acid.

See Chapter 12 in
RWNSG: *Pharmacology*

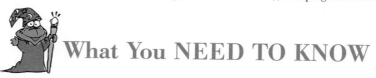

What You NEED TO KNOW

Clinical Manifestations

Because folate stores in the body are limited to 3 months, symptoms can be more pronounced than are those in vitamin B_{12} deficiency anemia. Signs and symp-toms include weakness, fatigue, pallor, dyspnea, and tachycardia. Irregular brown patchy pigmentation of the skin may be present, particularly in the folds of the skin and nail beds. No neurologic symptoms occur.

Prognosis

Most patients recover completely after the nutritional deficiency is corrected.

Answers: 1. 12, 3; 2. 24.

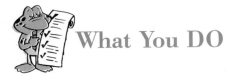

What You DO

Treatment

Treatment consists of oral folate therapy until hemoglobin or hematocrit levels are adequate. Nurses should provide nutritional counseling for patients to insure adequate folate intake in the future. Foods high in folate include liver, leafy green vegetables, broccoli, legumes, and brewer's yeast. Refer patients for counseling or therapy when alcoholism is suspected or known.

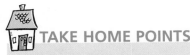

TAKE HOME POINTS

- Folate reserves in the body are limited to 3 months.
- Pregnant women should take folic acid supplements to prevent neural tube defects in the fetus.

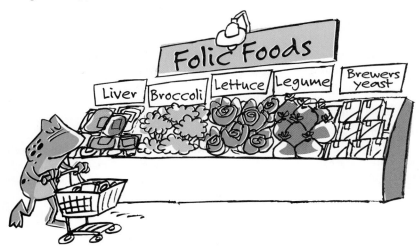

Nursing Responsibilities

The nurse should:

- Educate the patient about folate therapy.
- Counsel the patient on prevention of folate deficiency anemia in the future.
- When alcoholism, drug abuse, or a nutritional disorder is suspected, refer the patient to the appropriate specialist.

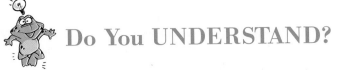

Do You UNDERSTAND?

DIRECTIONS: **Indicate in the space provided whether the statement is *true* or *false*. If false, draw a line through the false statements.**

_____ 1. Chocolate is high in folate acid.

_____ 2. Women should avoid taking folic acid supplements when they are trying to conceive.

_____ 3. Alcoholics tend to have increased absorption of nutrients in the gut.

Answers: There are no true statements.

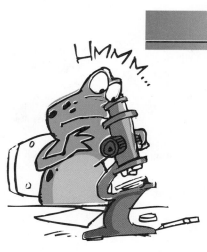

What IS Iron Deficiency Anemia?

Iron deficiency anemia is a microcytic anemia. The RBCs are smaller than are normal RBCs (**microcytic**) on examination under a microscope, and the MCV is decreased. The RBCs are also deficient in hemoglobin (**hypochromic**), and the RBCs appear pale under the microscope. A low serum iron and an elevated TIBC confirm the diagnosis. Iron deficiency anemia is the most common type of anemia and may be a result of an inadequate intake of iron, excessive blood loss, or poor absorption of iron.

Pathogenesis

Inadequate amounts of iron inhibit the synthesis of hemoglobin. Decreased levels of hemoglobin in the blood cause a decrease in the amount of oxygen that can be transported to the tissues.

At-Risk Populations

Iron deficiency anemia is also associated with blood loss from the gastrointestinal tract. Poor iron intake among young children or vegetarians can lead to anemia. The excessive use of antacids or gastrectomy can also lead to an inadequate absorption of iron. Additionally, iron deficiency anemia can be observed in patients with chronic renal failure who require hemodialysis.

See Chapter 12 in RWNSG: *Pharmacology*

What You NEED TO KNOW

Clinical Manifestations

Pica is a classic symptom of iron deficiency anemia in which patients have a craving for nonfood substances, such as ice, clay, or starch. Sore tongue and cracked lips (**cheilitis**) are common. The tongue may appear bright red and shiny, resulting from the loss of papillae. The nails can become soft and curl or "spoon" nails. The body is initially able to compensate for the loss of iron, but weakness, fatigue, pallor, dyspnea, tachycardia, and other symptoms of anemia occur with worsening disease. Extensive medical evaluation with complete gastrointestinal examinations may be indicated to locate bleeding sites, particularly in older patients. Treatment with oral iron preparations is usually adequate after the cause of the iron deficiency anemia is diagnosed.

Heavy menstruation is a common cause of iron deficiency anemia in women.

Prognosis

The prognosis for a full recovery is excellent if the underlying source of iron or blood loss is corrected and the patient receives iron supplementation.

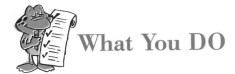

What You DO

Treatment

Medical and nursing care is directed toward correcting the underlying source of iron or blood loss whenever possible and replenishing iron stores in the body. Ferrous sulfate is commonly given by mouth in doses of 300 mg one to three times daily until blood tests reveal normal levels of iron and hemoglobin.

Nursing Responsibilities

The nurse should:
- Encourage patients to take iron preparations as instructed, and help them manage side effects, such as constipation or nausea.
- Caution patients to avoid using antacids or H_2-receptor blockers with iron.
- Counsel patients to decrease their activities and conserve energy until the anemia has improved. Offer assistance with daily activities as needed, and help the patient obtain assistance at home after discharge, when necessary.
- Dietary counseling is recommended. Foods high in iron include liver, fortified cereals and grains, dried apricots, raisins, meats, poultry, eggs, fish, and green leafy vegetables.

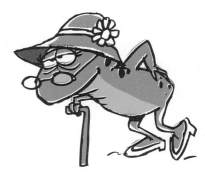

Older patients and those with co-morbid conditions should be monitored for cardio-pulmonary complications. Children, pregnant women, and patients with cardiac disease are most at risk to develop serious complications from anemia.

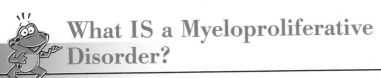

What IS a Myeloproliferative Disorder?

Myeloproliferative disorders are malignancies of the hemopoietic stem cells or immature blood cells. The hemopoietic stem cells, from which all blood cells originate, are normally found in the bone marrow. Various influences on stem cells normally cause them to differentiate or grow into RBCs, WBCs, or platelets.

Pathogenesis

Myeloproliferative disorders result from a lack of these cells (aplasia), the growth of these cells is exaggerated, or from ineffective proliferation (i.e., the cells are present in large numbers but fail to function properly). Because the most basic cell of the blood system is affected, these disorders can frequently evolve from one disorder to another, and symptoms can overlap.

The cause of myeloproliferative disease in most patients is never identified. Some association with the development of these diseases and previous exposure to radiation or chemotherapeutic treatment may be present.

At-Risk Populations

Although these diseases can occur in middle-age individuals, older patients are most at risk for developing myeloproliferative diseases.

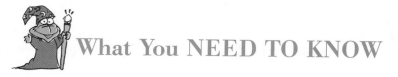

What You NEED TO KNOW

Clinical Manifestations

Clinical symptoms of these diseases are related to the cell line (RBC, WBC, or platelets) that is most affected. Diseases involving the RBCs will have symptoms reflective of low or high oxygen levels in the blood. These diseases frequently mimic megaloblastic anemias and occur mainly in the older population. When the WBCs are affected by disease, the symptoms reflect altered immunity, and persistent or unusual infections may occur. Platelets are involved in the clotting of blood, and a lack of platelets can result in bleeding. Excess platelets can lead to unusual and dysfunctional clotting, which will be reflected in the symptoms. An excess number of any types of cell can result in hyperviscosity or thick, sludgelike blood with associated symptoms. Although one cell line tends to be predominantly affected by a myeloproliferative disorder, the other cell lines are also affected, and a combination of symptoms will likely be present.

Prognosis

Without treatment, patients with myeloproliferative disorders will ultimately die of bone marrow failure. Currently, a bone marrow transplant is the only known cure for patients with this disorder, with disease-free intervals of up to 15 years having been recorded.

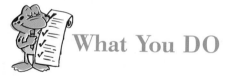

What You DO

Treatment

Supportive care and prevention of infections is the mainstay of therapy for this population. Patients with myeloproliferative disorders will require frequent transfusions of RBCs and platelets and will need to be monitored closely for signs of infection.

Nursing Responsibilities

The nurse should:
- Instruct patients carefully on methods of preventing infection and bleeding, as well as signs and symptoms that indicate the need for medical intervention.
- Administer RBCs and platelets, when ordered.

Older patients with cardiopulmonary or renal disease will require careful evaluation during repeated transfusions for symptoms of fluid overload and other complications.

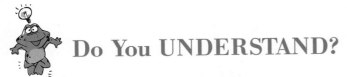

Do You UNDERSTAND?

DIRECTIONS: Circle all potential symptoms that may be observed in the
patient with a myeloproliferative disorder.

Bruises   Headache

Temperature elevations   Chest pain

Chills   Fatigue

Pallor   Dyspnea

Answer: All symptoms listed may be present
in the patient with a myeloproliferative
disorder.

Alterations in Blood Pressure and Blood Flow

This chapter provides information on the body's vascular system, including related diseases and disorders that can adversely affect the vital function of the heart and extremities. Without an effectively functioning vascular system, cardiac function can be compromised, and a potential exists for loss of limb and life. An understanding of both the normal and the abnormal hemodynamic and metabolic processes can help the nurse develop strategies for patients at risk and optimize their ability to recover from disorders affecting blood pressure and blood flow.

The vascular system is composed of three components: arterial, venous, and lymphatic conduits. Arteries carry oxygenated blood to organs under high pressure. Veins return unoxygenated blood to the heart within a low-pressure system, while lymphatic channels carry the waste products of metabolism back to the vascular system. Although each of these components has a distinct purpose, the normal function of other components can adversely affect each component.

SECTION A
DISORDERS OF THE ARTERIAL CIRCULATION

Arterial disorders generally result from a mechanical obstruction or increased resistance to blood flow. Although the causes are varied, atherosclerotic occlusive disease is the most common cause of arterial obstruction. A variety of nonatherosclerotic arterial disorders exists; however, these are less common. An understanding of some of these diseases and disorders is essential for the evaluation and care of the adult patient.

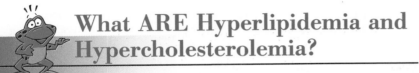

What ARE Hyperlipidemia and Hypercholesterolemia?

The terms hyperlipidemia and hypercholesterolemia refer to abnormally elevated blood levels of lipids and cholesterol.

Pathogenesis

Cholesterol is derived from two sources. The liver makes some cholesterol, and the rest is derived from eating animal products. Cholesterol and other fats cannot dissolve in the blood, thus they have to be transported by special carriers. These carriers are called lipoproteins—low-density lipoprotein cholesterol (LDL-C) or "bad" cholesterol and high-density lipoprotein cholesterol (HDL-C) or "good" cholesterol. HDL-C carries fats away from arteries. When deposited, these fats can cause clogging. HDL-C also has antioxidant and profibrinolytic properties, in addition to transporting key apolipoproteins, which mediate triglyceride metabolism.

Abnormalities in lipid metabolism can be manifested as a variety of clinical features. The most common clinical consequences of disorders of lipid metabolism include premature atherosclerosis, acute pancreatitis, and xanthoma formation (i.e., lipid deposits in the skin or tendons).

Causes of hyperlipidemia include both a genetic predisposition (primary) and several secondary disorders. Secondary disorders include hypothyroidism, nephrotic syndrome, obstructive liver disease, and diabetes mellitus. Additionally, chronic alcohol abuse, estrogen therapy, and some other drugs can cause secondary disorders.

At-Risk Populations

Total cholesterol levels above 240 mg/dl indicate a high risk for heart attack and stroke. Additionally, an HDL-C less than 40 mg/dl or LDL-C over 130 mg/dl are also associated with an increased risk of cardiovascular disease.

Because abnormal lipid metabolism tends to be hereditary, a positive family history should send up a red flag. Patients with sedentary lifestyles, morbid obesity, and diets high in fat are also at risk.

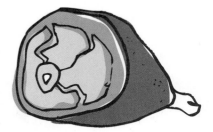

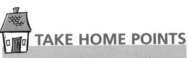

TAKE HOME POINTS

HDL-C plays an important role in reverse-cholesterol transport, carrying LDL-C to the liver, where it is biodegraded and excreted.

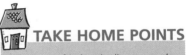

Abnormalities in lipid metabolism are commonly observed in industrialized societies because of the high fat content of the diet.

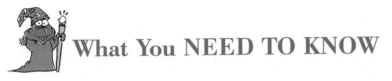

What You NEED TO KNOW

Clinical Manifestations

Frequently, no physical signs of hyperlipidemia or hypercholesterolemia are present, other than abnormally elevated serum markers found in conjunction with a routine physical examination. However, signs of atherosclerosis, such as angina or intermittent claudication in middle-age patients, can be the first warning of a problem.

TAKE HOME POINTS

Symptoms of ischemic disease can be the first indication of hyperlipidemia or hypercholesterolemia.

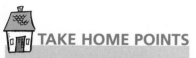

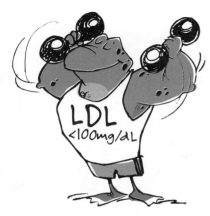

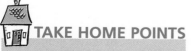

Acute pancreatitis and lipid deposits in the skin or tendons (**xanthoma**) can also be early symptoms, particularly in the patient who does not follow a wellness-focused program.

Prognosis

Early intervention focusing on primary prevention yields the best results. In most situations, aggressive treatment is commonly associated with the lowering of cholesterol and lipids and a slowing in the progression of atherosclerosis. However, adherence to a healthy lifestyle plays a key role.

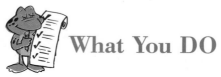

What You DO

Treatment

A diet low in saturated fat and cholesterol, in addition to regular exercise, is the mainstay of treatment. In patients who are overweight, reduced caloric intake to attain desired weight should also be included.

When diet and exercise fail in patients with risk factors for heart disease, more aggressive management using pharmacologic agents is always indicated. The goal is to reach low LDL-C and high HDL-C levels. However, the desired LDL-C level depends on the risk factor profile of each patient, including:

- Less than 160 mg/dl in patients with one or no risk factors for primary prevention.
- Less than 130 mg/dl in patients with two or more risk factors for primary prevention.
- Less than 100 mg/dl in patients for secondary prevention.

First-choice drugs for elevated LDL-C are HMG CoA reductase inhibitors—"statin" drugs. These drugs require medical follow-up and monitoring of liver function.

Nursing Responsibilities

A major focus of nursing responsibility is to promote an accurate understanding regarding the ways in which diet and exercise decrease total cholesterol and increase HDL-C. The nurse is in a strategic position to facilitate patient education and discussion regarding primary and secondary prevention of diseases associated with hypercholesterolemia. The nurse should:

- Counsel the patient about cardiovascular morbidity and mortality, providing information about specific problem areas including the following.
    1. *Obesity:* Maintain ideal weight; set realistic goals and remain active.
    2. *Smoking:* Reduce or eliminate nicotine use; participate in smoking cessation programs.
    3. *Hypertension:* Obtain regular blood pressure measurements; maintain diet, activity, and compliance with medication regimens.

4. *Diabetes mellitus:* Monitor blood glucose regularly; maintain diet, activity, and medication regimen as prescribed.
5. *Poor diet:* Follow reduced cholesterol and saturated fat diet; limit caffeine and alcohol intake.
6. *Stress:* Identify triggers for stressful situations and appropriate interventions to modify reactions.

🍎 Explain the purpose, administration guidelines, side effects, and special instructions regarding all prescribed medications.

• Determine methods of facilitating compliance with drug therapy. Monitor for adverse effects associated with cholesterol-lowering agents, especially decreased liver function and muscle weakness.

🍎 Counsel the patient on the importance of regular follow-up with health care providers and monitoring of serum cholesterol levels.

Older adult patients who are overweight may need a less restrictive diet to maintain adequate weight to improve overall health status.

Do You UNDERSTAND?

DIRECTIONS: **In the space provided, write the letter that corresponds to the word or phrase that completes each statement.**

_____ 1. A direct relationship exists between levels of _____ with the risk of coronary heart disease.
   a. LDL-C
   b. Triglycerides
   c. HDL-C
   d. LDL-C and total cholesterol

_____ 2. _____ plays an important role in reverse cholesterol transport.
   a. LDL-C
   b. Apolipoproteins
   c. HDL-C
   d. Nicotinic acid

_____ 3. The mainstay of treatment for hyperlipidemia is
   _____.
   a. Pharmacologic agents
   b. Diet
   c. Diet and exercise
   d. Dietary supplements

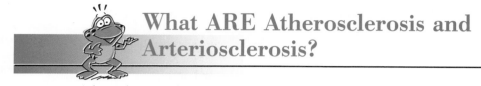

What ARE Atherosclerosis and Arteriosclerosis?

Atherosclerosis and arteriosclerosis are diseases that affect arterial blood vessels. Arteriosclerosis causes a thickening and loss of vessel wall elasticity that results in luminal narrowing. Atherosclerosis is a common form of arteriosclerosis.

Pathogenesis

Atherosclerosis is a complex condition that develops over a lifetime. Through a process called atherogenesis, fatty plaques (atheromas) are deposited on the artery walls, causing luminal narrowing (stenosis). When stenosis is severe and the body fails to adapt, the blood supply to tissues decreases, and the patient develops symptoms resulting from ischemia. Ischemia can also result from obstruction, resulting from embolization of microemboli or atheromatous debris distally.

Because of damage over time, fats, cholesterol, fibrin, platelets, cellular debris, and calcium are deposited in the intimal wall of the vessels. These substances stimulate intimal cells to produce other substances that contribute to further accumulation of plaque. As the intimal wall thickens, the diameter of the artery becomes further reduced to the extent that blood flow significantly decreases or stops.

At-Risk Population

The incidence of atherosclerosis has been reliably predicted based on certain risk factors:

- Age: for men, 45 years or older; for women, 55 years or older or those with premature menopause without estrogen replacement therapy
- Family history of premature atherosclerotic disease (father, brother, or son with history of heart attack before age 55 or mother, sister, or daughter before age 65)
- Cigarette smoking
- High blood pressure at 140/90 or higher measured on two or more occasions
- HDL cholesterol less than 40 mg/dl or LDL cholesterol over 130 mg/dl
- Diabetes mellitus: fasting blood sugar of 126 mg/dl or higher

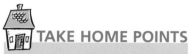

TAKE HOME POINTS

The exact cause of atherosclerosis is unknown, however, certain risk factors are thought to play an important role. These factors include:

- Elevated levels of cholesterol and lipids in the blood
- High blood pressure
- Cigarette smoking

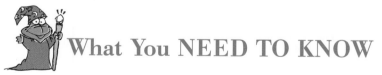

What You NEED TO KNOW

Clinical Manifestations

Signs and symptoms of atherosclerosis reflect tissue ischemia. Therefore when oxygen demands of tissue fail to be met, the following manifestations are likely to occur:

- Coronary arteries: angina, congestive heart failure, or myocardial infarction; atypical presentations of coronary ischemia may be manifested as dyspnea, fatigue, syncope, confusion, and abdominal or back pain
- Cerebrovasculature: transient ischemic attack (TIA) or stroke
- Extremities: intermittent claudication or gangrene

Prognosis

The prognosis for patients with atherosclerosis is highly individual and depends on underlying health, number of risk factors, and the severity of disease.

Early identification of persons at risk and modification of risk factors through compliance with treatment regimens generally create a positive influence. However, as the severity of disease progresses and more organs become involved, the prognosis becomes grave.

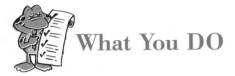 **What You DO**

Treatment

Treatment of atherosclerosis is directed at modification of risk factors and symptom management. Agents that inhibit platelet aggregation are frequently used to minimize thrombus formation, which frequently occurs because of plaque rupture.

Nursing Responsibilities

The nurse plays a key role in facilitating patient education focusing on primary prevention of atherosclerosis and secondary prevention of its sequelae. The nurse should:

- Educate the patient about risk-factor modification and associated reduction in cardiovascular morbidity and mortality.
- Provide direction and collaborate with the patient regarding realistic dietary and exercise prescriptions.
- Provide information about smoking cessation.
- Discuss the individual patient's ischemic symptoms, focusing on contributing events and interventions that are likely to lead to an improvement.
- Define situations in which emergency assistance using 911 should be used.
- Educate the patient about techniques on stress management.
- Discuss methods to facilitate compliance with medication regimens, such as cholesterol lowering agents and antihypertensives, and those that improve blood flow.
- Reinforce the importance of regular follow-up with health care providers and monitoring of appropriate laboratory tests (e.g., serum cholesterol levels, electrocardiogram data).

 Coronary artery disease in older adults may have an atypical presentation.

 American Heart Association
www.americanheart.org
National Institute of Neurologic Diseases and Stroke
www.ninds.nih.gov
Society for Vascular Nursing
www.svnnet.org

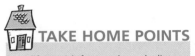 **TAKE HOME POINTS**

Modifying risk factors through diet, exercise, blood pressure control, and smoking cessation can improve prognosis. Prognosis for atherosclerosis is related to the severity of the disease.

 Older adult patients who are underweight may need a less restrictive diet to maintain adequate weight to improve overall health status.

Anxiety, frustration, depression, and fear of dying are frequently prevalent in homebound older adults.

See Chapters 4A, 4B, 6A, and 6B in
RWNSG: *Pharmacology*

Do You UNDERSTAND?

DIRECTIONS: **Match the statements in Column A with the appropriate responses in Column B.**

Column A

_____ 1. Treatment associated with minimizing microemboli

_____ 2. Responsible for atheroma

_____ 3. Primary prevention of atherosclerosis

_____ 4. Cause of gangrene

Column B

a. Cholesterol lowering drugs

b. Atherogenesis

c. Ischemia

d. Antiplatelet agents

e. Modification of risk factors

f. Cholesterol

What IS Raynaud's Phenomenon?

The term Raynaud's disease is used to imply a benign syndrome in which no demonstrable cause is present, although Raynaud's phenomenon is used in the presence of an underlying immunologic, pathologic source. Raynaud's phenomenon is a vasospastic disorder. Vasospasm refers to a sudden decrease in the internal diameter of a blood vessel. Raynaud's phenomenon almost exclusively occurs in women.

Pathogenesis

Raynaud's phenomenon is characterized by episodic vasospasm of the arteries of the fingers and toes in response to exposure to cold or emotional stress. Patients may have normal vessels with an exaggerated response to stimuli. However, approximately 60% of patients have a normal vasoconstrictive response to stimuli with underlying digital artery occlusion. Of this latter group, most individuals have an immunologic or connective tissue disorder, such as scleroderma.

The causes of Raynaud's phenomenon include the following:

- Exaggerated vasoconstrictive response to stimuli
- Underlying digital artery occlusion
- Excessive use of potent vasoconstrictive drugs (e.g., ergotamine tartrate)

At-Risk Populations

Women with the following disorders should be considered at risk:

- Peripheral arterial occlusive disease
- Connective tissue disorder, particularly scleroderma
- Migraine headaches treated with ergot agents

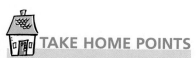

TAKE HOME POINTS

Raynaud's is frequently associated with scleroderma.

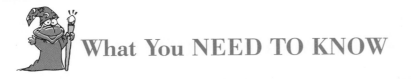

What You NEED TO KNOW

Clinical Manifestations

Raynaud's phenomenon is characterized by blanching of the digits and numbness with little pain. These signs and symptoms are followed by cyanosis after prolonged warming and, finally, reactive hyperemia with intense erythema and burning pain.

Prognosis

The prognosis is generally good. However, approximately 10% of patients with underlying occlusive disease eventually develop gangrene.

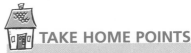

TAKE HOME POINTS

Symptoms of Raynaud's phenomenon are precipitated in response to cold or emotional stress.

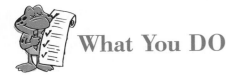

What You DO

Treatment

Treatment for Raynaud's phenomenon is primarily palliative, focusing on avoidance or removal of stimuli known to evoke symptoms.

Calcium channel blockers (**nifedipine**) can also provide benefit because of their vasodilatory effect. However, if pain and circulatory problems persist, then more aggressive treatment regimens (e.g., sympathectomy, spinal cord stimulation, acupuncture) can increase regional blood flow through sympathetic blockade.

Nursing Responsibilities

Nursing responsibilities for the patient with Raynaud's phenomenon include the following:

- Teach patients to avoid stimuli likely to provoke vasospasm, which includes protecting extremities from cold (e.g., wearing gloves, avoiding cold exposure) and effective stress-management programs to reduce catecholamine release.
- Encourage patients to avoid exposure to cigarette smoke because of the vasoconstrictor effect of nicotine.

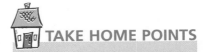

TAKE HOME POINTS

Treatment of Raynaud's phenomenon is directed at symptom control (i.e., limiting symptom triggers and calcium channel blockers).

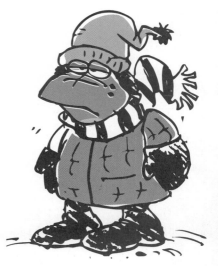

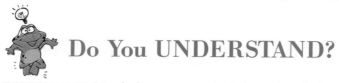

Do You UNDERSTAND?

DIRECTIONS: **Match the statements in Column A with the appropriate responses in Column B.**

Column A
_____ 1. Associated with redness and burning pain
_____ 2. Responsible for pallor and numbness
_____ 3. Benign vasospastic syndrome
_____ 4. Vasoconstrictive response associated with a connective tissue disease

Column B
a. Raynaud's phenomenon
b. Raynaud's disease
c. Hyperemia
d. Vasoconstriction
e. Scleroderma

What IS Peripheral Vascular Disease?

Peripheral vascular disease (PVD) is a term commonly used to designate atherosclerotic occlusive disease involving arteries that supply the extremities.

Pathogenesis

Atherosclerosis is a complicated process that develops over a lifetime. As a result of atherosclerotic deposits in the vessels, narrowing of the arterial lumen (stenosis) occurs. Generally, signs and symptoms do not develop until an artery has narrowed by 60% or more. Although any peripheral artery can be affected, the branches of large- or medium-sized vessels of the lower extremities are most commonly involved.

Atherosclerotic occlusive disease is the primary cause of PVD. Infrequently, an inflammatory process (e.g., vasculitis) triggers the localized development of atherosclerosis.

At-Risk Populations

Several risk factors increase the chances of developing PVD. The risk is compounded when more than one factor is present. Risk factors include the following:
- Hyperlipidemia and hypercholesterolemia accelerate atherogenesis and increase blood viscosity, thereby increasing the risk of occlusion.
- Cigarette smoking is associated with a profound acceleration in atherosclerosis. Smoking restricts blood flow by causing vasoconstriction and promoting coagulation.
- Diabetes mellitus complicates the clinical presentation of PVD. Not only is diabetes associated with accelerated atherogenesis, but also, the disease progression is atypical, with distal arteries being the first to manifest symptoms.
- Hypertension doubles the risk of symptomatic PVD.

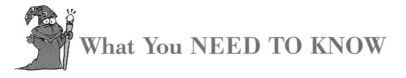

What You NEED TO KNOW

Clinical Manifestations

Early signs of PVD can include pain, changes in appearance, or changes in sensation in the foot or leg. Pulses can be diminished, weak, or absent. Pain generally falls into two categories: intermittent claudication or limb-threatening ischemia.

Intermittent claudication, the most common symptom, is characterized by muscle cramping or weakness triggered by exercise. Muscle cramping occurs distal to the obstruction, signifying insufficient blood flow to meet the demands of exercise. Increase in severity of symptoms indicates significant progression of disease. The activity that triggers intermittent claudication and the amount of rest that alleviates it are typically consistent in an individual patient.

Limb-threatening ischemia occurs when blood flow is insufficient at rest, the result of a severe arterial stenosis or complete obstruction. The patient typically develops burning pain, ulceration, or peripheral neuropathy, most commonly in the toes or the forefoot. Pain generally occurs when lying down, which can keep the patient awake at night (gravity increases blood flow to the feet when upright). This type of ischemic discomfort is called rest pain, which occurs acutely (**embolization** or **thrombosis**) or as a chronic progression of intermittent claudication.

Symptoms of PVD range from mild to severe and do not always correlate directly with the degree of stenosis. When arterial occlusion is acute, the signs and symptoms are obvious—pain, pallor, pulselessness, paresthesia, and paralysis (i.e., the 5 Ps).

Acute arterial occlusion requires emergency treatment. However, thrombosis of an arterial segment following years of progressive narrowing is usually associated with less severe symptoms because of the development of compensatory collateral pathways over time.

Chronic changes in appearance can include loss of hair over the lower legs, thickening of toenails, and muscular wasting. Changes may also occur in sensation, such as paresthesia or burning.

Prognosis

The prognosis for patients with PVD is highly individualized and depends on underlying health and the severity of disease. The severity of PVD has also been found to be a predictor of cardiovascular mortality. Early identification of individuals at risk and modification of risk factors through compliance with treatment regimens may slow progression of the disease.

TAKE HOME POINTS

Cramping or fatigue occurs in muscles distal to the diseased segment when oxygen demands exceed supply.

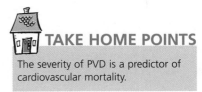

The 5 Ps signal an impending loss of limb. Pain, pallor, pulselessness, paresthesia, and paralysis usually indicate an acute thrombosis.

TAKE HOME POINTS

The severity of PVD is a predictor of cardiovascular mortality.

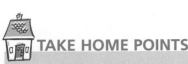

TAKE HOME POINTS

Modification of risk factors plays an essential role in the treatment of PVD.

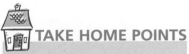

TAKE HOME POINTS

Aggressive management is generally reserved for limb loss situations or when quality of life is greatly compromised.

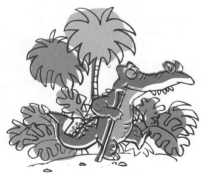

⚠ **The patient's blood supply is frequently sufficient to maintain tissue but not adequate to heal.**

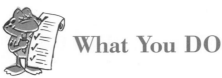

What You DO

Treatment

Similar to other atherosclerotic diseases, treatment is aimed at palliation and secondary prevention. Structured walking programs have been found to be beneficial because they tend to increase the pain-free walking distance over time.

Recent advances in potent antiplatelet agents with vasodilatory properties (**pentoxifylline** and **cilostazol**) now offer patients with intermittent claudication increased pain-free walking distances. Invasive techniques such as balloon angioplasty, stent placement, and bypass surgery are reserved for patients with symptoms that significantly affect quality of life and for patients in limb-loss situations.

Nursing Responsibilities

Primary goals in caring for the patient with PVD are directed at improving level of function and facilitating understanding of self-care measures. The nurse should:

- Educate the patient regarding the following:
  1. Modification of risk factors such as smoking cessation, weight control, control of hypertension and diabetes mellitus, and compliance with a low-fat, low-cholesterol diet
  2. Relaxation techniques, stress management, and fostering hope and spirituality
  3. Avoidance of leg crossing when sitting, prolonged sitting, and wearing of constricting garments
  4. Wearing of properly fitting footwear
  5. Daily inspection of feet and good hygiene, including the use of emollients
  6. Participation in a walking program (Exercise tolerance should be documented using specific measured distances. Walking distance should be increased in small increments with stops when pain occurs; resume after rest and pain relief. Walking should be timed [e.g., 20 to 30 minutes actual walking time] rather than using distance as a guide.)
  7. Notification of health care provider immediately when changes in color, temperature, sensation, or break in skin integrity are noticed

In assessing patients, an important point to remember is that PVD is a slow process. Therefore a sudden change in symptoms, such as the 5 Ps, should alert the nurse to an emergent situation.

Do You UNDERSTAND?

DIRECTIONS: In the space provided, write the letter(s) that correspond to the word or phrase that answers each question.

_____ 1. Instructions to a patient with PVD should include which of the following?
 a. Daily inspection of skin and feet
 b. Ways to participate in a walking program
 c. Avoidance of walking when pain occurs
 d. Immediate reporting of a decrease in pain-free walking distance

_____ 2. First line therapy for the patient with PVD includes which of the following?
 a. Balloon angioplasty, stent placement
 b. Bypass surgery
 c. Vasodilation and antiplatelet agents

SECTION B
DISORDERS OF THE VENOUS CIRCULATION

The venous circulation consists of peripheral and central components. The peripheral component, located primarily in extremities, contains valves that facilitate blood transport to the central venous system by modulating pressure effects under changing conditions. The central component includes veins from the intraabdominal and intrathoracic organs, which continuously return blood to the heart. This section deals primarily with disorders either directly related to disease involving the peripheral venous system or related to effects of the central venous system on the extremities.

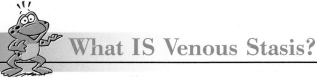

What IS Venous Stasis?

Venous stasis includes all conditions associated with slow flow or stagnation of blood within the venous system. These conditions include impairment in the mobility of extremities, congestive heart failure, extrinsic compression of veins by masses (e.g., tumors, abscesses, lymph nodes), and decreased arterial flow (e.g., severe hypotension or hypovolemic shock).

Pathogenesis

Venous stasis occurs in response to either an overabundance or decreased removal of fluid.

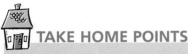 Pregnant women frequently experience temporary venous stasis in the second and third trimesters of pregnancy. This stasis frequently manifests itself visibly (varicose veins).

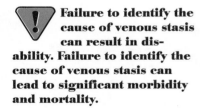

TAKE HOME POINTS

The patient confined to bed or chair is at increased risk for venous stasis.

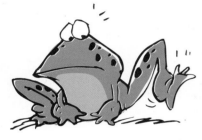

Failure to identify the cause of venous stasis can result in disability. Failure to identify the cause of venous stasis can lead to significant morbidity and mortality.

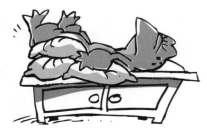

The following factors have been identified as common causes of venous stasis:

- Sedentary lifestyle
- Compression of blood vessels (i.e., obesity, abdominal mass)
- Congestive heart failure
- Chronic venous disease

At-Risk Populations

Patients with heart failure or a history of venous disease, such as varicose veins or chronic venous insufficiency and those with sedentary lifestyles are at risk for venous stasis. Additionally, obesity and pelvic masses are frequently associated with venous stasis because of compression of the great veins of the abdomen.

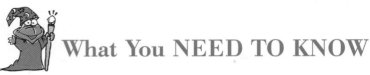

What You NEED TO KNOW

Clinical Manifestations

Mild ankle swelling is generally the first sign of venous stasis. With progression, the patient is likely to manifest dilatation of subcutaneous veins. Patients may complain of mild discomfort, described as lower extremity heaviness or painful varicosities.

Prognosis

When identified early and treated effectively, the prognosis is excellent. However, when the underlying cause is not addressed, the sequelae can be debilitating.

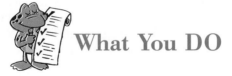

What You DO

Treatment

Treatment is directed at identifying the cause of venous stasis and management of swelling. Elevation and activity are the simplest methods to reduce extremity swelling. Pneumatic compression devices are commonly used in hospitals as primary prevention in those at risk, particularly for the surgical patient. Graduated compression stockings can also be used, particularly when the cause cannot be cured (**chronic venous insufficiency**).

Nursing Responsibilities

Because venous stasis is frequently preventable, health care providers should pay particular attention to body positioning and encourage physical activity.

The nurse should:

🐸 Be knowledgeable regarding the use of pneumatic compression devices and stockings.

🐸 Teach the patient primary prevention and symptom alleviation. Education should focus on:

1. Staying active (e.g., walking, structured exercise program)
2. Maintaining ideal weight or weight loss
3. Avoiding leg crossing when sitting, prolonged sitting, and wearing of constricting garments
4. Encouraging hygiene:
   - Checking skin daily for cracking or breakdown
   - Washing daily with mild soap
   - Using emollients, when necessary
   - Wearing clean stockings daily
5. Preventing injury
6. Providing guidelines about what to report to health care providers

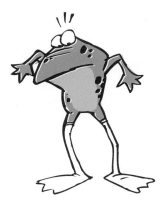

Do You UNDERSTAND?

DIRECTIONS: Indicate in the spaces provided whether the following statements are *true* or *false*.

_____ 1. Venous stasis can result from an ovarian tumor.

_____ 2. Lower extremity fatigue can be the first sign of venous stasis.

_____ 3. Walking is an effective method of preventing venous stasis.

_____ 4. Constipation can cause venous stasis.

_____ 5. Improperly fitted compression stockings can cause venous stasis.

What IS Chronic Venous Insufficiency?

Chronic venous insufficiency refers to the syndrome characterized by lower extremity edema, stasis dermatitis, and ulceration.

Pathogenesis

Chronic venous insufficiency results from abnormal changes that occur because of persistent high pressures in the deep venous system. These high pressures result from incompetent venous valves that are unable to facilitate normal flow from the periphery to the central venous system. This condition leads to congestion and an alteration in the microcirculation, which causes further changes in the skin and subcutaneous tissues. Hemoglobin and other protein waste mate-

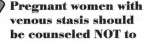 **Some brands of compression stockings contain latex, which can cause life-threatening allergic reactions in susceptible individuals.**

 Pregnant women with venous stasis should be counseled NOT to use compression or support hose during pregnancy.

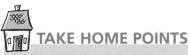 **TAKE HOME POINTS**

Elevation of the extremity above the level of the heart is the most effective position to decrease swelling.

Inappropriate use of pneumatic compression devices and stockings can cause serious injury, such as obstruction of venous or arterial circulation.

Answers: 1. true; 2. true; 3. false; 4. true; 5. true.

rials are deposited in subcutaneous tissue. These deposits subsequently result in increased pigmentation and increased oncotic pressure, which attracts additional fluid. Without treatment, obstruction of lymphatics further complicates the clinical course.

The majority of cases are related to the late aftermath of deep venous thrombosis. However, other factors, such as congenital absence or incompetent venous valves, can also be the cause.

At-Risk Populations

Patients with a history of deep venous thrombosis are at the greatest risk for venous insufficiency. However, individuals with varicose veins who have experienced repeated bouts of superficial thrombophlebitis should also be considered at risk.

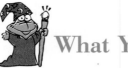

What You NEED TO KNOW

Clinical Manifestations

Nocturnal swelling is generally the first symptom of chronic venous insufficiency, but the condition usually becomes progressive and irreversible. A brawny (i.e., reddish-brown) pigmentation with stasis dermatitis of the lower leg can occur, along with secondary varicosities and ulceration. These ulcerations are not usually painful unless infected or involve deep tissues. Itching and burning sensations have been reported. Recurrent phlebitis and thrombosis are common.

Prognosis

Effective management of swelling and maintenance of skin integrity are possible when treated early. Recurrent phlebitis and thrombosis occur frequently and result in progressive deterioration. In rare cases, after many years, chronic ulceration can undergo malignant transformation. Lymphedema can be a late complication.

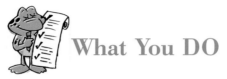

What You DO

Treatment

Compression therapy, periodic elevation of the legs, and avoidance of trauma are the mainstays of management. Good hygiene, including the use of emollients, is essential in preventing breaks in skin integrity. Careful attention to wound care must be included when the insufficiency is complicated by ulceration. When

TAKE HOME POINTS

Reddish-brown pigmentation with stasis dermatitis of the lower leg is commonly found in chronic venous insufficiency. Venous ulcers are usually not painful.

ulceration is present, compression therapy becomes a necessary adjunct to wound care, primarily because sustained pressures will prevent wound healing. Compression therapy may be ordered in the form of elastic bandages, graduated compression stockings, or a pneumatic compression pump.

Nursing Responsibilities

Patient education is essential in both the treatment and the prevention of complications associated with chronic venous insufficiency. The nurse should:

- Be knowledgeable about the use of pneumatic compression devices and compression stockings.
- Document skin appearance, characteristics of ulcers (when present), the current treatment regimen, and patient compliance during patient encounters.
- Educate the patient to facilitate primary prevention and symptom alleviation. Education should focus on:
  1. Staying active (e.g., walking, structured exercise program).
  2. Maintaining ideal weight or weight loss.
  3. Avoiding leg crossing when sitting, prolonged sitting, and wearing of constricting garments.
  4. Hygiene:
     - Check skin daily for cracking or breakdown.
     - Wash daily with mild soap using lukewarm water.
     - Avoid soaking legs in bathtub.
     - Use emollients, when necessary.
  5. Injury prevention:
     - Avoid bumping and bruising legs.
     - Do not go barefoot.
     - Avoid shaving with razor or hair-remover creams.
     - Avoid excess heat or cold exposure.
  6. Wound care instructions, including adverse effects.
  7. Compression therapy instructions, including adverse effects.
     - Wear clean stockings daily.
     - Always wear stockings while awake.
     - Apply stockings first thing in morning.
     - Discard stockings when elastic is lost (approximately every 6 months).
  8. Guidelines about what to report to health care providers:
     - Changes in skin (e.g., ulceration, dermatitis)
     - Changes in wound (e.g., pain, discharge, redness)

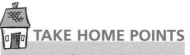

TAKE HOME POINTS

Compression therapy and wound care are both necessary to treat venous stasis ulcers effectively. Minor breaks in skin integrity frequently progress to ulceration.

Inappropriate use of pneumatic compression devices and stockings can cause serious injury, such as obstruction of venous and arterial circulation.

Do You UNDERSTAND?

DIRECTIONS: In the space provided, write the letter(s) that correspond to the word or phrase that completes each statement.

_____ 1. Compression therapy promotes healing of venous ulcers by:
   a. Promoting tissue oxygenation and nutrient exchange.
   b. Protecting the area from further injury.
   c. Removing waste products.
   d. Increasing venous pressure.

_____ 2. Interventions that minimize the sequelae associated with deep venous thrombosis include:
   a. Walking.
   b. Wearing compression stockings during the day.
   c. Avoiding sitting for prolonged periods.
   d. Soaking legs in a hot tub to relieve discomfort.

SECTION C
HYPERTENSION

Hypertension (HTN) is a disorder of blood pressure (BP) regulation. HTN refers to an abnormally elevated BP (above 140 mm Hg systolic or above 90 mm Hg diastolic) over a sustained period, which is associated with vascular damage and increased cardiovascular morbidity and mortality.

HTN is the most commonly treated disease that involves an abnormal function of blood vessels. However, in more than 80% of cases, the exact cause is unknown. In a smaller percentage of cases, diseases of the kidney, adrenal glands, and certain tumors are the cause.

American Society of Hypertension
www.ash-us.org
National Heart, Lung and Blood Institute
www.nhlbi.nih.gov/index.htm

What IS Essential HTN?

Essential or primary HTN refers to an abnormally elevated BP in which the exact cause cannot be defined.

Pathogenesis

HTN is a multifactoral condition in which one of the factors in the BP equation must change: peripheral resistance or cardiac output. Regulation of BP involves a complex interaction among the kidneys, the central nervous system and peripheral nervous system, and the vascular endothelium. A variety of organs, such as the adrenal and pituitary glands, also play a role. The heart responds to many of the changes mediated by these systems, secreting hormones both local-

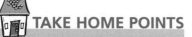

TAKE HOME POINTS

HTN represents three entities: a risk factor for atherosclerosis, a risk factor for cardiovascular disease, and a disease.

Answers: 1. a; 2. a, b, c.

ly and systemically. These hormones interact with substances produced elsewhere to regulate BP levels.

Hypotheses for the cause of HTN include:
- Increased renal reabsorption of sodium, chloride, and water related to natriuretic hormone, which is an inherited defect in sodium transport
- Increased activity of the renin-angiotensin-aldosterone system, resulting in extracellular fluid volume expansion and increased systemic vascular resistance
- Increased sympathetic nervous system activity related to autonomic nervous system dysfunction
- Decreased vasodilation of the arterioles related to vascular endothelium dysfunction
- Insulin resistance, which can be the reason for the common association of HTN, type 2 diabetes mellitus, glucose intolerance, obesity, and hypertriglyceridemia

Major risk factors for cardiovascular problems in the patient with HTN include tobacco abuse, hyperlipidemia, diabetes mellitus, advanced age, men and postmenopausal women, and a family history of premature cardiovascular disease (female relatives under age 65 and male relatives under age 55).

At-Risk Populations

Populations at risk for essential HTN include individuals with a positive family history, advanced age, obesity, and a sedentary lifestyle. Certain environmental factors have also been identified as contributing to the development of HTN. These factors include stress, excessive intake of sodium and alcohol, and the presence of sleep apnea.

The increased incidence of HTN in African Americans has been attributed to an increased prevalence of salt sensitivity.

What IS Secondary HTN?

Secondary HTN is the result of an identifiable abnormality.

Pathogenesis

The pathophysiologic nature of secondary HTN varies and is dependent on the specific abnormality. Although several types of disorders are responsible for causing HTN, the physiologic mechanisms all lead to increased vascular resistance and can be categorized as follows:
- Increased renin secretion
- Increased aldosterone production
- Increased stimulation of angiotension receptors
- Increased catecholamine production

Causes of secondary forms of HTN include the following:
- Renal vascular HTN: decreased renal perfusion stimulates the involved kidney to release renin
- Primary aldosteronism: excess aldosterone, usually a result of an adrenal tumor, causes sodium retention

- Pheochromocytoma: adrenal medulla tumor that secretes massive amounts of catecholamines
- Cushing's syndrome: excess cortisol production that stimulates increased angiotensin II and catecholamine release
- Hyperthyroidism: increased release of thyroid hormone, which stimulates catecholamine surge
- Estrogen-induced HTN: estrogen, which causes increased generation of angiotensin II

At-Risk Populations

Certain factors increase the risk for secondary HTN, which include alcohol consumption of more than three drinks per day, history of cocaine use, amphetamines, hormones, and immunosuppressive agents, history of genitourinary or renal disease, pregnancy, presence of a neurologic disorder such as increased intracranial pressure, quadriplegia and Guillain-Barré syndrome, and the presence of an endocrine disorder involving the adrenal, pituitary, thyroid, or parathyroid glands.

Both essential and secondary hypertensive patients at risk for target organ damage (TOD) and clinical cardiovascular disease (CCD). Patients in high-risk categories include those with a history of heart diseases (left ventricular hypertrophy, heart failure, angina, myocardial infarction, and prior coronary revascularization) and TIA or stroke (peripheral arterial disease, nephropathy, or retinopathy).

What You NEED TO KNOW

Essential HTN

Clinical Manifestations. HTN is generally an asymptomatic disease until a cardiovascular complication occurs. However, vague complaints, early morning occipital headache, fatigue, epistaxis, and dizziness can be early signs. Reproducible measurements of systolic BP over 140 mm Hg or diastolic over 90 mm Hg are consistent with a diagnosis of HTN. The Sixth Report of the Joint Committee on the "Detection, Evaluation, and Treatment of Hypertension" (JNC VI) summarizes the stages of HTN as: high-normal (130−139/85−89), stage 1 (140 to 159/90 to 99), stage 2 (160 to 179/100 to 109), and stage 3 (>180/>110).

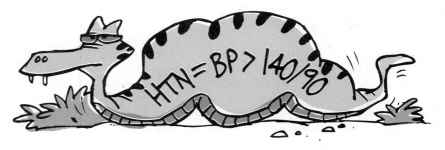

Prognosis. Effective control of BP in the asymptomatic phase significantly reduces overall cardiovascular morbidity and mortality. HTN is a leading cause of ischemic coronary and cerebrovascular disease, the second leading cause of end-stage renal disease, and the leading cause of congestive heart failure and hemorrhagic stroke in the United States. Additionally, a direct relationship exists between increasing systolic and diastolic BP levels with the incidence of coronary heart disease mortality.

Secondary HTN

Clinical Manifestations. Only 5% to 10% of patients with HTN present with a secondary cause. However, findings that are suggestive of secondary HTN include absence of family history and poor control on a 3-drug regimen with good compliance, or physical findings suggestive of drug abuse, neurologic, renal, or endocrine etiologic factors.

Prognosis. The prognosis is directly related to early identification of the secondary cause and effective treatment.

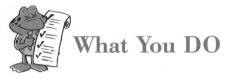

What You DO

Treatment

The goal of essential and secondary hypertensive management is to prevent death and complications by lowering and maintaining BP at 140/90 or lower. The JNC VI has defined a BP goal of 130/85 for patients with diabetes mellitus or with proteinuria greater than 1 g per 24 hours. In addition to treatment of the specific cause of secondary HTN, the same stepwise approach used to treat essential HTN is adopted. Management options for HTN are outlined in the following table.

Risk Stratification and Treatment

BP STAGES	RISK GROUP A[1]	RISK GROUP B[2]	RISK GROUP C[3]
High-normal	Lifestyle modification	Lifestyle modification	Lifestyle modification
Stage 1	Lifestyle modification (up to 12 months)	Lifestyle modification (up to 6 months)	Medication therapy[4]
Stages 2 & 3	Medication therapy[4]	Medication therapy[4]	Medication therapy[4]

BP, Blood pressure; *CCD,* cardiovascular disease; *TOD,* target organ damage.

[1]No risk factors and no TOD or CCD.
[2]At least one risk factor, not including diabetes; no TOD or CCD.
[3]TOD or CCD and/or diabetes, with or without other risk factors.
[4]Lifestyle modification should be adjunctive therapy for all patients on medication therapy.

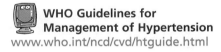

Hypertension, a journal by AHA
www.hyper.ahajournals.org

TAKE HOME POINTS

A direct relationship exists among increasing BP, risk factors, and TOD and CCD.

WHO Guidelines for Management of Hypertension
www.who.int/ncd/cvd/htguide.html

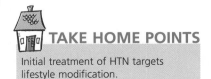

TAKE HOME POINTS

Initial treatment of HTN targets lifestyle modification.

Physical activity should begin at 10 to 15 minutes per day, 3 to 4 times per week, with gradual increase to 30 to 45 minutes, as tolerated in advanced age.

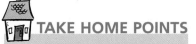 See Chapters 4A and 5A in RWNSG: *Pharmacology*

TAKE HOME POINTS

A strong association exists between dietary sodium intake and BP. A stepwise approach has been adopted for pharmacologic management of HTN.

Older adults should begin an exercise regimen under the supervision of a qualified health care provider. Exercise should be mild at first and gradually increased as the patient's tolerance improves.

Underweight older adults may require a less restrictive diet to maintain weight status.

Lifestyle modifications associated with lowering BP include reduction of body weight, decreased dietary sodium to no more than 100 mmol per day (2.4 g sodium or 6 g sodium chloride), increased consumption of fruits and vegetables (at least 4 servings per day), increased physical activity to 30 to 45 minutes for four times per week, moderation of alcohol consumption, stress management, and smoking cessation.

Many antihypertensive agents are available and may be used in combination. These include thiazide diuretics, beta-blockers, calcium channel blockers, ACE inhibitors, angiotensin II receptor blockers, alpha-beta ganglionic blockers, alpha-1 blockers, and central adrenergic inhibitors.

Nursing Responsibilities

Because compliance is essential to effective management, nursing responsibilities deal primarily with patient education including the following:
- Regular visits with a health care provider to monitor BP and adherence to treatment regimen:

> In 1 week if patient is in Stage 3
> In 1 month if patient is in Stage 2
> In 2 months if patient is in Stage 1
> In 1 year if systolic BP is 130 to 139 and diastolic BP is 85 to 89
> In 2 years if systolic BP is less than 130 and diastolic BP is less than 85

- Signs and symptoms of HTN
- Modifiable risk factors:

> Smoking cessation
> HTN—regular BP monitoring
> Diet—low sodium, low saturated fat and cholesterol, plenty of fresh fruits and vegetables; limited alcohol
> Exercise—goal of 30 to 40 minutes per day, 4 times per week
> Weight loss

- Medication regimen that includes purpose, dose, adverse effects, and special considerations

Guidelines to improve patient compliance to antihypertensive therapy include the following:

1. Integrate pill taking into routine activities of daily living.
2. Anticipate adverse effects; adjust therapy to prevent or minimize side effects.
3. Encourage positive attitude about achieving therapeutic goals and stress management.
4. Consider using nurse case management.

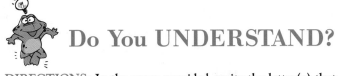

Do You UNDERSTAND?

DIRECTIONS: **In the space provided, write the letter(s) that correspond to the word or phrase that either answers the question or completes the statement.**

_____ 1. With BP measurements repeatedly in the range of 130 to 140 systolic and 86 to 90 diastolic, appropriate management of the patient with diabetes includes which of the following?
  a. Lifestyle modification and continued monitoring of BP in 1 month
  b. Lifestyle modification and antihypertensive medication
  c. Risk-factor modification and continued monitoring of BP
  d. Continued monitoring of BP

_____ 2. TOD as a result of HTN can be manifested as:
  a. Intermittent claudication.
  b. An aortic aneurysm.
  c. Superior vena cava syndrome.
  d. Renal failure.

DIRECTIONS: **Match the phrase in Column A with the appropriate term listed in Column B.**

Column A

_____ 3. Increased renin secretion
_____ 4. Increased stimulation of angiotensin II
_____ 5. Primary aldosteronism
_____ 6. Massive catecholamines

Column B

a. Pheochromocytoma
b. Adrenal tumor
c. Hyperparathyroidism
d. Estrogen therapy
e. Renal vascular HTN

What IS Malignant HTN?

Malignant HTN—occasionally called accelerated HTN—represents an urgent situation because of the risk of progressive TOD, particularly on the cardiovascular, renal, and central nervous systems. Although no specific numeric BP measurement is used to define malignant HTN, it rarely occurs at levels below 160/110.

Pathogenesis

Malignant HTN occurs when an acute or sustained elevation in BP causes rapid or progressive TOD, particularly in the cardiovascular, renal, and central nervous systems.

TAKE HOME POINTS

- Malignant HTN rarely occurs below BP levels of 160/110.
- In malignant HTN, BP is sufficiently elevated to cause acute vascular injury in vital organs.
- Renal vascular HTN is a common cause of malignant HTN.

Answers: 1. b; 2. a, b, d; 3. e; 4. d; 5. b; 6. a.

Malignant HTN frequently indicates a secondary form of HTN, which is particularly true when BP control is difficult to achieve despite patient compliance with an adequate and appropriate triple-medication regimen. Although noncompliance with antihypertensive medication therapy or any of the secondary forms of HTN can cause malignant HTN, renal vascular HTN is the most common etiologic factor.

Renal vascular HTN occurs in response to renal ischemia. Although renal ischemia is most commonly a result of renal artery stenosis, it may also occur because of dissection of the aorta adjacent to the kidneys. Renal vascular HTN results from increased peripheral vascular resistance induced when increased renin is released from an ischemic kidney. Suppression of renin secretion in the contralateral uninvolved kidney occurs as a compensatory response, thus serum renin levels remain normal.

At-Risk Populations

Individuals who are at increased risk for malignant HTN include young or middle-age patients with HTN and patients who suddenly cease antihypertensive medication therapy.

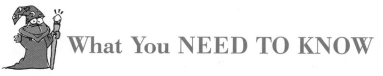

What You NEED TO KNOW

Clinical Manifestations

The clinical manifestations of malignant HTN include the following:
- Elevated BP, typically over 160/110
- Heart—chest pain, dyspnea
- Central nervous system—headache, fluctuating mental status
- Retinal—retinal hemorrhage, papilledema
- Gastrointestinal—nausea, vomiting
- Renal—azotemia, oliguria

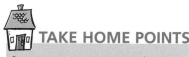
TAKE HOME POINTS

Symptoms can progress to a hypertensive crisis.

Prognosis

Without treatment, most patients die within 6 months. With effective treatment, 5-year survival rates of over 70% are possible. Acute causes of death include acute renal failure, hemorrhagic strokes, and heart failure.

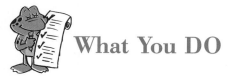

What You DO

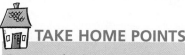
TAKE HOME POINTS

Treatment of malignant HTN focuses on reducing BP slowly using a combination of agents.

Treatment

The goal of treatment is to lower the BP slowly, over 6 to 24 hours. Although treatment is usually initiated with an intravenous antihypertensive agent, a combination of oral and parenteral agents is frequently used. The choice of agent is based on rapidity of action, ease in administration, and propensity for side effects. Addressing the secondary cause is equally important because antihypertensive medication therapy alone is frequently ineffective.

Nursing Responsibilities

Nursing care focuses on rapidly assessing the patient's baseline status, securing intravenous access, and facilitating admission to a critical care unit. Initial blood and urine specimens should be collected and antihypertensive medication therapy begun immediately. Abrupt falls in BP should be avoided with the goal to lower the diastolic pressure to approximately 110 mm Hg. Pressure reduction may need to be even less if signs of tissue ischemia develop, as evidenced by cardiac arrhythmias, chest pain, or changes in neurologic status.

Abrupt pressure reduction can result in stroke or myocardial infarction.

Do You UNDERSTAND?

DIRECTIONS: **Indicate in the spaces provided whether the following statements are *true* or *false*.**

_____ 1. Diastolic BP is more important than is systolic elevation in malignant HTN.

_____ 2. Renal artery revascularization is an important component of managing renal vascular HTN.

_____ 3. Dropping the systolic BP from 280 to 160 mm Hg in a 30-minute period in an 80-year-old patient is likely to cause a TIA or stroke.

What IS a Hypertensive Crisis?

A hypertensive crisis is a situation in which a severe elevation in BP and a rapid or progressive deterioration in the function of the central nervous system, heart, kidneys, or hematologic system occur simultaneously.

Pathogenesis

In this condition, the BP is elevated to the extent that immediate vascular damage is threatened. A persistent diastolic pressure above 140 mm Hg is associated with acute vascular damage in most individuals. However, the rapidity of the rise can be a more important factor than is the absolute level itself. If the pressure is not reduced rapidly, then cerebral edema worsens and can result in acute herniation.

Causes of hypertensive crisis include hypertensive encephalopathy, increased intracranial pressure, increased systemic peripheral vascular resistance, and excessive circulating catecholamines.

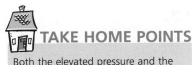
TAKE HOME POINTS

Both the elevated pressure and the rapidity in rise indicate the severity of vascular injury.

Answers: 1. false; 2. true; 3. true.

At-Risk Populations

Circumstances that place patients at risk for a hypertensive crisis include the following:

- Malignant HTN
- Intracerebral hemorrhage
- Head injury
- Ischemic stroke
- Acute aortic dissection (particularly when renal arteries are involved)
- Acute left ventricular failure
- Conditions that cause increased catecholamine circulation (e.g., pheochromocytoma, hyperthyroidism)

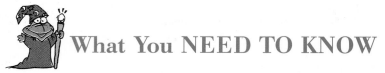

What You NEED TO KNOW

Clinical Manifestations

Symptoms are usually dramatic, however, some patients are relatively asymptomatic, despite markedly elevated BP levels and extensive organ damage. However, when pressures are sufficiently high to cause encephalopathy, the following clinical features are frequently present:

- Central nervous system: confusion, decreased level of consciousness, headache, visual disturbances, weakness, seizures, and nystagmus
- Cardiac: prominent apical pulse and heart failure
- Renal: oliguria and azotemia
- Gastrointestinal: nausea and vomiting
- Hematologic: hemolytic anemia and intravascular coagulation

Prognosis

Without treatment, patients die quickly from brain damage.

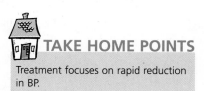

TAKE HOME POINTS

Treatment focuses on rapid reduction in BP.

 Failure to rapidly lower BP is associated with death.

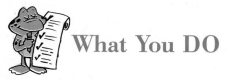

What You DO

Treatment

In a hypertensive crisis, the BP must be rapidly reduced within 1 hour. Because of the risk to life, an intravenous agent is always used. Sodium nitroprusside and nitroglycerin are two of the more commonly used agents; however, other agents are available.

Nursing Responsibilities

Nursing responsibility focuses on rapidly assessing the patient's baseline status, securing intravenous access, and facilitating critical-care monitoring. Initial blood and urine specimens should be collected and antihypertensive therapy begun simultaneously. Pressure reduction must be accomplished as rapidly as possible, preferably within 1 hour.

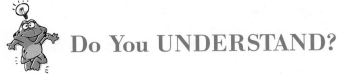

Do You UNDERSTAND?

DIRECTIONS: **Indicate in the spaces provided whether the following statements are *true* or *false*.**

_____ 1. Dissection of the infrarenal abdominal aorta is likely to cause a hypertensive crisis.

_____ 2. A combination of intravenous and oral agents are used to treat hypertensive crisis.

_____ 3. Dropping the diastolic BP slowly over 3 hours from 180 to 100 mm Hg is an acceptable plan.

5 Cardiovascular Disorders

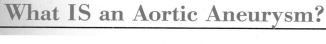

SECTION A
DISORDERS RESULTING FROM STRUCTURAL DEFECTS

What IS an Aortic Aneurysm?

An aneurysm is a defect causing dilation or ballooning of either a blood vessel or a heart chamber. Aneurysms can occur anywhere within the aorta and are classified according to their location. An aneurysm that occurs within the ascending aorta or within the aortic arch is known as a thoracic aneurysm. An aneurysm that occurs within the descending aorta in the abdominal area is known as an abdominal aneurysm.

Pathogenesis

The aorta is susceptible to aneurysms because the vessel is under constant pressure. A true aneurysm involves weakening of all three layers of the vessel wall. The three layers of the aorta include the innermost layer (tunica intima), the middle layer (tunica media), and the outermost layer (tunica adventitia). A false aneurysm involves weakening of one or two layers of the aortic wall. Many false aneurysms result from trauma during which a tear occurs in one or two vessel layers.

A dissecting aneurysm occurs when blood accumulates in the vessel layers. The most common cause of an aortic aneurysm is atherosclerosis. The accumulation of plaque or calcium weakens the walls of the aorta, causing them to tear and bulge, which forms an aneurysm. Hypertension is also a contributing factor because the high pressure further stresses the aorta. Other causes include syphilis and any type of infection that can affect the aorta.

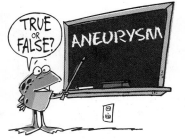

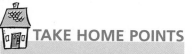

TAKE HOME POINTS

An aneurysm is a defect that causes dilation or ballooning of either a blood vessel or a heart chamber.

At-Risk Populations

Several associated risk factors contribute to aneurysms. Atherosclerosis and hypertension are the highest risk conditions associated with aortic aneurysms and are found in 50% of individuals with an aortic aneurysm. Other risk factors include Marfan's syndrome, congenital defects, and coarctation of the aorta. Marfan's syndrome is a genetic disorder characterized by a breakdown of the collagen fibers of the aorta; a fusiform aneurysm develops, which affects the thoracic ascending aorta.

> A dissecting aneurysm becomes a life-threatening condition. As blood accumulates within the layers, the layers separate and tear away from each other, spreading down the entire aorta.

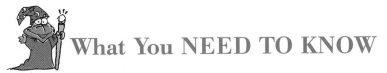 What You NEED TO KNOW

Clinical Manifestations

The signs and symptoms of aortic aneurysms vary, depending on the location of the defect. Most patients with an aneurysm are asymptomatic until the aneurysm begins to tear and leak. A large thoracic aneurysm can cause hoarseness (stridor) when it presses on the trachea. An abdominal aortic aneurysm can cause a pulsating abdominal mass that can be visualized or felt.

A tear that occurs in one of the layers of the arterial wall is known as a dissection, a major complication of an aneurysm. Blood leaks in between the layers of the aneurysm and expands along an area of the aorta. The thoracic ascending area is the most common place for a dissecting aortic aneurysm, primarily because this area is under the greatest pressure from the left ventricle ejecting blood.

Clinical manifestations of a dissecting aneurysm occur suddenly. A dissecting thoracic aneurysm produces a sudden onset of severe chest pain that radiates to the neck and back. Initially, the blood pressure is elevated; then it will drop rapidly from the sudden loss of blood as the aorta dissects. The patient develops signs and symptoms associated with hemorrhagic shock, such as tachycardia, hypotension, cold and clammy skin, decreased urine output, and weak or thready peripheral pulses. When the body experiences a decrease in the circulating volume, the baroreceptors located in the carotid arteries and the aorta stimulate the sympathetic nervous system thus producing the symptoms of hemorrhagic shock. These receptors sense the low blood pressure and stimulate the sympathetic nervous system. The sympathetic nervous system causes constriction of all the arterioles in the body to shunt blood flow to the brain and heart. Because blood flow to the kidneys is also shunted away, the vasoconstriction produces the cool skin, weak pulse, and decreased urine output. Paralysis of the lower extremities can occur when an aneurysm dissects into the area of the abdominal aorta in which the spinal arteries branch. A dissecting thoracic ascending aortic aneurysm near the aortic valve can tear and damage the aortic valve or cause a myocardial infarction from bleeding, sending clots through the coronary arteries because the coronary arteries originate from the base of the aorta.

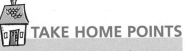 TAKE HOME POINTS

Causes of aneurysms include myocardial necrosis that is secondary to an infarction and atherosclerosis.

Prognosis

The prognosis depends on the location and size of the aneurysm. Dissecting aortic aneurysms can cause paralysis of the lower extremities as a result of impaired blood flow to the brain or spinal cord. Sudden rupture of an aneurysm can be fatal, particularly when the aneurysm is large. Emergency surgery after a rupture carries a mortality rate in excess of 50%.

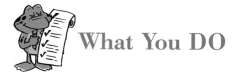

What You DO

Treatment

Treatment for an aneurysm is surgical repair. The aneurysm is excised and a synthetic graft is sewn in its place. Surgery is usually performed when the aneurysm is greater than 5 cm; smaller aneurysms are usually not at risk for dissection or rupture. Other indications for surgery include the following:

- Progressive increase in size
- Symptoms causing cerebral or coronary ischemia
- Pain
- Pericardial tamponade (i.e., blood leaking into the pericardial sac)
- Leaking, threatened, or actual rupture
- Visceral ischemia

Nursing Responsibilities

Prompt treatment and emergency surgery are required. The nurse must remain with the patient and administer intravenous fluids, such as normal saline or Ringer's lactate. Blood transfusions must be performed to maintain the systolic blood pressure between 100 and 120 mm Hg. A systolic blood pressure in this range maintains adequate tissue perfusion (oxygen and nutrients to the tissues) and helps prevent further dissection or rupture of the aneurysm. A urine output of at least 30 ml per hour should also be maintained; if urine output falls, then acute renal failure can result. Additionally, the patient should not be given anything by mouth to prepare for surgery. Several nursing interventions are required in caring for a patient with an aneurysm. The nurse should:

- Avoid palpating an abdominal pulsating mass to prevent rupture of the aneurysm.
- Report any signs and symptoms of dissection immediately to the health care provider, and prepare the patient for emergency surgery.
- Evaluate circulation in all extremities by assessing for color, temperature, capillary refill, and quality of pulse. A leaking thoracic aneurysm will decrease circulation to all extremities; an abdominal aneurysm will impair circulation to the lower extremities.
- When a patient with an aneurysm is hypertensive, administer antihypertensive agents. When antihypertensive agents by mouth are ineffective, intravenous agents that dilate arteries may be given. Common agents include nitroprusside (Nipride), nitroglycerin (Tridil), and labetalol (Trandate).

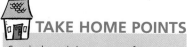

TAKE HOME POINTS

Surgical repair is necessary for aneurysms greater than 5 cm because of the risk of dissection and rupture.

A dissecting aneurysm is an emergency situation and represents the most critical aspect of nursing care for a patient, largely because the patient looses blood quickly, resulting in immediate death. An aneurysm located in the thoracic ascending aorta or aortic arch are sites that produce the greatest signs and symptoms of hemorrhagic shock. Occasionally, the patient has symptoms that mimic an acute myocardial infarction because patients with thoracic ascending aortic aneurysms have severe chest pain.

See Chapter 3A in **RWNSG:** *Pharmacology*

Do You UNDERSTAND?

DIRECTIONS: In the space provided, write the letter that corresponds to the phrase that answers each question.

_____ 1. A patient who is diagnosed with a thoracic aneurysm suddenly complains of severe chest and neck pain and is anxious. What is the first nursing intervention for this patient?
  a. Administer pain medication
  b. Assess vital signs
  c. Administer intravenous fluids
  d. Call the health care provider

_____ 2. The following information pertains to a patient who has a dissecting abdominal aneurysm: blood pressure, 150/70; pulse, 120; urine output, 35 ml/hr. What is the most important intervention for this patient?
  a. Administer intravenous fluids
  b. Administer a vasoconstrictor to increase the blood pressure
  c. Administer a vasodilator to decrease the blood pressure
  d. Place the patient supine

_____ 3. Maintaining a urine output more than 30 ml/hr for a patient with a dissecting aneurysm is important for what reason?
  a. To prevent acute renal failure
  b. To prevent renal hemorrhage
  c. To reduce pressure on the aneurysm
  d. To prevent further bleeding from the aneurysm

_____ 4. What type of aneurysm will produce profound shock?
  a. Descending aortic
  b. Abdominal aortic
  c. Abdominal saccular
  d. Ascending aortic

What IS Cardiomyopathy?

Cardiomyopathy is a group of disorders that affect the heart muscle (**myocardium**). Cardiomyopathy impairs the heart's ability to fill and eject blood efficiently. The myocardium should normally be able to stretch and fill with enough blood and then contract strongly enough to eject blood out of the chambers. The three basic types of cardiomyopathy are dilated, hypertrophic, and restrictive cardiomyopathy. The types of cardiomyopathy can be further grouped as either primary or secondary.

Answers: 1. b; 2. c; 3. a; 4. d.

Pathogenesis

The cause of primary cardiomyopathy is unknown (**idiopathic**). Secondary types are a result of other cardiac or noncardiac causes. The causes of secondary cardiomyopathy are:

- Ischemic (coronary artery disease)
- Valvular disease
- Severe hypertension
- Alcohol abuse
- Autoimmune disease
- Drugs (some chemotherapy agents)

The two most common types of secondary cardiomyopathy result from ischemia and hypertension. Ischemic cardiomyopathy occurs from either a massive myocardial infarction (MI) or from multiple MIs. Ischemia from an infarction causes necrosis of the myocardium. When a significant amount of the myocardium is affected, the muscle is unable to fill and contract as efficiently as it should. Chronic severe hypertension causes cardiomyopathy as a result of the high pressure within the arterioles. Without treatment, the left ventricle has to pump against the high vascular pressure for years. Eventually, the left ventricle will enlarge and weaken from being overworked, and the myocardium will fail.

Dilated cardiomyopathy consists of severe dilation, which reduces ventricular contractility. The reduction in contraction by the ventricles, particularly the left ventricle, decreases cardiac output and causes heart failure. Most cases of dilated cardiomyopathy are idiopathic, with the other cases resulting from ischemia, cardiotoxic drugs, alcohol, and postpartum conditions. Dilated cardiomyopathy in the postpartum patient usually develops 3 to 4 months after delivery for unknown reasons. Hypertrophic cardiomyopathy involves an abnormal thickening of the interventricular septum. The septum becomes greatly thickened to the extent that the left ventricle chamber size is significantly decreased. Occasionally, the septum enlarges asymmetrically within the left ventricle and blocks the outflow of blood from the left ventricle into the systemic circulation (**idiopathic hypertrophic subaortic stenosis [IHSS]**). Usually, survival for hypertrophic cardiomyopathy is long term.

Restrictive cardiomyopathy occurs when the myocardium becomes rigid and loses compliance, which presents a problem during diastole, primarily because the ventricles are unable to stretch adequately while filling with blood. As a result, the left ventricle fills with a reduced amount of blood thus decreasing cardiac output. Typically, infiltrative diseases of the myocardium cause restrictive cardiomyopathy, such as amyloidosis, hemochromatosis, and glycogen storage disease. Prognosis is poor and death usually results from either arrhythmias or heart failure.

At-Risk Populations

Cardiomyopathy can develop in anyone with cardiovascular disease or certain autoimmune disorders, such as lupus and rheumatic fever. Risk factors for cardiovascular disease include smoking, obesity, hyperlipidemia, and hypertension.

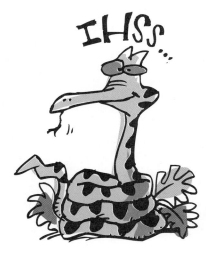

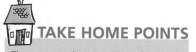

TAKE HOME POINTS

The term cardiomyopathy refers to a group of disorders that affect the myocardium, resulting in decreased ability of the heart to fill and eject blood efficiently.

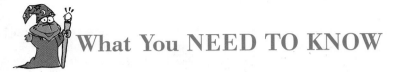

What You NEED TO KNOW

Clinical Manifestations

Clinical manifestations of all types of cardiomyopathy are those associated with heart failure, including loss of breath (**dyspnea**), fatigue, dyspnea on exertion, pulmonary crackles, and peripheral edema. Abnormal heart rhythms (**arrhythmias**) are common in all types of cardiomyopathy.

Prognosis

The prognosis for dilated cardiomyopathy depends on the degree of left ventricular function, because left ventricular failure is the primary cause of death. Most deaths occur within 5 years after diagnosis.

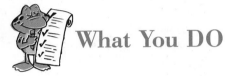

What You DO

Treatment

Treatment varies with each type of cardiomyopathy and is aimed at optimizing cardiac output (i.e., the amount of blood the left ventricle pumps to the systemic circulation). For dilated cardiomyopathy, digoxin, dobutamine, and amrinone are used to increase the myocardial contractility, and diuretics are used to reduce excess fluid. Angiotensin-converting enzyme (ACE) inhibitors are used to dilate the systemic arteries, resulting in decreased pressure within the arteries.

> **See Chapters 4A, 5A, and 9A in RWNSG:** *Pharmacology*

The reduced pressure decreases the workload of the left ventricle because the left ventricle now has less pressure against which to pump during systole. Nitroglycerin is used because it dilates both arteries and veins. Veins return blood from the body to the heart. When veins are dilated, blood pools in the peripheral veins, which decreases the amount of blood returning to the heart. The workload of the myocardium is reduced because the heart now has less blood to pump than is normal.

Treatment for hypertrophic cardiomyopathy includes the use of beta-adrenergic blockers. These agents inhibit the beta-receptors of the heart and cause a decrease in heart rate. The decreased rate gives more time for the ventricles to fill, which ultimately increases cardiac output.

> **See Chapter 5A RWNSG:** *Pharmacology*

No definite treatment for restrictive cardiomyopathy exists, other than treating any symptoms of heart failure. Beta-adrenergic blockers are occasionally used to increase ventricular filling time, as is the case with hypertrophic cardiomyopathy.

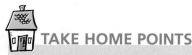

⚠ **Sudden cardiac arrest can result if the obstruction persists.**

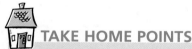

TAKE HOME POINTS

Dobutamine
- Infusion only
- Dose: 250 mg to 500 mg/250 ml D5W (dextrose 5% in water) or NS (0.9% NS) at 2.5 to 10.0 mcg/kg/min
- Action: Stimulates B₁ receptors
- Precautions: Increases workload of myocardium; worsens myocardial ischemia

Milrinone (Primocor)
- Action: Positive inotrope; relaxes vascular smooth muscle
- Dose: Bolus 50 mcg/kg over 10 minutes followed by infusion 10 mg in 40 ml D5W or NS at 0.5 mcg/kg/min
- Precautions: Arrhythmias, angina, thrombocytopenia

Nursing Responsibilities

Knowing which type the patient has is important for the nurse caring for a patient with cardiomyopathy because treatment will vary. The most important aspects of nursing care required for a patient with any type of cardiomyopathy are monitoring and treating heart failure.

- Place the patient in a semi-Fowler's to a high-Fowler's position. When the head of the bed is up, venous return to the heart is decreased thus reducing the workload of the heart.
- Report any episodes of acute heart failure, such as worsening of dyspnea, pulmonary crackles, increased heart rate, and jugular vein distention. Pulmonary edema, which is an emergency situation requiring prompt treatment, should be reported immediately.

Some special considerations for patients with IHSS are present. Medications such as vasodilators (drugs that dilate blood vessels) and inotropic agents (drugs that increase contractility)—treatments of choice for most cardiomyopathies—can be dangerous for patients with IHSS. Drugs that reduce venous return to the heart (e.g., nitroglycerin) and drugs that increase contractility (e.g., digoxin, dobutamine, amrinone) should be avoided in patients with IHSS. These agents cause an obstruction of the outflow tract (i.e., area from the left ventricle through the aorta), and blood from the left ventricle is blocked and restricted from leaving the left ventricle.

Negative inotropic drugs (i.e., drugs that decrease contractility) can be used to prevent obstruction of blood from the left ventricle through the aorta. The most commonly used drug is disopyramide (Norpace).

Intravenous inotropic agents are used for most types of cardiomyopathies except IHSS. The nurse must be familiar with preparation, safe dose ranges, action, and precautions for the drugs. The most common intravenous inotropic agents used are dobutamine (Dobutrex) and milrinone (Primocor).

Do You UNDERSTAND?

DIRECTIONS: **Fill in the blanks, using the italicized scrambled words. (Not all the words may be used.)**

1. Dobutamine should be used with caution because it can worsen myocardial _____.
2. Drugs that increase _____ should be avoided in patients with IHSS.
3. Vasodilating agents are helpful in the treatment of cardiomyopathy because they decrease _____.

   mischea   *clicartitnoty*
   prouefis   *reacadc kradolow*

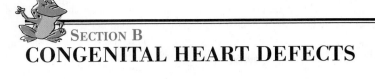

CONGENITAL HEART DEFECTS

What IS Valvular Heart Disease?

Valvular heart disease is damage to the structure of one or more of the heart valves resulting from a variety of diseases and conditions. Valvular heart disease usually affects the mitral or aortic valve. Valvular heart disease can affect the tricuspid and pulmonic valve, but it is rare and is usually congenital when it occurs. A variety of congenital or acquired conditions can cause valvular heart disease including:

- Ischemia (MI)
- Infection (endocarditis)
- Inflammation (rheumatic fever)
- Calcification
- Trauma

Because rheumatic fever frequently causes valvular heart disease, further discussion is warranted. Rheumatic fever is an abnormal immune or inflammatory response that reacts to group A beta-hemolytic streptococcus. Typically, this type of streptococcal infection occurs in either the skin or the throat ("strep throat"). Rheumatic fever has a 3% chance of developing as a result of a streptococcal infection. Toxins that are produced from the streptococcus stimulate the immune system. The antibodies produced by the immune system to attack the bacteria also attack the connective tissues of the heart. All layers of the heart can be affected, resulting in inflammation of the endocardium (**endocarditis**), the myocardium (**myocarditis**), or the pericardium (**pericarditis**). The valves are affected when endocarditis occurs because of the inflammation of the innermost layer of the heart where the heart valves are located. One or more of the valves become inflamed, and vegetative lesions develop on the valve leaflets. Eventually, as the inflammatory response resolves, the affected valve or valves develop scar tissue, which alters the shape of the valve. When the valve leaflets become rigid and deformed, the condition is then referred to as rheumatic heart disease. This condition develops after an acute episode of rheumatic fever or after repeated attacks of rheumatic fever. Episodes of rheumatic fever can recur and will typically occur within 5 years after the initial episode.

Pathogenesis

Two types of general structural damage can occur in valvular heart disease: stenosis and incompetence. When a valve has stenosis, narrowing within the orifice of the valve occurs when the valve is opened. Narrowing presents a

In children, rheumatic fever can affect the heart, joints, skin, and central nervous system. During the acute stages, the patient may have inflammation of the valves, myocardium, and pericardium, as well as cardiac enlargement (cardiomegaly) and heart failure. Narrowing of the valves (stenosis) may eventually require surgical intervention.

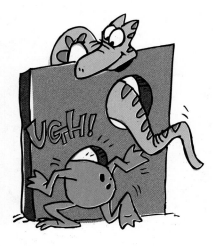

All four of the valve disorders will ultimately lead to heart failure without treatment or when the condition worsens.

problem because blood from behind the valve is restricted through the valve. Narrowing also creates resistance against which the heart chamber must pump. The chamber pumping through the stenosed valve must work harder than is normal to push blood through the narrow opening. As a result, excess blood remains in the chamber behind the valve. Eventually the walls of the chamber behind the stenosed valve become thickened and enlarged (hypertrophy) as a result of the excess blood remaining in the chamber and because of having to pump with an increased force.

An incompetent valve is one in which the leaflets "flap back" when the valve should be closed. The problem with a valve that partially opens when it should be closed is that blood from the chamber in front of the valve leaks back into the chamber behind the valve. Insufficiency and regurgitation are the terms used to describe the back flow of blood from the incitement valve. Excess blood builds up in the chamber behind the valve and the chamber eventually thickens (hypertrophies).

All types of valvular heart disease will eventually lead to heart failure and pulmonary congestion as the conditions worsen. The most common types of valvular heart disease are summarized in the following text.

Mitral Stenosis. During diastole, as the left ventricle is filling, blood flow from the left atrium to the left ventricle decreases, causing a decrease in cardiac output because the left ventricle ejects less blood to the body than is normal. Blood backs up from the left atrium to the pulmonary system and can cause pulmonary edema or pulmonary hypertension as a result of the increased pressure in the pulmonary system.

Because of the high pressure in the pulmonary system, the left atrium eventually enlarges, and right ventricular failure results.

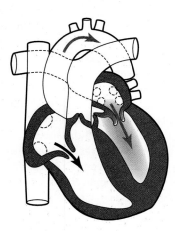

MITRAL STENOSIS

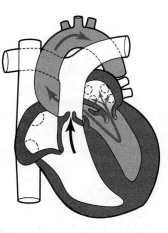

MITRAL INSUFFICIENCY

Mitral Insufficiency or Regurgitation. During systole, as the left ventricle ejects blood, some of the blood from the left ventricle regurgitates into the left atrium, resulting in a decrease in cardiac output because the left ventricle ejects less blood than is normal. Because blood backs up from the left atrium to the pulmonary system, pulmonary congestion and right ventricular failure can result. Eventually, left ventricular hypertrophy and left atrial enlargement occurs.

A prolapsed mitral valve is a type of mitral insufficiency and occurs when one or both of the valve cusps flap into the left atrium during systole.

Aortic Stenosis. During systole, the left ventricle is unable to eject all of the blood through the narrow opening of the aortic valve, causing a decrease in blood flow to the systemic circulation. Because not all of the blood is able to pass through the narrowed aortic valve, cardiac output decreases. Left ventricular hypertrophy results because of the excess blood remaining in the ventricle and because the left ventricle has to pump harder to get blood through the narrow opening in the aortic valve. Blood eventually backs up into the left atrium and then into the pulmonary system, and right ventricular failure can result because of the increased pressure within the pulmonary system.

Aortic Insufficiency or Regurgitation. During diastole, as the left ventricle is filling, blood regurgitates back from the aorta into the left ventricle, resulting in a decrease in cardiac output because not all of the blood passes through the aorta into the systemic circulation. Left ventricular hypertrophy, increased pulmonary congestion, and right ventricular failure can result.

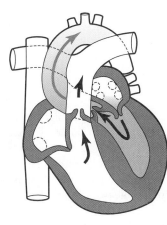

AORTIC STENOSIS

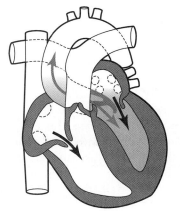

AORTIC INSUFFICIENCY

At-Risk Populations

Any individual with a valvular defect is at risk for cardiac complications. Patients with minor structural defects may be asymptomatic until they develop a coexisting illness or stressor that adversely affects cardiac function.

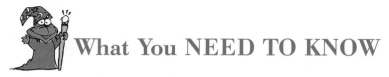

What You NEED TO KNOW

Clinical Manifestations

Clinical manifestations for a patient with valvular heart disease depend on the nature and severity of the particular valve disorder. Patients can be asymptomatic when only mild stenosis or insufficiency of the valve occurs. Symptoms associated with valvular heart disease are primarily symptoms associated with left ventricular failure, such as dyspnea on exertion, crackles in the lungs, a nonproductive cough, weakness, and fatigue. As the condition worsens, pulmonary edema can develop. Eventually, if right ventricular failure results, then symptoms such as jugular vein distention, hepatomegaly, and peripheral edema will occur. Patients with mitral stenosis can develop atrial arrhythmias (i.e., abnormal cardiac rhythms originating from the atria) because of the enlarged left atrium. A patient with detectable valvular heart disease usually has a murmur that can be auscultated.

Prognosis

The prognosis for recovery from valvular disease depends on the severity of the defect, the presence of coexisting diseases that can adversely affect cardiac function, and the patient's access to prompt and appropriate medical care.

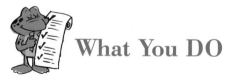

What You DO

Treatment

Several medications are available that can be used to treat valvular heart disease. Treatment includes primarily the management of heart failure. Digoxin is given to increase myocardial contractility. Diuretics are used to reduce excess fluid, thus the weakened ventricles will have less blood to pump. An ACE inhibitor is also used because it dilates the systemic arterioles, which decreases the pressure within the vessels. This decrease in pressure decreases the resistance against which the weakened left ventricle has to pump during systole.

See Chapters 4A, 5A, and 9A in RWNSG: *Pharmacology*

Valve surgery is the treatment of choice for patients experiencing symptoms of heart failure or when the left ventricle is at risk for failure. Valves can be either replaced or repaired. Three types of reconstructive surgery can be performed. Open commissurotomy is typically performed for mitral stenosis, which involves incising fused leaflets and removing calcium deposits on the valve. An annuloplasty is typically performed for mitral insufficiency, which involves the insertion of a ring to reduce the size of a dilated mitral valve. A valvuloplasty involves a variety of techniques used to repair valves, such as patching damaged portions of a valve or removing excess tissue or calcium deposits on a valve. Valve replacement surgery is performed for a severely damaged valve that cannot be repaired. The valve is removed and replaced with either a tissue or prosthetic valve.

Nursing Responsibilities

The nurse must be aware that any valvular heart disease can cause a decrease in cardiac output and lead to heart failure. A patient with severe damage to a valve can develop pulmonary edema suddenly and at any time. Others with long-term valve damage can develop heart failure slowly over years.

The nurse should be able to recognize basic murmurs when caring for a patient with valvular heart disease. A murmur is an abnormal heart sound that is auscultated when a patient has valvular heart disease. The sound is usually a swishing and somewhat loud sound. A murmur is heard because turbulent blood flow occurs when it is passing through a stenosed valve or is regurgitating through an incompetent valve. A murmur can be auscultated either during the first heart sound (**systole**) or during the second heart sound (**diastole**).

A murmur that is heard during systole is referred to as a systolic murmur, and a murmur that is heard during diastole is referred to as a diastolic murmur. A systolic murmur can represent either aortic stenosis or mitral insufficiency. The murmur can be aortic stenosis because, during systole, the left ventricle is ejecting blood through the aortic valve. A systolic murmur can be a result of mitral insufficiency because, during systole, the mitral valve should be closed. However, when the valve is incompetent, the blood from the left ventricle will regurgitate through the mitral valve during systole. A diastolic murmur can indicate either mitral stenosis or aortic regurgitation. The murmur can be mitral stenosis because, during diastole, blood is leaving the left atrium into the left ventricle. A diastolic murmur can also be a result of aortic insufficiency because, during diastole, the aortic valve should be closed. However, when the valve is incompetent, the blood regurgitates from the aorta back into the left ventricle.

The nurse who is caring for a patient with valvular heart disease should be able to recognize the basic heart murmurs associated with the specific disorder. Auscultating for murmurs is a difficult skill and must be practiced. The best way to become familiar with murmurs is to always auscultate heart sounds on patients with known valvular heart disease. For example, if you read in the history and physical examination that the patient has aortic stenosis, then auscultate the heart sounds and listen for the murmur. Become familiar with the circulation of blood through the heart and know which valves should be opened and closed during systole and diastole.

The following list highlights simple steps in auscultating for murmurs:

- Listen for the first or systolic heart sound and then for the second or diastolic heart sound.
- Determine whether the murmur occurs during the first or second heart sound and whether it is a systolic or diastolic murmur.

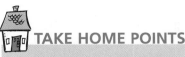

TAKE HOME POINTS

Valvular heart disease is treated with medications. Surgery to repair or replace the valve is indicated for patients experiencing symptoms of heart failure.

Patients who develop a severe case of endocarditis or a massive MI can develop sudden valvular heart disease and heart failure quickly with pulmonary edema. This condition is usually an emergency situation and may require valve replacement surgery.

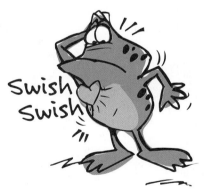

Swish Swish

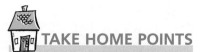

TAKE HOME POINTS

Auscultation of each particular valve can be best heard over the following areas:

Type of murmur	Location to auscultate
Aortic	2nd intercostal space, right sternal border
Pulmonic	2nd intercostal space, left sternal border
Tricuspid	5th intercostal space, left sternal border
Mitral	5th intercostal space, midclavicular line

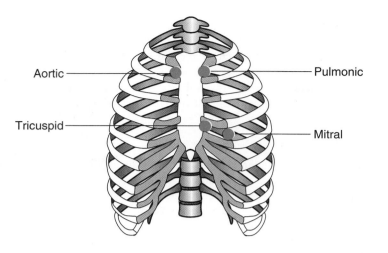

- Listen over the four points where each valve is best heard. If you hear the murmur louder in the area over a particular valve, then that valve is likely to be damaged.
- Determine whether the valve has stenosis or insufficiency by assessing whether the murmur is systolic or diastolic.

  Example of using steps:
  1. Auscultate both heart sounds.
  2. Listen for a murmur during the first heart sound to know that the murmur is systolic.
  3. Listen over the four areas of heart sounds, and hear the murmur loudest over the aortic area.
  4. The patient likely has aortic stenosis because (a) the murmur is systolic and (b) the left ventricle is pumping blood through the aorta during systole.

A patient with valvular heart disease requires several special nursing care imperatives, including the following:

- Teach patients and family members about early treatment of skin and throat infections. When group A beta-hemolytic streptococcus causes the infections, rheumatic fever can result. Antibiotic therapy is a mainstay of treatment. Penicillin is the drug of choice. Erythromycin or clindamycin can be used when the patient is allergic to penicillin. Teaching must include the importance of completing antibiotic therapy as prescribed. Patients must also understand the need to continue with prophylactic antibiotic therapy for at least 5 years to prevent endocarditis.

Appropriate antibiotic therapy is particularly important for children to decrease the risk of cardiac complications in adulthood.

- Assess for signs and symptoms of heart failure and report these immediately to the health care provider; symptoms can indicate worsening of the valve dysfunction. The patient may require emergency valve surgery or repair.

Signs and symptoms include shortness of breath, crackles auscultated in the lungs, dyspnea on exertion, jugular vein distention, peripheral edema, and weight gain.

- When the patient develops hypotension or when the skin is cool and clammy, notify the health care provider. These symptoms indicate an emergency situation, indicating that the left ventricle is failing and insufficient blood is being pumped to the body.
- Report any signs and symptoms of pulmonary edema, because it is an emergency situation that can cause respiratory failure. Signs and symptoms include severe labored breathing, tachycardia, crackles in all lung fields, and pink, frothy sputum.
- Report any fever to the health care provider immediately. Turbulent blood flow through damaged valves increases the risk for patients to develop endocarditis.

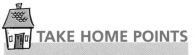

TAKE HOME POINTS

Patients with valvular heart disease should receive prophylactic antibiotics before any invasive procedure, including dental work, to prevent endocarditis.

Do You UNDERSTAND?

DIRECTIONS: **In the space provided, write the letter that corresponds to the phrase that answers each question.**

_____ 1. Which statement by a patient with rheumatic fever indicates that further teaching is required?
   a. "I will need to take antibiotics for 10 days and for 5 years."
   b. "I only need to take antibiotics for 10 days."
   c. "I will need to take a dose of an antibiotic for 5 years to prevent the infection from returning."
   d. "I should not miss any doses of the antibiotics."

_____ 2. Which one of the following statements refers to an incompetent valve?
   a. Has a narrow opening
   b. Is fused and is unable to open
   c. Has leaflets that flap back when the valve should be closed
   d. Has leaflets that flap in when the valve should be open

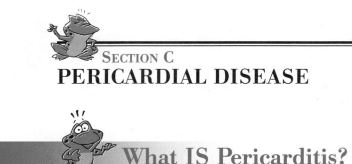

SECTION C
PERICARDIAL DISEASE

What IS Pericarditis?

Pericarditis is inflammation that occurs within the pericardium. The pericardium is a double-walled membranous sac that surrounds the heart. The area between the outer layer **(parietal pericardium)** and the inner layer **(visceral pericardium)** is the pericardial cavity or sac. This cavity contains approximately 10 to 30 ml of fluid **(pericardial fluid)** that creates a smooth and frictionless atmosphere for the pumping heart.

Pathogenesis

The inflammatory response in pericarditis causes fibrin to be deposited in the pericardium with the subsequent development of edema and thickening of the pericardial membrane. Pericarditis can be an acute or chronic condition. Acute pericarditis is a condition that suddenly occurs, usually secondary to an infection, an MI, or trauma. Acute pericarditis usually responds to treatment and is resolved without problems. However, some patients can develop recurrent episodes of acute pericarditis. Chronic pericarditis is a slow and progressive process during which the pericardium transforms into scar tissue. The pericardium becomes extremely thick with the layer up to 10 times the normal thickness of the pericardium. The scar tissue of the pericardium limits or constricts the movement of the pericardium; thus chronic pericarditis is frequently referred to as constrictive pericarditis.

Pericardial disease is usually secondary to another disorder. The two most common pericardial disorders are pericarditis and pericardial effusion. A pericardial effusion is a condition in which fluid, exudate, or blood accumulates within the pericardial sac. A pericardial effusion can occur from any of the conditions that cause pericardial disease and can be associated with either acute or chronic pericarditis. A pericardial effusion can develop suddenly, as with chest trauma, or slowly, as with chronic pericarditis. Pericardial effusions associated with trauma involves blood leaking into the pericardial sac and usually occur with chest trauma secondary to a motor vehicle injury from the steering wheel or after any type of cardiac surgery. Pericardial effusions associated with pericarditis involve the accumulation of fluid in the pericardial sac. Small pericardial effusions usually do not present a problem.

Conditions that can affect the pericardium include connective tissue disorders, cancer, infections (particularly of the heart and lungs), trauma, amyloidosis, drugs, acute MI, and end-stage renal failure. Common causes of chronic pericarditis include tuberculosis, cancer, and amyloidosis.

At-Risk Populations

Pericarditis is not limited to an age group or population and may occur at any time as a consequence of other conditions and disease processes.

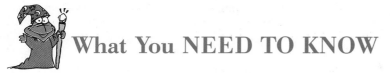 What You NEED TO KNOW

Acute Pericarditis Clinical Manifestations

Chest pain is the main clinical manifestation of acute pericarditis. The patient is typically uncomfortable and restless. Differentiating pericardial chest pain from ischemic chest pain is important. Chest pain associated with pericarditis is usually persistent and unrelieved by nitroglycerin or opioids. The pain is relieved only by an antiinflammatory agent, such as a nonsteroidal antiinflammatory drug (NSAID). Inspiration or cough frequently aggravates the chest pain and can be relieved after the patient sits up. Most patients will also have fever. Patients who have had an MI can develop pericarditis, usually within 24 to 48 hours after the infarction (**Dressler's syndrome**). These patients complain of persistent chest pain and nitroglycerin is ineffective. An electrocardiogram (ECG) may show S-T segment elevation on all or most leads. This widespread S-T elevation represents inflammation of the pericardium.

A pericardial friction rub may be auscultated when assessing heart sounds in a patient with acute pericarditis. A "creaky" or "leathery" sound is usually heard with each heartbeat. A pericardial friction rub should not be confused with a pleural friction rub, which indicates inflammation of the pleura. When auscultating heart sounds, feel the patient's pulse at the same time; when the rub is heard with the pulse, the sound is a pericardial friction rub. Another way to differentiate a pericardial friction rub from a pleural friction rub is to have the patient stop breathing for a few seconds; if you still hear the rub, then the sound is a pericardial friction rub.

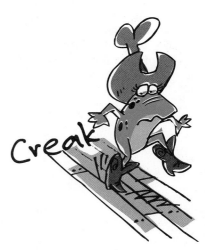

Creak

Chronic Pericarditis Clinical Manifestations

Chronic pericarditis involves the formation of scar tissue that constricts the movement of the pericardium. This constriction presents a problem during diastole when the ventricles are filling with blood. During diastole, the ventricles must stretch to fill with an adequate amount of blood. In chronic pericarditis, the scar tissue of the pericardium prevents the ventricles from stretching and the ventricles fill with less blood than is normal. This reduction in ventricular filling reduces cardiac output because the left ventricle ejects less blood to the body than is normal. This type of heart failure is frequently called diastolic heart failure.

Clinical manifestations of chronic pericarditis are those associated with heart failure, such as peripheral edema, pulmonary crackles, fatigue, and shortness of breath. Jugular vein distention, dyspnea on exertion, generalized edema, and hepatomegaly are frequently observed in chronic pericarditis.

A large pericardial effusion presents a problem in that if the pericardial sac fills with too much fluid or blood, the heart's movement is restricted and is unable to fill and contract, which results in the ejection of less blood than is normal. When the amount of fluid or blood severely impairs the heart's movement, the condition is referred to as a cardiac tamponade. This condition is an emergency situation because cardiac output is severely diminished and cardiogenic shock results because the left ventricle is unable to eject sufficient blood to supply oxygen to the tissues.

Pericardial Effusion Clinical Manifestations

Clinical manifestations of a pericardial effusion depend on the amount of fluid or blood in the pericardial sac. Typically, the patient is asymptomatic until the fluid impairs cardiac output. When the cardiac output is impaired, the patient will have signs and symptoms associated with heart failure. In severe cases, when cardiac tamponade develops, signs and symptoms are distinct. Clinical manifestations of cardiogenic shock are present, such as hypotension, tachycardia (usually 120 or greater), weak and thready peripheral pulses, cool and clammy skin, and diminished or absent urine output. Severe jugular vein distention is present with a cardiac tamponade. Heart sounds are muffled and frequently cannot be auscultated. Pulsus paradoxus is also a classic sign of cardiac tamponade. Pulsus paradoxus is a condition in which the cardiac output and blood pressure is decreased more during inspiration than it is during expiration. This condition occurs because venous return to the right ventricle is increased during inspiration. This increase in volume adds further pressure to the left ventricle, along with the pericardial fluid.

Prognosis

Any form of pericarditis can result in a pericardial effusion. Eventually, the accumulation of fluid will restrict the heart's ability to fill with blood if it is not recognized and treated appropriately.

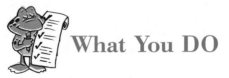

What You DO

Acute Pericarditis Treatment

Treatment of acute pericarditis is aimed at reducing the inflammation. NSAIDs, particularly indomethacin, are the drugs of choice and improvement is usually rapid. If no response to NSAIDs is forthcoming and no infection is present, then steroids are used. When bacterial pericarditis is suspected, intravenous antibiotics are administered.

See Chapters 1A and 11 in RWNSG: *Pharmacology*

Chronic Pericarditis Treatment

Treatment for chronic pericarditis involves surgery. The surgical procedure is a pericardiectomy, which involves excision of the pericardium to allow movement of the pericardium. Some centers perform laser pericardiectomy, during which laser slits are made in the pericardium.

Pericardial Effusion Treatment

Treatment of a pericardial effusion involves removal of the fluid or blood when the fluid produces symptoms. A pericardiocentesis is a nonsurgical procedure that is performed to evacuate the pericardial fluid. The procedure involves inserting a needle into the pericardial sac. The heart may be visualized with the use of either an echocardiogram or a cardiac catheterization to facilitate correct placement of the needle. Surgical drainage is typically performed on patients with trauma or a tumor because the surgery allows for repair of any damage from trauma, and a biopsy can be obtained from tumors.

When a cardiac tamponade occurs with pericardial effusion, emergency removal of the fluid or blood must be performed immediately or the condition will be fatal.

Nursing Responsibilities

The nurse must know several important aspects when caring for patients with pericardial disease. The nurse should:

- Be able to recognize signs and symptoms of increasing pericardial effusion and cardiac tamponade. These signs and symptoms must be reported to the health care provider immediately. If treatment is not implemented promptly, then the condition can be fatal. Patients susceptible to sudden cardiac tamponade are those with chest trauma and those with recent cardiac surgery.
- Be on alert for signs and symptoms of cardiogenic shock, jugular vein distention, and pulsus paradoxus. The nurse can assess for pulsus paradoxus by taking the patient's blood pressure during inspiration and again during expiration. Pulsus paradoxus is present when the systolic blood pressure during inspiration is 10 mm Hg or lower than during expiration.
- Monitor for the occurrence of acute pericarditis following an acute MI and following cardiac surgery. These patients usually complain of continuous chest pain 24 to 48 hours after the infarct or surgery and are extremely uncomfortable. The pain is unrelieved by nitroglycerin and opioids. Measures that can alleviate pain include administering NSAIDS as ordered, giving with food to prevent gastrointestinal ulcers, and keeping the patient in an upright position.

Pulmonary complications, such as atelectasis and pneumonia, can result because the intensified pain with inspiration prevents the patient from taking deep breaths. To optimize breathing:

- Assist the patient with the use of an incentive spirometer and with deep-breathing exercises.
- Maintain the patient in a high-Fowler's position to promote lung expansion, and administer pain medications as ordered.

To prevent cardiac complications, watch for clinical manifestations of increasing pericardial effusion or a cardiac tamponade.

> **Signs and symptoms of cardiac tamponade include faint muffled heart sounds, distention of the jugular veins, and pulsus paradoxus. These symptoms must be reported to the health care provider immediately. Other signs and symptoms include a pericardial friction rub and heart failure.**

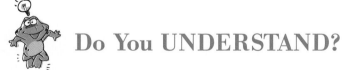

Do You UNDERSTAND?

DIRECTIONS: Fill in the blanks.

1. The condition that causes the formation of scar tissue within the pericardium is known as _____ pericarditis.
2. Chest pain associated with acute pericarditis can be differentiated from pain associated with myocardial ischemia in that it is not relieved by _____.
3. A patient after cardiac surgery develops hypotension, jugular vein distention, tachycardia, cold and clammy skin, and muffled heart sounds. The patient most likely has developed cardiac _____.
4. Chronic pericarditis diminishes cardiac output because it causes _____.
5. A pericardial friction rub can be auscultated when a patient is _____.

Answers: 1. chronic; 2. nitroglycerine; 3. tamponade; 4. a reduction in ventricular filling; 5. holding the breath.

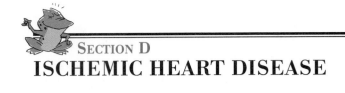

SECTION D
ISCHEMIC HEART DISEASE

What IS Coronary Artery Disease?

Yale University School of Medicine Heart Book
http://www.med.yale.edu/library/heartbk/http://www.med.yale.edu/library/heartbk/
Journals of the American Heart Association
http://www.ahajournals.org/
American Heart Association
http://www.americanheart.org/

Coronary artery disease (CAD) is the leading cause of death from heart disease. CAD affects the coronary arteries by causing narrowing within the lumen of the artery.

Pathogenesis

CAD is a progressive condition in which fat and fibrin are deposited along arterial walls. These deposits of fat and fibrin are known as plaque. Vessels eventually become thickened and hardened. The lumens of the vessels become narrow and restrict blood flow through the lumen. As a result, the tissue that is distal to the narrowing becomes ischemic from a decrease in blood flow. CAD causes two ischemic heart conditions: angina and MI. All arteries can be affected, in addition to the coronary arteries, such as the cerebral, carotid, renal, and peripheral arteries.

Three stages have been theorized in the development of plaque in atherosclerosis. The first stage is the fatty streak stage during which streaks of fat form on the vessel walls. The second stage is the fibrous plaque stage during which plaque is formed and lipids are accumulated. The third stage is the advanced stage during which the plaque becomes hardened or calcified.

At-Risk Populations

CAD incidence is higher in men compared with premenopausal women. After female menopause, the occurrence rate is not significantly different for either gender. A close blood relative with an MI or stroke before the age of 60 is a risk factor for CAD development.

A variety of risk factors are associated with CAD. Nonmodifiable risk factors include age, gender, family history, and race. Modifiable risk factors include elevated serum lipids, hypertension, smoking, impaired glucose tolerance, diets high in saturated fat, cholesterol, calories, sedentary lifestyle, obesity, oral contraceptive use, psychological stress, personality type, and coping skills.

Cholesterol levels have a significant correlation with CAD. Persons with levels greater than 270 mg/dl have four times the risk of developing CAD than do those with lower levels. Elevated triglycerides also contribute to CAD. Substances known as lipoproteins transport cholesterol and triglycerides in the body by substances called lipoproteins. Very low-density lipoproteins (VLDL) carry triglycerides to the vessels where they accumulate. Low-density lipoproteins (LDL) carry cholesterol to vessels, and the cholesterol accumulates within the arterial walls. High-density lipoproteins (HDL), conversely, are "good" lipoproteins because they carry cholesterol away from tissues to the liver where it is metabolized. This process prevents cholesterol from building up within the arteries. Elevated HDL levels are associated with a lower risk of developing CAD.

CAD incidence is higher in African-American and Hispanic populations of both genders than it is in Caucasians.

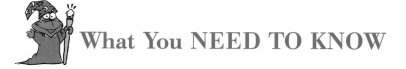

What You NEED TO KNOW

Angina Clinical Manifestations

Angina is a symptom of CAD and occurs when a coronary artery becomes temporarily occluded. Blood flow is blocked to the area of the myocardium (heart muscle) distal to the location in which the coronary artery is supplying blood. The occlusion associated with angina causes the myocardium to become ischemic but does not cause necrosis.

Clinical manifestations of angina include pain in the chest, neck, arms, jaw, or back. The pain results from the ischemia and typically lasts from 30 seconds to 30 minutes. Women tend to have more atypical pain and stomach (epigastric) pain than do men. Factors that can precipitate angina include exercise, exertion, cold weather, emotional upset, and sexual activity.

Stable angina begins gradually, reaches maximal intensity in minutes, and then dissipates. Stable angina can be precipitated by activity or hypertension. Unstable angina is more intense than is stable angina and is described as pain rather than discomfort. Usually, treatment requires more than nitroglycerin alone. Unstable angina can remain in a stable pattern or result in a new onset of severe angina. Unstable angina can also be precipitated by activity or hypertension.

Variant, or Prinzmetal's angina, is a result of coronary vasospasm, a spasm that occurs within the coronary artery, temporarily closing off the artery. This type of angina may or may not have an atherosclerotic lesion. Variant angina frequently occurs at rest. Smoking, alcohol, sudden temperature change, and cocaine use can precipitate a variant angina attack.

Silent ischemia is myocardial ischemia without the patient experiencing symptoms of angina and may be associated with less severe ischemia. The silent ischemia patient may have a higher pain threshold.

> **Silent ischemia is associated with an increased risk of MI and sudden cardiac death.**

Angina Prognosis

The prognosis for angina is positive if the patient is willing to modify behaviors and thus decrease the chances of further angina attacks. Severe angina attacks can be relieved with nitroglycerin.

MI Clinical Manifestations

MI occurs when a coronary artery is completely blocked (occluded). Plaque rupture, which causes the formation of a clot within the coronary artery, is the most common cause of an MI. Less common causes include spasms of the artery and dissection, which occurs when the arterial wall is torn from a cardiac catheterization procedure and the torn piece blocks the coronary artery.

Three stages, frequently referred to as zones, of myocardial damage take place during an MI. Zone of ischemia occurs when the myocardium becomes ischemic and injured cells are viable. Zone of injury occurs when cells have a significant reduction in blood flow. Zone of infarction is characterized by cellular death and muscle necrosis. Damage in the zone of infarction is irreversible.

Irreversible myocardial damage occurs 6 hours after the onset of the infarction or occlusion. The myocardium becomes distended, pale, and cyanotic after an infarction. The infarcted area of the myocardium forms into scar tissue over 3 to 4 weeks; the healing process of the myocardium is complete after 6 weeks.

Two basic types of MIs have been identified: transmural and subendocardial. A transmural infarction causes necrosis of all three layers of the heart, including the endocardium, myocardium, and epicardium. A subendocardial infarction involves only the endocardium. MIs can also be classified as either a Q wave or a non-Q wave infarct. A Q wave infarct occurs when the ECG shows S-T segment elevation during the infarct, and then Q waves appear after the infarct. A non-Q wave infarct occurs when the ECG shows S-T segment depression, and Q waves do not appear after the infarct.

An MI can affect any surface area of the myocardium, depending on which coronary artery is occluded. The areas of the myocardium that can be affected include the front of the heart (**anterior wall**), side of the heart (**lateral wall**), the undersurface of the heart (**inferior wall**), and the back of the heart (**posterior wall**). The coronary arteries and the areas of the heart that an infarct would occur when the vessel becomes blocked are listed below.

The main clinical manifestation of an MI is pain in the chest, arms, neck, jaw, or epigastric area. The pain is different from angina in that it is not temporary and it is not relieved by nitroglycerin. Profuse sweating (**diaphoresis**) is present in almost all MI cases. Nausea is frequently present, and vomiting indicates a severe infarction because blood is being shunted from the gastrointestinal tract as a result of a significant decrease in cardiac output.

Several complications can occur from an MI. Arrhythmias occur in 95% of all MIs. Inflammation of the pericardium (**pericarditis**) can and usually will occur 24 to 48 hours after the infarct. Rupture of the ventricular septum and papillary muscle rupture can occur and will cause death in most cases.

MI Prognosis

The prognosis for recovery depends on the area and extent of damage to the myocardium, the presence of preexisting organ disease, and access to prompt medical care.

Anterior wall infarcts have occlusion of the left anterior descending artery and are associated with twice the mortality of inferior wall infarctions. Anterolateral wall infarcts have occlusion of the circumflex branch. Inferior wall infarcts have occlusion of the right coronary artery. Posterior wall infarcts have occlusion of the circumflex branch.

TAKE HOME POINTS

The ECG will show the following:
- Zone of ischemia: T wave inversion
- Zone of injury: S-T segment elevation
- Zone of infarction: Deep Q waves, which reflect a lack of depolarization in scar tissue

Heart failure, cardiogenic shock, and pulmonary edema can result if a significant part of the myocardium is damaged and the myocardial contractility is decreased (see Section E in this chapter).

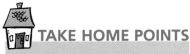

TAKE HOME POINTS

The signs and symptoms of MI include pain in the chest, arms, neck, jaw, diaphoresis, nausea, and vomiting.

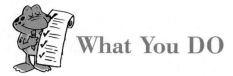

What You DO

Treatment

Treatment of angina and an MI is aimed at increasing coronary perfusion (coronary blood flow and oxygen) and decreasing the myocardial workload. The myocardial workload (myocardial oxygen demand or MVO_2) is a general term used to describe the extent to which the myocardium must work to pump blood. The harder the myocardium has to pump, the more oxygen it requires. When angina occurs, the myocardial oxygen demand is reduced because oxygen to the myocardium is already compromised.

Nitroglycerin is the drug of choice in treating angina because it increases coronary perfusion and reduces the myocardial oxygen demand. Nitroglycerin increases coronary perfusion because it dilates the large coronary arteries. Additionally, nitroglycerin reduces the myocardial oxygen demand because it dilates veins and arteries. By dilating the veins, preload is reduced; by dilating the arteries, afterload is also reduced. A reduction in preload decreases the myocardial oxygen demand because the ventricles do not have to eject as forcefully as when they are filled with less blood. A reduction in afterload decreases the myocardial oxygen demand because a reduction in arterial pressure reduces the resistance against which the left ventricle must pump.

Other drugs used to reduce the myocardial oxygen demand are calcium channel blockers, beta-adrenergic blockers, and ACE inhibitors. Calcium channel blockers block the flow of calcium into the myocardium thus myocardial contractility is reduced. The force of contraction is directly proportional to the myocardial oxygen demand. Beta-adrenergic blockers decrease the heart rate and force of contraction, thereby reducing the myocardial oxygen demand. As the heart rate increases, the myocardial oxygen demand also increases. ACE inhibitors dilate arteries, which reduces the afterload, thereby reducing the myocardial oxygen demand.

Other drugs are used to prevent clot formation in the area of the coronary artery that has plaque. A complication of angina occurs when the plaque eventually ruptures, causing bleeding within the arterial wall. The bleeding causes the formation of a clot, and the coronary artery is completely occluded, resulting in an MI. Because most of the clot is made up of platelets, antiplatelet aggregation drugs are used. Antiplatelet drugs inhibit platelets from agglutinating or "clumping." Intravenous heparin is used as an anticoagulant to help prevent clot formation.

Treatment of an acute myocardial infarction (AMI) involves reestablishing blood flow to the myocardium, particularly during the "6-hour window." Some of the damage to the myocardium can be reversed if blood flow is returned within 6 hours after the onset of symptoms. One way to establish blood flow is to dissolve the clot within the coronary artery that is producing the complete occlusion. Administering a thrombolytic agent accomplishes this task. Thrombolytics dissolve clots throughout the body, including the clot causing the MI. Common

See Chapter 4A in RWNSG: *Pharmacology*

See Chapter 5A in RWNSG: *Pharmacology*

See Chapter 3A in RWNSG: *Pharmacology*

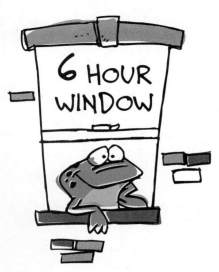

agents used are tissue plasminogen activator (t-PA), streptokinase, and Retavase. An emergency percutaneous transluminal coronary angioplasty (PTCA) can also be performed if personnel and equipment are available within 1 hour. This procedure involves taking the patient to the cardiac catheterization laboratory. The cardiologist places a catheter into the coronary artery and inflates a balloon on the end of the catheter until the coronary artery is open. If the patient with an MI has multiple vessel disease, then an emergency coronary artery bypass graft (CABG) surgery may be performed. The surgery should take place within the 6-hour window because complications of a CABG surgery significantly increase after that time.

Nursing Responsibilities

Nurses must be aware of several important points when caring for a patient with angina or an MI. The nurse should:

* Maintain the systolic blood pressure less than 140 mm Hg to decrease the afterload, which, in turn, will decrease the myocardial oxygen demand. Many of the medications used for ischemic heart disease such as nitroglycerin, beta-adrenergic blockers, and ACE inhibitors decrease blood pressure.
* Watch for signs and symptoms of heart failure in more extensive MIs. Signs and symptoms include dyspnea, pulmonary crackles, jugular vein distention, and tachycardia.
* Monitor for cardiogenic shock that can occur with a massive infarct. Signs and symptoms of cardiogenic shock include hypotension, tachycardia, cool and clammy skin, weak peripheral pulses, and decreased urine output.
* Give medications for treatment of angina and MI as ordered and be certain that doses are not omitted. Medications such as nitroglycerin preparations, ACE inhibitors, and beta-adrenergic blockers will decrease the systolic blood pressure and can cause hypotension. Administer morphine sulfate for relief of ischemic pain that is not relieved by nitroglycerin. The drugs should be held only when the systolic pressure is less than the parameter ordered by the health care provider, such as 100 or 110 mm Hg. When a patient is ordered not to receive anything by mouth (NPO) for surgery or a procedure, check with the health care provider about administering the medications with small sips of water. The patient may develop acute angina or infarction in surgery or during a procedure if the medications are not given.
* Obtain a 12-lead ECG when a patient with ischemic pain does not obtain relief with nitroglycerin. The 12-lead ECG should be examined for S-T segment elevations, which indicates an AMI. A 12-lead ECG is needed because it records conduction throughout the heart 12 different ways that represent the different surface areas of the heart. A single-lead cardiac monitor, which is frequently used in telemetry units or in the cardiac care units, records conduction traveling only one way in the heart, thus only one surface area of the heart is reflected. If an infarction occurs in another area not represented by the lead, no changes will be observed.

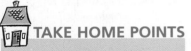

TAKE HOME POINTS

Treatment of angina and MI is aimed at increasing coronary perfusion and decreasing the cardiac workload.

The nurse should report hypotension immediately thus medication doses may be adjusted. Additionally, watch for bradycardia with beta-adrenergic and calcium channel blockers. A heart rate that is less than 60 beats per minute should be reported to the health care provider.

Several important nursing interventions are needed for a patient with angina or an MI. These interventions include the following:

- Bed rest with bedside commode privileges, which presents less straining with a commode compared with a bedpan
- Semi-Fowler's position to decrease preload
- Clear liquid diet during acute anginal attacks and for the first 24 hours after AMI Food increases the gastrointestinal [GI] tract's demand for oxygen. The weakened myocardium will have to pump harder to get blood flow to the GI tract.
- Quiet environment and administration of antianxiety agents when the patient is anxious. Anxiousness and an increase in heart rate increase the myocardial oxygen demand.
- Patient education directed toward maintaining optimal cardiovascular health after discharge, including activity restrictions, dietary modifications, and the need for continuing health care and evaluation

Do You UNDERSTAND?

DIRECTIONS: Unscramble the letters to form the word or words that complete each sentence.

1. High levels of _____ reduces the occurrence of coronary artery disease. (DHL)
2. The type of angina that frequently occurs at rest and usually results from coronary vasospasms is known as _____ angina. (travian)
3. _____ _____ can result when the contractility of the myocardium is significantly diminished after an MI. (iodraccenig cohsk)
4. A patient with unstable angina complains of chest pain to the nurse. After administering nitroglycerin, the patient does not obtain relief. The most important intervention is for the nurse to _____ _____ _____. (binato na gec)

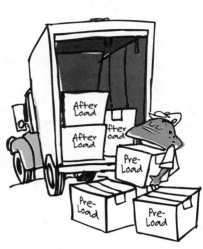

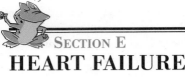

SECTION E

HEART FAILURE

To understand heart failure, the nurse must understand the cardiac cycle, including the concepts of preload and afterload. Before discussing heart failure, a review of the cardiac cycle is warranted.

The cardiac cycle is made up of two phases. During the first phase of the cardiac cycle (diastole) the ventricles fill with blood from the atria. The amount of blood in the ventricles at the end of diastole is known as preload.

The more important concern is with preload of the left ventricle, because the left ventricle pumps blood to the tissues throughout the body. Preload refers to the amount of stretching imposed on myocardial fibers at the end of diastole immediately before contraction. The blood that the left ventricle ejects to the tissues is known as cardiac output. Specifically, cardiac output is the amount of blood that is ejected in liters per minute. Normal cardiac output in the adult is 4 to 8 liters per minute. Preload is important because it affects cardiac output.

During the second phase of the cardiac cycle (systole), the ventricles eject blood. The left ventricle ejects blood through the aorta into the systemic arteries and the right ventricle ejects blood through the pulmonary artery into the pulmonary arteries in the lungs. These arteries create resistance that the ventricles must overcome. The resistance depends on the diameter of the vessels. If the vessels are dilated, pressure decreases. If the vessels are constricted (narrowed), pressure increases. Afterload is the resistance the ventricles have to overcome during systole. Left ventricular afterload is important because it directly affects the cardiac output.

What IS Heart Failure?

Heart failure is a condition that occurs when the heart muscle (myocardium) fails to pump a sufficient amount of blood to meet the metabolic needs of the body. Heart failure is the most common cause of mortality in cardiac disease and is responsible for one third of deaths as a complication of MI. Heart failure can be either an acute or a chronic condition. Acute heart failure occurs suddenly. Retention of sodium and water does not occur during the initial period. In chronic heart failure, the onset is progressive and develops slowly. Retention of sodium and water occurs in a progressive manner. Persons with chronic heart failure can develop episodes of acute heart failure when treatment is ineffective or when a sudden illness develops.

Several conditions can result in heart failure: atherosclerosis, hypertension, MI, valvular heart disease, cardiomyopathy, arrhythmias, and circulatory overload.

Pathogenesis

Two basic types of heart failure have been identified: left ventricular failure and right ventricular failure. The most common type of heart failure is left ventricular failure. In most cases, primary left ventricular failure will cause secondary right ventricular failure. These patients are said to have biventricular failure because both ventricles fail.

To better understand the pathologic aspects of heart failure, a review of the chambers and vessels of the heart and a familiarity with how blood circulates into and out of the heart is recommended. In left ventricular failure, the left ventricle is weak and is unable to pump all of its blood into the systemic circulation. A reduction in cardiac output results because of the decreased amount of blood the left ventricle ejects. The weak left ventricle is unable to empty all of its blood from the chamber, thus an increase in left ventricular preload is present. The residual volume of blood makes emptying all of the left atrium's blood into the left ventricle during diastole difficult. The left atrium now over fills and the pulmonary veins are unable to return all of the blood from the pulmonary arteries into the left atrium. The buildup of blood in the pulmonary arteries causes congestion and increases pressure within the vessels. The high pressure eventually forces fluid from the pulmonary arteries into the alveoli, and fluid enters the lungs. At this point, the patient develops pulmonary symptoms such as crackles, dyspnea, and an increase in respiratory rate.

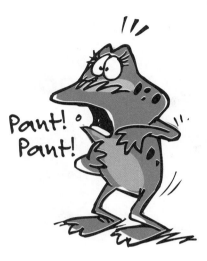

Right ventricular failure follows left ventricular failure. The right ventricle becomes affected because the high pressure and congestion within the pulmonary system prevents the right ventricle from emptying all of its blood through the pulmonary artery. The right ventricle over fills with blood and now the right atrium is unable to empty all of its blood into the right ventricle. The veins throughout the body that return blood to the heart via the superior and inferior vena cava into the right atrium are unable to return all of the blood, and venous congestion results. The patient now develops systemic symptoms, such as jugular vein distention and peripheral edema. High pressure and excess fluid in the veins causes edema because high pressure forces fluid into the space between the vascular space and tissue (interstitial space).

When heart failure occurs, the body compensates to resolve the problem of low cardiac output. These compensatory attempts actually worsen heart failure, which causes vasoconstriction of the arteries to increase the left ventricular afterload, making the already weakened left ventricle work harder to pump against the high pressure. Decrease in blood flow to the kidneys also causes more vasoconstriction by stimulating the renin-angiotensin system to produce more angiotensin II, a potent vasoconstrictor. The decrease in blood flow to the kidneys also stimulates the release of the hormone aldosterone from the adrenal gland. Aldosterone causes the reabsorption of sodium and water. The body retains water in an attempt to increase cardiac output, but this mechanism worsens heart failure because the failing myocardium is unable to handle any additional fluid.

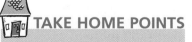

TAKE HOME POINTS

Cardiac output equals the amount of blood ejected by the heart in liters per minute. Changes in preload and afterload can adversely affect cardiac output.

At-risk Populations

A variety of diseases and conditions can place people at risk for heart failure. These conditions include MI, arrhythmias, cardiomyopathy, and valvular heart defects. Other conditions that adversely affect the pumping action of the heart include systemic hypertension, chronic obstructive pulmonary disease, and thyrotoxicosis.

What You NEED TO KNOW

Clinical Manifestations

Clinical manifestations of heart failure are related to the low cardiac output and the presence of left or right ventricular failure. The worse the cardiac output is, the stronger the sympathetic response will be. Signs and symptoms of the sympathetic response include tachycardia, decreased urine output, dark amber urine, weak pulses, and cool skin. As mentioned, pulmonary symptoms indicate left ventricular failure and systemic symptoms indicate right ventricular failure. If both pulmonary and systemic symptoms are present, the person is in biventricular failure.

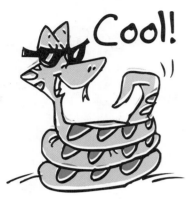

Heart Failure

LEFT VENTRICULAR FAILURE PULMONARY SYMPTOMS	RIGHT VENTRICULAR FAILURE SYSTEMIC SYMPTOMS
• Tachypnea, dyspnea • Pulmonary crackles • Restlessness (from hypoxemia)	• Jugular vein distention • Peripheral edema • Hepatomegaly

The two most dangerous complications of heart failure are pulmonary edema and cardiogenic shock. Pulmonary edema is an emergency situation and if treatment is not implemented immediately, respiratory arrest will follow.

Pulmonary edema occurs from acute left ventricular failure. Fluid builds up in the pulmonary vessels to the extent that the fluid forces its way from the capillary bed into the alveoli. The fluid literally "drowns" the patient. Clinical manifestations of pulmonary edema include extreme dyspnea and tachypnea, tachycardia, restlessness or agitation, senses of impending doom and panic, severe crackles in all lung fields, and pink, frothy sputum. The sputum is pink because some blood enters the alveoli from the capillary vessels. Pulmonary edema can be reversed when appropriate treatment is initiated in a timely manner. An immediate intravenous dose of a loop diuretic, such as furosemide (Lasix) or bumetanide (Bumex), will reverse pulmonary edema if administered in time.

Cardiogenic shock is a complication of heart failure with a 75% to 95% mortality rate. This situation occurs at either the end stage of chronic heart failure or suddenly after a massive MI. In cardiogenic shock, less than 20% of the myocardium is contracting normally. The left ventricle is unable to eject sufficient blood to deliver oxygen to the body (low tissue perfusion). This condition is a state of shock because shock, by definition, is a decrease in circulating volume insufficient to provide oxygen and nutrients to the tissues. Clinical manifestations of cardiogenic shock will include hypotension (systolic blood pressure under 90 mm Hg) and sympathetic symptoms, such as tachycardia, cold and diaphoretic skin, weak, thready pulse, and low or no urine output.

Prognosis

Despite recent treatment advances, patients with heart failure have poor survival rates. Of those who survive the first acute episode of failure, 50% die within 5 years. Mortality rates are increased in men, older adults, and those who have underlying heart disease.

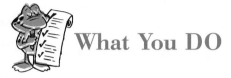

What You DO

Treatment

A variety of medications are used to treat heart failure and are aimed at reducing preload and afterload and increasing contractility. Loop diuretics are used to pull fluid from the alveoli and reduce the circulating volume, thereby reducing preload. Nitroglycerin is also used to reduce preload because it dilates veins. When veins are dilated, less blood returns to the heart and thus the ventricles fill with less blood. ACE inhibitors are used to reduce afterload because they dilate arteries. When arteries are dilated, the pressure is decreased within the systemic arteries, resulting in a decrease in resistance or left ventricular afterload. ACE inhibitors have helped decrease the mortality of heart failure by 60%. Inotropic agents are used to increase myocardial contractility. For end-stage heart failure, beta-adrenergic blockers are occasionally used because they decrease the heart rate, giving the ventricles more time to fill and improve cardiac output.

Nursing Responsibilities

The nurse must know several important aspects of heart failure. The nurse should be aware that all patients with chronic heart failure have the potential to develop acute heart failure. The nurse must be alert to early signs and symptoms of an acute episode, which include worsening of symptoms (e.g., increasing dyspnea), increasing heart rate, and development or worsening of crackles. These crackles are best auscultated in the posterior bases of the lungs because fluid gravitates to the lowest areas of the lungs.

The nurse must also immediately report when the patient's urine output averages less than 30 ml per hour, which indicates the cardiac output is decreased to the point of diminishing organ perfusion. When the cardiac output drops, blood flow to the kidneys is immediately shunted away. Urine output is the best and most sensitive indicator of cardiac output when performing a physical assessment. Urine output declines before changes in blood pressure or pulse are observed. When tissue perfusion is sufficient, blood flow to the kidneys is also sufficient thus urine output is maintained. Nursing care centers on preventing acute episodes and preventing complications.

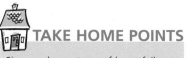

TAKE HOME POINTS

Signs and symptoms of heart failure include tachycardia, decreased urine output, dark amber urine, weak pulse, and cool skin.

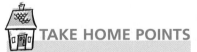

See Chapters 4A, 5A, and 9A in RWNSG: *Pharmacology*

TAKE HOME POINTS

Treatment of heart failure involves pharmacologic measures such as diuretics, ACE inhibitors, inotropic agents, and beta-adrenergic blockers.

When the crackles are auscultated higher than the posterior bases of the lungs, an acute episode of heart failure has occurred, and a diuretic is needed immediately to prevent pulmonary edema.

The nurse should:

- Maintain the head of the bed in a semi-Fowler's to a high-Fowler's position to reduce preload. Venous return is reduced with the head in an upright position.
- Give medications as ordered and do not omit doses. Medications such as nitroglycerin preparations, ACE inhibitors, and diuretics decrease the systolic blood pressure and can cause hypotension. These drugs should be withheld only when the systolic pressure is less than the parameter ordered by the health care provider, such as 100 or 110 mm Hg. If a patient is kept NPO for surgery or a procedure, the nurse should check with the health care provider about administering the medications with small sips of water. The patient may develop acute heart failure or pulmonary edema in surgery or during a procedure if the medications are not administered.
- Check the potassium level before administering a loop diuretic, which causes an increase in the excretion of potassium. Hypokalemia can be dangerous because it can cause abnormal cardiac rhythms within the ventricles (ventricular arrhythmias).
- Limit fluid intake by mouth and minimize intravenous fluids used for medications to reduce preload.
- Monitor strict intake and output. The intake should balance with the output, or the output should exceed the input if the patient has acute heart failure.
- Daily weights are necessary to assess whether the patient is retaining fluid. A weight gain of more than 2.5 pounds in 1 day indicates fluid retention. A low-sodium diet should also be maintained to help prevent fluid retention.

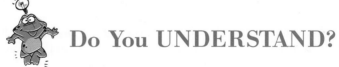 # Do You UNDERSTAND?

DIRECTIONS: **Fill in the blanks.**

1. Heart failure occurs when the _____ fails to pump sufficient blood to meet the needs of the body.
2. A weak left ventricle will result in an increase in left ventricular _____.
3. A congested left ventricle will eventually cause the person to experience _____ because of congestion within the pulmonary vessels.

SECTION F

CARDIAC ARRHYTHMIAS

To understand arrhythmias, the way in which a normal rhythm of the heart is produced must be examined. For the atria and ventricles to fill and contract optimally, proper timing and synchronization must exist between the atria and the ventricles. The conduction system of the heart is responsible for facilitating proper timing and synchronization. The conduction system is made up of specialized cells that produce electrical impulses throughout the atria and the ventricles. These electrical impulses produce perfect timing of contractions between the atria and ventricles.

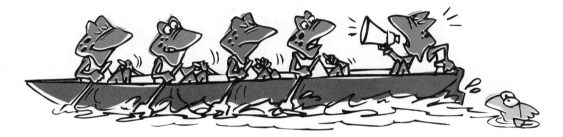

Specialized cells that make up the conduction system are present throughout the heart. Pacemaker cells initiate electrical impulses. The sinoatrial (SA) node of the right atrium is the normal pacemaker of the heart, which produces a rate of 60 to 100 beats per minute. Conducting cells carry the electrical impulses from the SA node to the left atrium and through the ventricles. The conduction cells then stimulate the muscle cells, and these cells cause contraction of the myocardium. The normal pathway of the conduction system is illustrated on page 152.

Conduction of the electrical impulses through the heart produces a normal heart rhythm called a normal sinus rhythm (NSR), as well as normal heart rate and stroke volume.

The heart rate is the number of times the heart contracts per minute; the stroke volume is the amount of blood the left ventricle ejects with each contraction. When the heart rate is too slow, the left ventricle will not pump as much blood as needed by the body. The formula for cardiac output is:

Heart rate (HR) × stroke volume (SV) = cardiac output

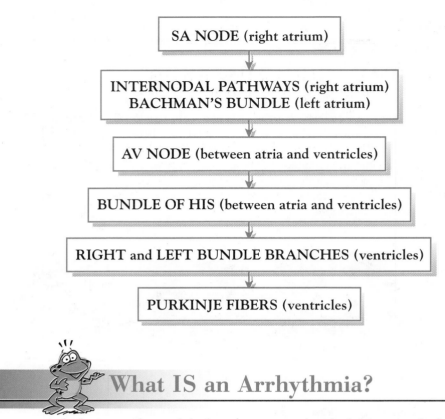

What IS an Arrhythmia?

Arrhythmias are abnormal rhythms that occur within the heart or any rhythm that is not an NSR. Some arrhythmias can be faster or slower compared with the NSR. Other arrhythmias are abnormal rhythms produced by conducting cells that produce electrical impulses outside of the normal conduction system. These abnormal conducting beats are referred to as ectopic beats.

A variety of arrhythmias exist. Four common types of arrhythmias are sinus tachycardia, sinus bradycardia, atrial fibrillation, and premature ventricular contraction.

Sinus Tachycardia Pathogenesis

Sinus tachycardia is a normal rhythm, but the rate is greater than 100 beats per minute and usually less than 150 beats per minute. The cause of sinus tachycardia is not from a conduction problem with the heart, but rather, from various problems outside of the conduction system. Any condition that increases the pulse rate will cause sinus tachycardia.

Sinus Tachycardia At-Risk Populations

Many conditions stimulate the sympathetic nervous system, which results in sinus tachycardia. Common conditions include heart failure, hypoxemia, fever, pain, shock, hemorrhage, hypovolemia, and anxiety. Several medications can cause sinus tachycardia, including theophylline and any drug that stimulates the sympathetic nervous system, such as alpha- and beta-adrenergic drugs. Adrenergic drugs include over-the-counter decongestants, epinephrine, norepinephrine, dopamine, dobutamine, and Neo-Synephrine. Atropine can also cause sinus tachycardia.

Sinus Bradycardia Pathogenesis

Sinus bradycardia is a normal rhythm, but the rate is less than 60 beats per minute. Causes of sinus bradycardia include medications, severe hypoxemia, and AMI. Stimulation of the vagus nerve can also cause sinus bradycardia. The vagus nerve is a parasympathetic nerve, thus when it is stimulated, the heart rate decreases. Common factors that cause vagal stimulation include vomiting, retching, bearing down, and bowel movements. Usually, after the action is stopped, the vagus nerve is no longer stimulated, and the heart rate increases to a normal rate.

Sinus bradycardia can be a normal condition for athletes or persons who exercise regularly. A person who exercises regularly increases venous return to the heart. Eventually, this increase in venous return causes the left ventricle to strengthen and enlarge. The increase in size allows the left ventricle to hold more blood thus increasing the stroke volume. Because the stroke volume is increased, a normal heart rate is unnecessary to have an adequate cardiac output, thus the heart rate slows.

Sinus Bradycardia At-Risk Populations

Patients who are at the highest risk for developing sinus bradycardia include those who have had an AMI, particularly an inferior wall infarct, and those taking various cardiac medications. The most common cardiac medications associated with sinus bradycardia include digoxin, beta-adrenergic blockers, calcium channel blockers, and any antiarrhythmic drug. Severe hypoxemia can cause a sudden bradycardia, which usually leads to cardiopulmonary arrest. Immediate action is therefore required to resolve the hypoxemia.

Atrial Fibrillation Pathogenesis

Atrial fibrillation is an abnormal rhythm that originates from an ectopic in the atria. The atrial ectopic becomes the primary pacemaker of the heart and conducts at an extremely fast rate, making the atria quiver rather than contract. The rhythm of a patient with atrial fibrillation is irregular; an irregular pulse can be palpated. Common causes of acute atrial fibrillation include stimulants such as coffee, tobacco, myocardial ischemia, acute heart failure, cardiomyopathy, chronic obstructive pulmonary disease, drugs (e.g., theophylline, isoproterenol), and cardiac surgery.

Atrial Fibrillation At-Risk Populations

The most common causes of atrial fibrillation are ischemic heart disease, rheumatic fever, and hyperthyroidism. In atrial fibrillation, the atrium does not contract normally during diastole. As a result, the atrium is unable to empty all of its blood into the ventricles. This pooling of blood in the atria forms clots. These clots can eventually break loose and cause a pulmonary embolus, a stroke,

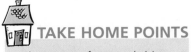

TAKE HOME POINTS

- Always assess for an underlying cause of sinus tachycardia, such as fever, hypotension, pain, drugs, and so on.
- Watch patients with angina or MI who develop sinus tachycardia because the increased heart rate makes the heart require more oxygen, which can cause chest pain.

▼ **Sinus bradycardia can be a dangerous rhythm if the heart rate is insufficient to provide an adequate cardiac output.**

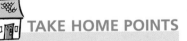

TAKE HOME POINTS

- Sinus bradycardia can be an emergency situation when the patient has symptoms. Atropine should be available.
- When severe hypoxemia causes bradycardia, cardiopulmonary arrest will usually follow immediately, unless the hypoxemia is corrected. High-risk patients include those with a tracheostomy and those with any type of respiratory disorder.

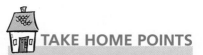

 PVCs can be dangerous when the beats reduce the force of ventricular contraction or fail to produce ventricular contraction. Some patients with PVCs may not have a pulse with the beat or may have a weak pulse with the beat.

or a bowel infarct. Atrial fibrillation can be an acute problem or a chronic rhythm and is the most common type of chronic arrhythmia.

Premature Ventricular Contraction Pathogenesis

Premature ventricular contractions (PVCs) are abnormal beats that originate from an ectopic beat found in the ventricles. Common causes of PVCs include an AMI or ischemia, hypoxemia, and medications that can irritate the heart.

PVC At-Risk Populations

The causes of PVCs in patients are numerous. Any form of heart disease can cause PVCs, such as ischemic heart disease and cardiomyopathy. The most common metabolic causes include hypoxemia, hypokalemia, acidosis, and a low magnesium level. Drugs that can cause PVCs include digitalis toxicity, theophylline, adrenergic drugs, and antiarrhythmic drugs, such as quinidine, procainamide, and disopyramide.

What You NEED TO KNOW

Sinus Tachycardia Clinical Manifestations

The clinical manifestations of sinus tachycardia are palpitations and a rapid pulse rate.

Sinus Tachycardia Prognosis

The prognosis for sinus tachycardia is usually good, because after the underlying problem is corrected, the sinus tachycardia is resolved.

Sinus Bradycardia Clinical Manifestations

A patient with sinus bradycardia may not have any symptoms if the cardiac output is sufficient. Patients with reduced cardiac output frequently experience weakness, dizziness, fainting, chest pain, hypotension, diaphoresis, cool and clammy skin, and decreased level of consciousness.

Sinus Bradycardia Prognosis

The prognosis for bradycardia can be poor when the heart rate is not sufficient to produce an adequate cardiac output. Tissues will not receive sufficient oxygen if the heart is not pumping at the required rate.

Atrial Fibrillation Clinical Manifestations

Most patients with atrial fibrillation are asymptomatic. The nurse will palpate an irregular pulse or auscultate an irregular apical pulse.

Atrial Fibrillation Prognosis

The prognosis for atrial fibrillation is fair to poor because of the risk for clot formation. These patients are at risk for stroke, pulmonary embolus, and ischemic bowel.

PVC Clinical Manifestations

Most patients with PVCs have no symptoms. Some may complain of feeling a "skipped beat." When a patient is having frequent PVCs, the nurse can palpate an irregular pulse.

PVC Prognosis

The prognosis for PVCs is usually good, as long as the PVCs do not progress to more lethal ventricular arrhythmias. Usually, when metabolic conditions are corrected or irritating drugs are discontinued, the PVCs will stop.

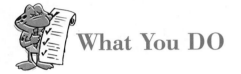 # What You DO

Sinus Tachycardia Treatment

The treatment for sinus tachycardia involves determining and treating the underlying cause. For example, if the patient has hypoxemia, then oxygen should be given to the patient. Sinus tachycardia usually does not in and of itself present a problem, unless the patient has ischemic heart disease. An increase in heart rate increases the myocardial oxygen demand and the ischemic myocardium can become overworked. These patients will develop chest pain or acute heart failure with sinus tachycardia.

Sinus Bradycardia Treatment

Treatment of sinus bradycardia is performed only when the person is symptomatic or fails to tolerate the slow rate. Signs and symptoms of a person who is not tolerating sinus bradycardia include hypotension, chest pain, cool and clammy skin, dizziness, fainting, or confusion. Treatment for sinus bradycardia includes administration of intravenous atropine or a pacemaker. Atropine inhibits the parasympathetic response thus the heart rate increases. A pacemaker is an electronic device used to artificially stimulate conduction within the heart. Pacemakers can be temporary or permanent.

Atrial Fibrillation Treatment

Treatment for atrial fibrillation includes use of antiarrhythmics and synchronized cardioversion. Common antiarrhythmic drugs include diltiazem, procainamide, digoxin, amiodarone, verapamil, and adenosine. Synchronized cardioversion is used when the heart rate is greater then 120 beats per minute and antiarrhythmic drugs are ineffective. Synchronized cardioversion is a procedure in which an electrical voltage is sent through the heart that is synchronized with ventricular contraction. The voltage is sent from electrical paddles placed on the chest.

> ⚠️ The nurse should assess the blood pressure immediately and determine whether the systolic pressure has decreased since the arrhythmia started. The nurse should assess for the presence of chest pain and symptoms of decreased cerebral blood flow, such as dizziness, fainting, confusion, or change in the level of consciousness.

TAKE HOME POINTS

Steps for assessing a patient who develops any of the four arrhythmias:

- Checking vital signs—pulse and blood pressure
- Assessing for chest or cardiac ischemic pain
- Assessing for decrease in cerebral perfusion
- Assessing for decrease in tissue perfusion

PVC Treatment

Treatment of PVCs is performed only when the patient is symptomatic, such as the presence of hypotension, chest pain, cool and clammy skin, dizziness, fainting, or confusion. Treatment includes use of antiarrhythmics, such as lidocaine, amiodarone, and procainamide.

Nursing Responsibilities

The nurse should have some familiarity with interpreting basic arrhythmias on an ECG. The ECG device measures electrical currents of the heart. Electrical impulses are picked up by electrodes placed on the skin and are recorded on graphic paper. The nurse must be aware that an ECG is a diagnostic test that measures only electrical conduction. The nurse must also be aware that a wide range of normal ECG patterns exists. In other words, a normal sinus rhythm can appear slightly different to each person.

When a patient develops any of the arrhythmias, the nurse should:
- Evaluate the patient's tolerance of the abnormal rhythm.
- Assess for signs of decreased tissue blood flow (perfusion), such as cool and clammy skin, weak or thready pulses, decrease in urine output, and capillary refill greater than 3 seconds.
- Report any signs of intolerance to the health care provider immediately.

Sinus Tachycardia Nursing Responsibilities

The nurse should:
- Determine the underlying cause, such as drugs, fever, anxiety, acute heart failure, and so on.
- Carefully monitor patients with ischemic heart disease because the increase in heart rate can cause chest pain or precipitate an MI.

SINUS TACHYCARDIA

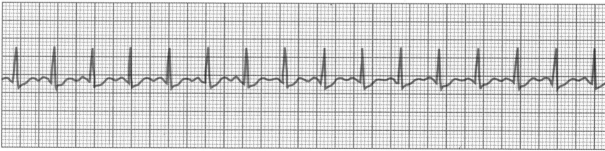

Sinus Bradycardia Nursing Responsibilities

The nurse must be aware that sinus bradycardia should be treated only when the person is symptomatic, especially when the person has any type of ischemic heart disease. If atropine is given to a patient with ischemic heart disease who is not symptomatic, the increase in heart rate can increase the myocardial oxygen demand too much and ischemia can result. An important point to remember is that the faster the heart rate is, the more oxygen the heart will require. A person with ischemic heart disease may be unable to supply the additional oxygen needed.

The nurse should:

- Immediately assess the patient's tolerance of the slow rate, and prepare for emergency treatment because sinus bradycardia can progress to a cardiac arrest.
- Keep atropine at bedside even when the patient is asymptomatic in case the person suddenly becomes symptomatic.
- Always check the pulse rate before giving cardiac drugs that commonly cause bradycardia, such as beta-blockers, calcium channel blockers, and digoxin.

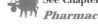 See Chapter 5B in **RWNSG:** *Pharmacology*

See Chapter 5A in **RWNSG:** *Pharmacology*

SINUS BRADYCARDIA

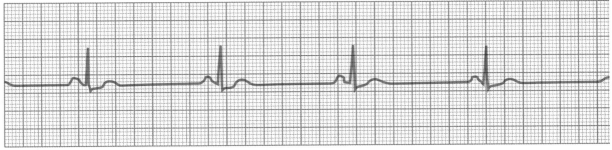

Atrial Fibrillation Nursing Responsibilities

The nurse must also be on alert for thrombotic episodes ("throwing clots") in patients with atrial fibrillation. The person may also develop a cerebral vascular stroke or "brain attack" if a clot enters the cerebral arteries. Clinical manifestations include weakness or paralysis of extremities on one side of the body, slurred speech, facial droop, aphasia, or unresponsiveness in severe strokes. The person can also develop an ischemic bowel from a clot entering the mesentery. Clinical manifestations include abdominal distention, abdominal pain, hypoactive or absent bowel sounds, and shock.

A pulmonary embolus can occur when a clot from the atria breaks loose and lodges in a branch of the pulmonary artery. The clinical manifestations include a sudden onset of chest pain, dyspnea, tachycardia, and hypoxemia.

ATRIAL FIBRILLATION

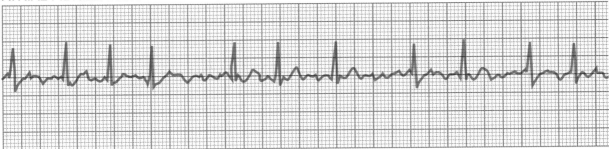

The nurse should:

- Suspect atrial fibrillation when a patient has an irregular pulse.
- Immediately report when a patient with atrial fibrillation also has tachycardia (pulse greater than 100 beats per minute). The fast heart rate along with the atrial fibrillation increases the risk for clot formation and decreases cardiac output.
- Administer anticoagulants as ordered to prevent clot formation. The most common drug used is warfarin. Report any signs of bleeding.

See Chapter 3 in **RWNSG:** *Pharmacology*

- Watch patients after cardiac surgery for sudden development of atrial fibrillation. The pulse rate is usually fast in these patients (150 to 200 beats per minute).

PVC Nursing Responsibilities

The nurse should:
- Report frequent occurrences of PVCs, such as more than 5 episodes per minute, particularly in the patient with an AMI. The PVCs can cause a lethal rhythm called ventricular fibrillation in which the ventricles quiver and the patient has no pulse.
- When a patient suddenly develops PVCs, determine possible causes, such as hypoxemia, drugs, or acute myocardial ischemia or AMI.

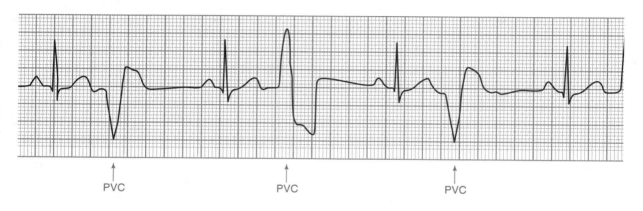

PVC   PVC   PVC

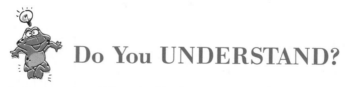

Do You UNDERSTAND?

DIRECTIONS: **Fill in the blanks. Not all words may be used.**

1. The _____ _____
   is the pacemaker of the heart.
2. The _____ _____
   are responsible for contraction of the ventricles.
3. Sinus tachycardia can be hazardous when the patient has
   _____ _____ disease.
4. Sinus bradycardia can be normal for _____.

ischemic heart	atrioventricular node
Purkinje fibers	sinoatrial node
athletes	

6 Respiratory Disorders

SECTION A
RESTRICTIVE LUNG DISEASES

Respiratory disorders can adversely affect quality of life and impair a person's ability to provide personal care, work, and socialize. This chapter provides an overview of the various disease and disorders that commonly affect the lungs and respiratory system.

What IS Sarcoidosis?

Sarcoidosis is a disorder that currently has no known cause. This disease can affect every part of the body, but the most commonly affected areas include the lungs, skin, eyes, and lymph nodes. The disease is thought to be the result of an increased cellular immune response to a persistent antigen that the body is unable to destroy. This illness is characterized by the accumulation of T lymphocytes (a specialized type of white cell that is active in the immune response), mononuclear phagocytes, granulomas in epithelial tissues, and changes in the structure of affected organs. A granuloma is an accumulation of inflamed cells. Depending on the degree of involvement, these accumulations of abnormal cells (lesions) ultimately interfere with normal organ function, particularly the lungs.

Research indicates that the disease likely has both immunologic and genetic components. In approximately 15% of patients, the disease appears to be genetic. Causative agents can be infectious or noninfectious. Various infectious organisms are considered as contributing factors, including mycobacteria, fungi, and spirochetes. Environmental compounds that may contribute to the disease include beryllium, organic dusts (e.g., peanut or wheat dusts), and inorganic compounds (e.g., clay).

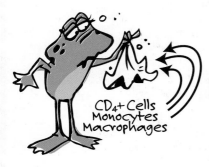

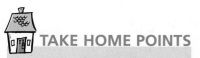

CD4+ Cells
Monocytes
Macrophages

Pathogenesis

The disease begins with an accumulation of CD4+ cells, monocytes, and macrophages within the targeted tissue. These cells secrete cytokines that maintain and promote the inappropriate inflammatory process. Monocytes and macrophages begin to differentiate and form a ring around the inflamed areas, eventually evolving into granulomas.

At-Risk Populations

Sarcoidosis has been found in both sexes and nearly all ages and races throughout the world. Women appear to be slightly more at risk for the disease than do men.

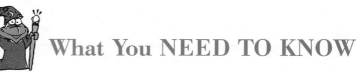

What You NEED TO KNOW

TAKE HOME POINTS

Granulomas can form anywhere in the body. The most commonly affected areas are the blood vessels, lungs, lymph nodes, heart, liver, skin, and eyes.

Clinical Manifestations

Sarcoidosis can be acute, subacute, or chronic in form. Patients with sarcoidosis tend to have depressed cell-mediated immunity with a decreased number of circulating T lymphocytes. Many patients are asymptomatic and are diagnosed incidentally with a chest x-ray film.

When symptoms occur, they tend to be related to the organ system that is involved. Wheezing, breathlessness, cough, and chest pain are commonly observed when lungs are involved. Nodules, papules, and plaques are frequently present with skin involvement. When the disease affects the eyes, patients experience a sensitivity to light, excessive tearing, and visual changes. Involvement of the peripheral lymph nodes is common, particularly in the cervical, axillary, epitrochlear, and inguinal areas. These nodes tend to be mobile, with a firm, rubbery texture when palpated.

Constitutional symptoms include fever, fatigue, anorexia, chills, and night sweats. The disease tends to be unpredictable and can follow either a chronically progressive course, or it can have periods of exacerbation interspersed with periods of remission.

Sarcoidosis tends to appear most frequently in people who are in their 20s and 30s, although cases have been diagnosed in children as young as 1 year and in middle-age women.

Prognosis

Even individuals with subacute or fluctuating forms of the disease generally experience some residual organ dysfunction. The prognosis for the disease depends largely on the clinical manifestations and behavior of the disease. Acute pulmonary sarcoidosis can present with or without symptoms of pulmonary dysfunction or demonstrable abnormalities on radiologic examination. This form of the disease may subside without treatment, or it may respond well to a comparatively brief course of steroids. Disease that persists for 2 years or longer is considered chronic. Patients with the chronic form frequently experience progressive pulmonary dysfunction. The prognosis of pulmonary sarcoidosis appears to be correlated with the presence or absence of other symptoms.

In the United States, African Americans are more frequently affected with sarcoidosis than are Caucasians, and these individuals tend to be younger than are Caucasians with the disease. In Europe, the disease is most common among people in Sweden and among Irish women. On a worldwide basis, nearly 80% of patients with the disease are Caucasian.

Patients who have erythema nodosum, arthritis, and fever at the time of diagnosis tend to have a better prognosis than do those who have skin lesions, splenomegaly, or bone involvement.

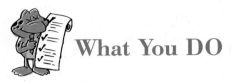

What You DO

In children, the disease is usually self-limiting and can resolve within 2 to 3 years.

Sarcoidosis appears to have a poorer prognosis for African-American patients and for those who are diagnosed after the age of 40.

Treatment

Goals of therapy are directed toward decreasing inflammation that impairs organ function, preventing pulmonary damage, and decreasing distressing symptoms. When the patient presents with mild symptoms and normal pulmonary function tests, they are typically placed under ongoing medical observation to monitor for disease progression.

When patients have organ involvement, particularly of the eyes, skin, heart, lungs, and central nervous system, treatment is indicated. To preserve organ function, corticosteroids are administered to suppress the acute inflammation. Patients may need a low dose of prednisone for up to 1 year to prevent a recurrence of symptoms.

Patients who fail to respond to corticosteroids or who cannot tolerate the side effects of these drugs may require alternate therapy with immunosuppressive agents. Some of the drugs that have proven useful in the treatment of sarcoidosis include methotrexate, azathioprine, and pentoxifylline, although these agents also have significant side effects and require close monitoring by a health care provider.

See Chapters 1C, 7B, and 11 in RWNSG: *Pharmacology*

Nursing Responsibilities

In the acute-care setting, nurses must be prepared to monitor and evaluate for evidence of progressive disease. The nurse should:
- Establish a baseline physical assessment, and then evaluate for changes in status, particularly of the respiratory, cardiac, and neurologic systems. Careful physical assessment is particularly important when the patient is undergoing a steroid taper.
- Design a plan of care to alleviate distressing symptoms. Patients who have severe dyspnea and hypoxia may require oxygen and aggressive respiratory therapy with aerosolized bronchodilators. Plan patient care activities to minimize oxygen demands, and help the patient conserve energy as much as possible.
- Administer prescribed steroids accurately and on time. Minimize toxicities and side effects associated with steroid therapy as much as possible. Inspect the patient's mouth daily for evidence of oral candida, particularly when therapy is being given with nebulized corticosteroids. Give steroids with meals to decrease gastric irritation. Seek an order for an antiulcer agent before the patient begins to complain of stomach pain.
- Monitor the patient for possible hyperglycemia, particularly when a family history of diabetes is present.

- Inform the patient about the desired therapeutic effects and potential side effects and toxicities associated with treatment.
- Help the patient learn to manage side effects competently before discharge.
- Explain and be certain that the patient understands that even when the disease appears to be in remission, a potential for recurrence is always present.
- Alert the patient about possible signs and symptoms of recurrence that require medical evaluation and follow-up.

Do You UNDERSTAND?

DIRECTIONS: **In the space provided, write the letter that corresponds to the phrase that answers each question.**

_____ 1. Sarcoidosis is thought to be a result of which of the following?
   a. Decreased immune response
   b. Defective genes
   c. Infectious organisms
   d. An overactive immune response

_____ 2. In the United States, sarcoidosis has the highest incidence in which population?
   a. Native Americans
   b. Asians
   c. African Americans
   d. Caucasians

_____ 3. A symptom that is typically associated with skin involvement in sarcoidosis is which of the following?
   a. Vesicles
   b. Plaques
   c. Local pain
   d. Pruritus

_____ 4. Drugs that are used in the treatment of sarcoidosis include which of the following?
   a. Antineoplastics
   b. Glucocorticoids
   c. Cytotoxic agents
   d. Interferon

What IS Pulmonary Fibrosis?

The term _pulmonary fibrosis_ is used to describe a group of lung diseases characterized by thickening and scarring of interstitial tissue in the lungs. The interstitium is the wall between the alveoli of the lungs. Damage to this tissue decreases the ability of oxygen to travel from the alveoli across the damaged

Answers: 1. d; 2. c; 3. b; 4. b.

membrane into the bloodstream. Other terms used to describe this process include interstitial lung disease, idiopathic pulmonary fibrosis, usual interstitial pneumonia, acute interstitial pneumonia, and cryptogenic fibrosing alveolitis. Pulmonary fibrosis is associated with many different diseases and conditions; however, it can also arise without any apparent cause or explanation.

Pathogenesis

Pulmonary fibrosis is the result of an exaggerated inflammatory response in lung tissue. As the inflammatory response progresses, pulmonary tissue becomes infiltrated by lymphocytes and plasma cells. Mononuclear cells begin to accumulate in the alveoli. The alveolar sacs become thickened, scarred, and are eventually destroyed, leading to the formation of large cysts within the lungs and enlarged bronchioles.

Pulmonary fibrosis can result from many different causes and conditions and is frequently observed with connective tissue disorders, such as scleroderma, rheumatoid arthritis, and systemic lupus erythematosus. Drugs and certain medical therapies can also cause this condition, as will exposure to certain organic and inorganic agents in the environment. Dilantin, amiodarone, and some antineoplastic agents are examples of drugs that can cause pulmonary damage. In some cases, the cause of pulmonary fibrosis is unknown. This group of disorders can also have a genetic component.

At-Risk Populations

Individuals with connective tissue diseases and autoimmune disorders have an increased risk for pulmonary fibrosis. Additionally, anyone who experiences long-term exposure to air-borne agents that are inhaled (e.g., coal dust, glass particles, wheat chaff) is at high risk for lung disease.

Many occupations are well known to carry an increased risk of lung disease, including coal mining, farming, and those involving steel and heavy metal industries. Individuals who have high-risk occupations and are exposed to air pollution have a high cumulative risk for developing pulmonary disease. This disorder is thought to occur in approximately 5 per 100,000 people in the United States.

People who work in occupations that are known to have respiratory hazards must be provided with the appropriate protective devices to safeguard their health. Examples of these protective measures include special air-filtering systems and particulate respirator masks. Workers in hazardous environments may also need to have their work schedule modified to reduce the duration of their exposure and will benefit from training in safety measures to decrease their risk of exposure. Anyone exposed to occupational hazards will require vigilant screening by a qualified health care provider to detect early signs and symptoms of pulmonary changes when the disease is most likely to respond to treatment.

TAKE HOME POINTS

Pulmonary fibrosis is a disease that causes permanent damage to lung tissue and ultimately results in respiratory failure.

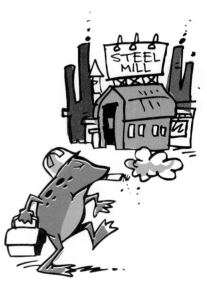

Idiopathic pulmonary fibrosis (pulmonary fibrosis of an unknown cause) is diagnosed most frequently in patients 40 to 60 years of age.

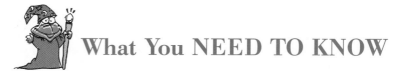

What You NEED TO KNOW

Clinical Manifestations

Gradually increasing breathlessness is the most common presenting complaint in the patient with pulmonary fibrosis. Some patients also complain of fever, fatigue, weight loss, and diffuse muscle and joint pain. Other symptoms include a dry, nonproductive cough; rapid, shallow breathing (tachypnea); clubbed finger tips; inspiratory crackles; and severe dyspnea during exertion.

In early stages of pulmonary fibrosis, chest x-rays usually have a characteristic "ground glass" appearance, which is frequently described as diffuse interstitial infiltrates. As the disease progresses, cysts form within lung tissue and cause a honeycombed appearance on x-rays, which typically indicates a poor prognosis.

Prognosis

The prospect varies to some extent, depending on the probable cause of the disorder and the amount of lung damage sustained. When the initial inflammatory response that damaged the lungs can be halted or controlled, some patients experience a stabilization of their disease but will require life-long treatment.

Patients who have interstitial lung disease that is associated with other diseases such as lupus may respond favorably to steroids. After scarring of pulmonary tissue has occurred, the process is irreversible. The prognosis for patients with idiopathic pulmonary fibrosis is poor, with a mean survival of 5 to 7 years after diagnosis.

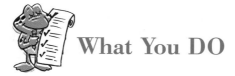

What You DO

Treatment

Corticosteroids are the primary treatment available for this disorder, but they appear to help only 10% to 20% of patients and, in some cases, may even be harmful. These drugs are given in an attempt to suppress the inflammatory process and prevent further lung damage. Patients most likely to respond to this therapy include those with limited lung damage or those who have coexisting diseases, such as lupus or mixed connective tissue disorders. Other pharmacologic measures that appear to benefit some patients include immunosuppressant drugs, such as cyclophosphamide and azathioprine. In cases in which the causative agent can be identified, the patient must be removed from that environment immediately to decrease the risk for further lung damage.

Generally, supportive measures such as supplemental oxygen and respiratory therapy will be required to help maintain respiratory function. For patients who fail to respond to conventional therapy and show progressive disease, lung transplant may be a lifesaving alternative.

See Chapters 1C and 7B in RWNSG: *Pharmacology*

Nursing Responsibilities

The nurse should:

- 🍎 Help the patient learn ways to cope with progressive respiratory disease and to maintain optimal respiratory function. The patient must be protected from factors such as infection that can further compromise respiratory function.
- 🍎 Advise the patient with pulmonary disease that influenza and pneumococcal vaccinations are desirable to prevent respiratory infection.
- 🍎 Teach patients who are receiving medical therapy for their respiratory disease the proper way to self-administer medications and managing potential side effects of corticosteroid therapy.
- Carefully assess respiratory function on a routine basis.
- Document and report evidence of declining respiratory status, including abnormal (adventitious) breath sounds, increased respiratory rate, cyanosis, complaints of increased breathlessness, and decreased oxygen saturation levels. Patients with severe respiratory involvement must also be evaluated for evidence of cardiac compromise, including gallops (an abnormal heart rhythm) and peripheral edema.
- Organize group activities and nursing care to minimize the patient's oxygen demands.
- Offer assistance with personal care as necessary.
- Promote relaxation, rest, and comfort, because stressors such as anxiety and pain can increase the patient's oxygen requirements.
- Position the patient to promote maximal lung expansion and removing noxious agents from the environment that may cause further respiratory compromise.
- 🍎 Prohibit visitors from smoking in the patient's environment. Instruct family and caregivers that highly aromatic aerosolized compounds such as cleaning solutions and perfumes can exacerbate respiratory distress.

Patients who are experiencing severe respiratory distress may require frequent respiratory treatments and high doses of oxygen. Some breathless patients obtain partial relief from a fan blowing across their face. Low doses of parenteral morphine can help relieve the sensation of air hunger that many patients with end-stage disease experience.

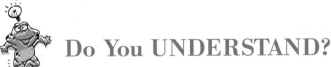

Do You UNDERSTAND?

DIRECTIONS: Fill in the blanks.

1. _____ is an early symptoms of pulmonary fibrosis.
2. Patients with pulmonary disease should be immunized with _____ and _____ vaccines.
3. List three measures that can be used to help a patient who is experiencing respiratory distress.

   _____
   _____
   _____

Answers: 1. tachypnea, 2. influenza, pneumococcal; 3. position in high Fowler's to promote lung expansion, place a fan such that it blows on the patient, administer low doses of parenteral morphine.

What IS a Pleural Effusion?

The pleural space contains 5 to 10 ml of serous fluid, which serves as a lubricant between the visceral and parietal pleura. This lubrication allows the layers of the pleura to slide smoothly across one another, facilitating expansion of the lungs with respiration. Ordinarily, this fluid enters the pleural space from the capillaries that line the parietal pleura. The fluid is then reabsorbed by the capillaries in the visceral pleura and is also taken up into the lymphatic system. The term pleural effusion refers to an excess accumulation of fluid within the pleural space, which can ultimately restrict the movement of the lungs within the chest cavity.

Patients who have experienced chest trauma or undergone surgery to the lungs may experience an accumulation of blood within the pleural cavity (hemothorax). When the pleural fluid has a high white blood cell count and is purulent, evidence of a severe infection exists, thus the fluid must be drained and the condition treated (empyema). In cases of obstruction or trauma to the thoracic duct, pleural fluid can be thick and white. This leakage of lymph (chyle) from the thoracic duct is called a chylothorax.

Pathogenesis

Four possible mechanisms behind pleural effusions have been identified:
- Increased hydrostatic pressure
- Reduced capillary pressure
- Increased capillary permeability, resulting from infection or trauma
- Impaired lymphatic function and drainage, usually from obstruction by tumor

Pleural effusion occurs as a consequence of a variety of diseases and disorders. Transudative effusions are frequently observed in conjunction with heart failure (HF), cirrhosis of the liver, and nephritic syndrome. All of these diseases tend to cause increased venous and hydrostatic pressure. The hypoalbuminemia that is associated with hepatic and renal disease can also cause decreased oncotic pressure.

Exudative effusions occur as a result of a change in permeability of the pleural capillary membranes. These effusions tend to occur in conjunction with infectious and inflammatory processes, such as pneumonia and tuberculosis. Other causes include lung abscesses subsequent to surgery, pancreatitis, esophageal rupture, rheumatologic diseases, and malignancies.

At-Risk Populations

Any individual with the diseases and disorders previously listed is at risk for a pleural effusion. In cases of malignancy, patients with certain types of tumors, especially of the lungs, breast, and lymphatic tissue, appear to have an increased risk for developing malignant pleural effusions.

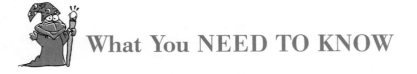

What You NEED TO KNOW

Clinical Manifestations

Small effusions can be asymptomatic. Early symptoms of effusion include decreased strong vocal vibrations (tactile fremitus) and dull or flat percussion notes when examining the chest. Patients may also complain of chest pain with deep inspiration. Large effusions tend to restrict chest expansion, causing complaints of dyspnea during exertion and a nonproductive cough. Uneven chest expansion may be noted and breath sounds are usually decreased.

Prognosis

Recovery from a pleural effusion depends on the nature of the event that caused the effusion and the overall status of the patient. When the underlying disease process that caused the effusion can be reversed or cured, many patients recover. Without treatment, pleural effusions can lead to fibrosis and scarring, with subsequent respiratory compromise.

Effusion resulting from rupture of the esophagus can be serious because of the tendency of organisms from the gastrointestinal tract and mouth to colonize in the lung and set up local inflammation and infection. Prompt treatment is required with surgical closure of the esophageal defect.

For patients with a primary diagnosis of cancer, pleural effusions are usually a result of advancing disease. Malignant effusions frequently recur and may require repeated drainage and treatment to maintain respiratory function.

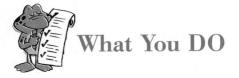

What You DO

Treatment

Small pleural effusions (150 ml of fluid or less) may resolve without treatment. Larger effusions are likely to cause respiratory distress and require prompt treatment. Large effusions must be drained to improve the patient's respiratory status. Microscopic examination of the pleural fluid also provides valuable information about the cause of the effusion and is helpful in establishing a diagnosis.

To provide immediate relief, the health care provider may perform a thoracentesis and remove up to 1500 ml of pleural fluid. This procedure involves inserting a long, thin catheter into the pleural cavity and draining the accumulated fluid. For larger or recurrent effusions, a chest tube may be inserted and connected to gentle suction to drain the fluid and promote reexpansion of the lung.

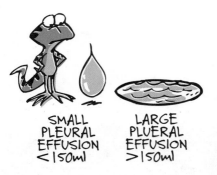

SMALL PLEURAL EFFUSION <150ml

LARGE PLUERAL EFFUSION >150ml

See Chapters 2A, 2B, 5A, and 9A in RWNSG: *Pharmacology*

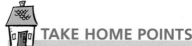

TAKE HOME POINTS

Medical treatment is directed toward resolving the underlying cause or causes of the effusion. Measures to provide symptom relief include thoracentesis, insertion of chest tubes, and, occasionally, pleurodesis. Nursing care emphasizes maintaining optimal respiratory function for the patient, assessing for changes in respiratory function, and assisting with therapeutic procedures.

Depending on the cause of the effusion, concurrent management and treatment of underlying disease processes must also take place. For example, the patient with cardiac disease may require oxygen, diuretic therapy, and vasoactive drugs to improve and stabilize cardiac function.

In patients with underlying malignancies, effusions tend to recur, unless the pleural space is obliterated. This treatment is called pleurodesis and is performed by instilling an irritating agent into the pleural cavity. Various agents have been used, including nitrogen mustard, sterile talc, bleomycin sulfate, and doxycycline. These drugs are usually instilled through a large-bore chest tube and allowed to remain in place for 2 to 4 hours, depending on the preference of the health care provider. During this time, the patient must be helped to turn from side to side and positioned in Trendelenburg and reverse Trendelenburg position thus helping the drug to coat all the pleural surfaces.

Nursing Responsibilities

The nurse should:

- Frequently assess and evaluate the patient's lungs:
  1. Listen to the patient's lungs carefully for decreased breath sounds or a pleural rub.
  2. Percuss the lungs and assess for decreases in tactile fremitus, which can indicate an expanding pleural effusion.
  3. Use a pulse oximeter to obtain capillary oxygen levels, and notify the health care provider of declining trends in readings.
- Plan activities and nursing care to minimize oxygen demands.
- Provide supplemental oxygen, when indicated.
- Place frequently used objects within convenient reach of the patient, and offer assistance with personal care, such as hygiene and toileting.
- When the patient requires drainage of the effusion, explain the procedure to the patient and gather the appropriate equipment.
- For a thoracentesis, the patient may be positioned either leaning over a tray table or in a side-lying position, depending on the status of the patient, the location of the effusion, and the health care provider's preference.
- When a chest tube insertion is performed, place the patient in either a supine or a side-lying position, and administer analgesics for the procedure as ordered. Be prepared to help maintain sterile technique for the procedure and receive specimen tubes as fluid is removed.
- After insertion of a chest tube, monitor the amount and characteristics of the pleural drainage. The chest tube must be secured with a heavy occlusive bandage to prevent air from entering the chest cavity and should be securely taped to prevent the tube from becoming accidentally dislodged. Document drainage from the chest tube on the patient's intake and output records.
- Perform regular assessments of the patient's respiratory status. Assess the integrity of the chest tube and suction at least every 2 hours and with each patient contact. Remember to assess the patient's level of comfort routinely after the chest tube is inserted. Patients with poor pain control after chest tube placement tend to have inadequate lung expansion and are consequently at risk for further respiratory complications.

- For patients who require pleurodesis, prepare to assist with the procedure and rotate the patient according to the directions of the health care provider. Because the procedure involves instillation of an irritating substance, the patient should be medicated with the appropriate analgesic before the procedure and assessed for adequate pain control on an ongoing basis. As mentioned, maintaining adequate pain control is imperative to help the patient regain optimal respiratory function.

Do You UNDERSTAND?

DIRECTIONS: **Indicate in the space provided whether each statement is**
true or _false._

1. _____ The pleural space normally contains 5 to 10 ml of pleural fluid.
2. _____ Blood within the chest cavity is called an empyema.
3. _____ Chest tubes must be secured with a heavy bandage to prevent accidental dislodging of the chest tube and air from entering the chest cavity.

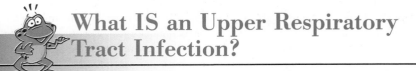

SECTION B

INFECTIOUS LUNG DISEASES

The respiratory tract is one of the most frequent sites for infection because every breath taken exposes an individual to potential pathogens. These agents may be carried on dust, smoke, or droplets from other individuals with infectious illnesses. This section will discuss some of the most common infections of the upper and lower respiratory tract.

What IS an Upper Respiratory Tract Infection?

Upper respiratory tract infections (URI), frequently referred to as common colds, are the most common type of infections that affect humans. The infection can attack any or all of the upper respiratory tract, including the nose, sinuses, throat, larynx, and trachea.

Pathogenesis

In most cases, a virus causes the common cold. Viral infections can be spread through the air or contracted by touching contaminated surfaces. Because of the many different viral strains, developing complete immunity to viral infections is nearly impossible. Occasionally, bacterial organisms can also cause URIs but are much less common as causative agents. URIs usually occur more frequently in the fall and winter, primarily because this is the time during which people congregate indoors.

Answers: 1. true; 2. false; 3. true.

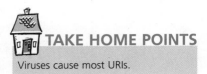

TAKE HOME POINTS

Viruses cause most URIs.

Because of their decreased immune status, the very young and the very old have an increased risk for respiratory infections. Young children are likely to "catch" a cold because of their poor hand-washing habits and their tendency to put things in their mouth.

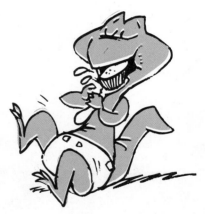

TAKE HOME POINTS

In most cases, a viral respiratory infection is self-limiting and subsides within 48 to 72 hours.

 See Chapters 6A, 6B, and 12 in RWNSG: *Pharmacology*

At-Risk Populations

Anyone can contract a URI, although some individuals are more susceptible than are others. Individuals who smoke, have a previous history of lung disease, hematolymphatic disorders, or are undergoing immunosuppressive therapy are all highly susceptible to respiratory infections.

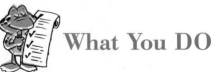

What You NEED TO KNOW

Clinical Manifestations

The pathogen triggers an inflammatory response with subsequent swelling of the mucous membranes. These membranes secrete a serous or mucopurulent exudate. Purulent discharge in the nose, mouth, or throat is suggestive of a bacterial rather than a viral infection. Other symptoms of a URI include sneezing, nasal stuffiness, a sore and irritated throat, fatigue and malaise, and a low-grade fever.

Prognosis

Debilitated or susceptible individuals may experience longer periods of infection, or they may have secondary complications, including bronchitis, sinusitis, and pneumonia.

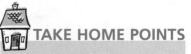

What You DO

Treatment

No cure for the common cold is available. The risk of contracting a viral infection can be decreased through good hand-washing practices. Because the disease is self-limiting, most health care providers recommend rest, a sensible diet, and maintaining adequate hydration. A variety of over-the-counter and prescription drugs, including decongestants, antihistamines, and anticholinergic preparations, may be used to make the cold sufferer more comfortable. Some research indicates that zinc lozenges can shorten the duration of a viral infection. Antibiotics are inappropriate for colds, unless the patient has a secondary bacterial infection, in addition to the cold virus.

Nursing Responsibilities

Most colds can be managed at home. However, the nurse should:
- Encourage the patient with a cold to rest, keep warm, and drink plenty of liquids.
- Remind the patient to practice meticulous hand washing, to cover the nose and mouth when coughing or sneezing, and to use disposable tissues rather than a handkerchief.
- Advise patients with a medical history of hypertension, thyroid disorders, or cardiovascular disease to consult with their health care provider or pharmacist before using over-the-counter cold remedies.

Do You UNDERSTAND?

DIRECTIONS: **Indicate in the space provided whether each statement is**
true or _false_.

1. _____ Most viral infections of the respiratory tract cause purulent nasal discharge.
2. _____ The very young and very old are at increased risk for viral respiratory infections.

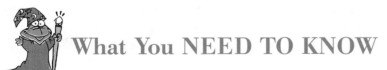

What IS Bronchitis?

Pathogenesis

Acute bronchitis is an inflammation of the bronchial tree caused by an infectious organism or irritating agents such as smoke, dust, pollen, or chemical irritants. Chronic bronchitis is characterized by repeated attacks of acute bronchitis, lasting for at least 3 months over a 2-year period. Both types of bronchitis are the result of an inflammatory process. An inflammatory response in the bronchial tubes leads to swelling and mucus production. Excess accumulations of mucus within the airways provides a favorable environment for bacterial growth.

At-Risk Populations

Patients who have had a recent URI, influenza, or other infectious diseases can develop bronchitis. Smokers, individuals who are exposed to respiratory irritants, or those who are debilitated, malnourished, or with a compromised immune system are also at risk for this disorder.

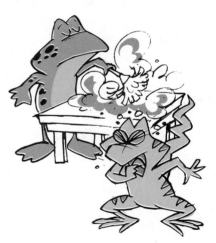

What You NEED TO KNOW

Clinical Manifestations

Signs and symptoms of bronchitis include fever, painful persistent cough that may or may not be productive, chest congestion and tightness, and general malaise. Symptoms can be present for up to 10 days, but the cough can persist for several weeks.

Prognosis

With appropriate care, persons without other underlying diseases will recover fully without residual lung damage. In weakened or debilitated individuals, bronchitis can evolve into pneumonia. Chronic bronchitis tends to have more serious long-term consequences and can cause chronic obstructive pulmonary disease (see Section C in this chapter).

Answers: 1. false; 2. true.

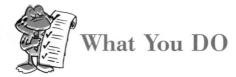

What You DO

Treatment

Acute viral bronchitis is treated with rest and palliative measures. Patients may benefit from inhaling moist air and increased intake of liquids to help dilute thick, sticky (viscous) respiratory secretions. Prescription or over-the-counter expectorants or antitussive agents can also be helpful, depending on the patient's condition. Patients with documented bacterial infections or those who are extremely debilitated may require antibiotic and respiratory therapy. No cure for chronic bronchitis is available. Patients with this disorder will require supportive care and must be instructed to avoid contagious respiratory illnesses and environmental irritants that can exacerbate their condition.

See Chapters 1A, 6A, and 6C in
RWNSG: *Pharmacology*

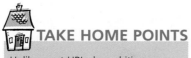

TAKE HOME POINTS

Unlike most URIs, bronchitis may require treatment with antibiotics.

Nursing Responsibilities

Nursing measures for the patient with bronchitis are directed toward relieving symptoms, improving comfort, and decreasing the risk for future recurrences. The nurse should:

- Encourage the patient to maintain adequate hydration to dilute respiratory secretions.
- Administer expectorants and mucolytic agents to promote mobilization of secretions.
- Position the patient to promote effective coughing, and monitor the color and character of pulmonary secretions. Inhalation of warm or cold steam can help loosen secretions.
- Administer antibiotics on time.
- Ensure that the patient understands the importance of taking antibiotics for the prescribed length of time.
- Teach patients to avoid exposure to environmental irritants and contagious people with colds or influenza. The patient who smokes should be urged to stop and referred to a smoking cessation program for further assistance.

Do You UNDERSTAND?

DIRECTIONS: **Fill in the blanks.**

1. Bronchitis can occur after an _____ respiratory tract infection.
2. Chronic bronchitis can lead to _____ _____ _____.
3. Hydration is important for the bronchitis patient to _____ respiratory secretions.

What IS Pneumonia?

Pathogenesis

Pneumonia is an inflammatory process that can involve all or part of the lungs and is a consequence of infection within the respiratory tract. Many different pathogens, including bacteria, viral, and fungal organisms, can cause pneumonia. Affected tissues become edematous, altering the ability of the lungs to maintain oxygenation.

Pneumonia is frequently classified as either a community-acquired pneumonia (CAP) or a hospital-acquired pneumonia (HAP). CAP is defined as an infection that became symptomatic before the patient was hospitalized or within 2 days after hospitalization. HAP occurs 2 or more days after admission to the hospital setting.

Pneumonia is the sixth leading cause of death in the United States.

At-Risk Populations

Pneumonia is more likely to cause complications in people with underlying chronic diseases. People with compromised immune systems, such as patients undergoing transplant or cancer chemotherapy, are at risk. Other risk factors include cystic fibrosis, diabetes mellitus, bronchial obstruction, and altered levels of consciousness. Pneumonia can also occur from a blood-borne infection from an infected site elsewhere in the body (hematogenous spread).

People who have experienced a stroke, seizure, general anesthesia, and alcohol intoxication lack the normal cough or gag reflexes that serve to protect the airway and, consequently, have an increased risk for aspiration and bronchial obstruction.

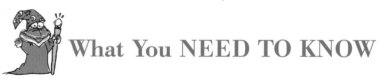

What You NEED TO KNOW

Clinical Manifestations

The signs and symptoms vary, depending on the individual, the severity of the infection, and the causative agent. Common complaints include high fever of abrupt onset, cough, malaise, and breathlessness. Patients may also complain of chills, sweats, pleuritic chest pain, and purulent, blood tinged, or rust-colored sputum. A physical examination may reveal rales and dull tones with chest percussion.

Older individuals may show few of the symptoms commonly associated with pneumonia but may have changes in behavior and mental status.

Prognosis

The outcome of this disease is highly variable and depends on the immune status, age, and underlying health of the patient, as well as the timeliness and availability of appropriate treatment. Frail, immunocompromised, or debilitated individuals are most likely to succumb to this infection.

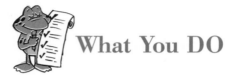

What You DO

 See Chapter 1A in **RWNSG:**
Pharmacology

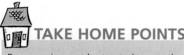 Individuals who are otherwise in good health and under 60 years of age can be successfully treated on an outpatient basis with macrolide antibiotics, such as erythromycin or azithromycin.

Treatment

Antibiotics are the mainstay of therapy for pneumonia. People with co-morbid illnesses, such as cardiovascular disease, may require hospitalization and treatment with intravenous antibiotics. Currently, no effective treatment for viral pneumonia is available, other than supportive care. Supportive measures to improve oxygenation include nebulized respiratory therapy, chest physiotherapy, and supplemental oxygen. Acutely ill patients may require respiratory support with a mechanical ventilator.

Nursing Responsibilities

Nursing care for the patient with pneumonia places priority on maintaining oxygenation and treating the underlying cause of the infection. The nurse should:

- Assess the patient carefully for evidence of respiratory distress, and report abnormal respirations and oxygen saturation levels promptly to the health care provider.
- Position the patient to optimize lung expansion, and encourage the patient to turn, cough, and deep breathe frequently.
- Administer antibiotics as scheduled, and monitor for therapeutic response to treatment.
- Collaborate with respiratory therapists to help the patient obtain maximal benefit from treatments.
- Schedule activities requiring exertion after treatments.
- Mobilize the patient as much as possible to avoid further respiratory complications associated with inactivity.
- Teach the patient (before discharge) the proper way to correctly self-administer medications and about the symptoms that indicate the need for medical intervention.
- Assess the patient for risk factors, such as a smoking history or occupational exposure to respiratory irritants, that may need to be modified or eliminated.

TAKE HOME POINTS

Pneumonia must be treated promptly with the appropriate therapy to decrease the risk of dying from this illness.

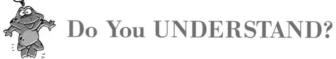

Do You UNDERSTAND?

DIRECTIONS: Indicate in the space provided whether each statement is *true* or *false*.

1. _____ Patients with decreased levels of consciousness are not at risk for pneumonia.
2. _____ Pneumonia can be lethal, particularly when the individual is frail or debilitated.
3. _____ Patients with pneumonia should always be kept on strict bedrest to decrease oxygen demands.

Answers: 1. true; 2. true; 3. false.

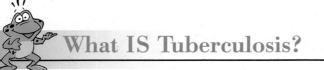

What IS Tuberculosis?

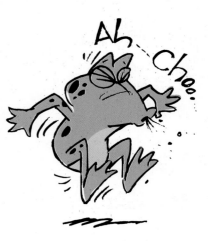

Tuberculosis (TB) is an infectious organism that is caused by *Mycobacterium tuberculosis*. This organism can affect any area of the body, but usually invades the lungs. TB is spread via aerosolized droplets from a person with the infection. The droplets are spread by activities such as laughing, coughing, and sneezing. TB is not spread by hand-to-hand contact nor contact with infected items in the environment.

Pathogenesis

After the droplets are inhaled, they are picked up by macrophages in the lungs and moved to hilar lymph nodes. Macrophages can engulf and contain the organism and may interact with T lymphocytes to form granulomas. The residual effect of the initial infection is a healed, hardened lesion called a Ghon complex. These patients then demonstrate a positive TB skin test. As these lesions heal, the infection may either progress or become dormant. Bone and joints may be involved, as well as the kidneys and adrenal glands. Reactivation of TB can occur years later if the patient has decreased immune function.

At-Risk Populations

Patients with human immunodeficiency virus (HIV) are highly vulnerable to tuberculosis. Other risk factors include homelessness, living in crowded conditions (e.g., prisons, mental hospitals), or living in countries with poor housing and sanitation.

TB is prevalent in native American populations and near the border of Mexico.

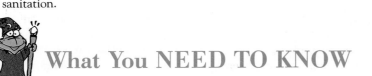

What You NEED TO KNOW

Clinical Manifestations

Most patients are asymptomatic during the early stages. As the disease progresses, patients can experience weight loss, night sweats, fever, cough, chest pain, and bloody sputum (hemoptysis).

Prognosis

Most patients recover fully from the disease when they receive adequate treatment, particularly during the early stages of the disease. In patients with HIV, tuberculosis tends to progress rapidly without treatment.

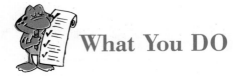

What You DO

Treatment

Medical management of this disease involves the use of drug therapy. Because a growing worry over drug-resistant TB exists, a combination of four drugs is usually required to treat the disease. First-line drugs used in the treatment of TB include isoniazid, rifampin, pyrazinamide, streptomycin, and ethambutol. To cure the disease, therapy must be continued consistently for at least 6 to 9 months. Patients who have a known exposure to TB may undergo preventive therapy (chemoprophylaxis) to keep them from developing the disease. In most cases, this therapy may be accomplished with daily doses of isoniazid. Usually, TB therapy can be successfully accomplished on an outpatient basis.

See Chapter 1A in **RWNSG:** *Pharmacology*

Nursing Responsibilities

The nurse should:

- Impress on all patients the importance of taking anti-TB therapy on time and for the duration ordered. Patient noncompliance with therapy is thought to be a major factor in developing drug resistant tuberculosis. Directly observed therapy may be necessary for patients at risk for noncompliance, which means that the patient must take their medication in the presence of a qualified health care worker.
- Help the patient identify measures to cope with the therapy and minimize side effects. Many antituberculous drugs have side effects and are poorly tolerated.
- Place the hospitalized patient in respiratory isolation for at least 2 weeks after the start of therapy. Patients who are coughing and with active disease may require placement in a negative pressure room that filters and exchanges the air with outside air. Isolation should be maintained until the patient demonstrates clinical improvement and has had three negative sputum cultures on 3 different days. Conventional face masks are not adequate protection when caring for the patient with active disease.

Personnel caring for the patient with active TB must wear an individually fitted, disposable particulate respirator mask.

Do You UNDERSTAND?

DIRECTIONS: **Provide short answers to the following statements.**

1. Identify the two major differences between pneumonia and tuberculosis.

2. Summarize safety measures that should be used when caring for a TB patient with active disease.

Answers: 1. Tuberculosis can affect other tissues and organs in the body, as well as the lungs. Tuberculosis requires significantly longer treatment than does pneumonia; 2. Negative-pressure isolation rooms with air filtration system. All personnel in direct contact with the infected patient should wear a particulate respirator mask.

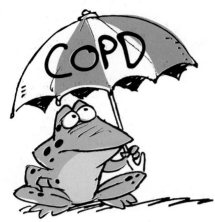

SECTION C
OBSTRUCTIVE RESPIRATORY DISORDERS

Chronic obstructive pulmonary disease (COPD) is a respiratory disorder characterized by gradual reduction in the ability to exhale air. COPD is frequently used as an umbrella term to refer to a variety of respiratory diseases that cause obstruction of the airways. Other terms that may be used to refer to this disorder include chronic obstructive airway disease (COAD) and chronic obstructive lung disease (COLD). A variety of diseases can lead to this condition, including chronic bronchitis, asthma, and emphysema. This section will provide an overview of these diseases.

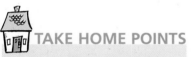

What IS Chronic Bronchitis?

Pathogenesis

Chronic bronchitis is characterized by excessive production of mucus with a chronic cough that lasts 3 months of the year for 2 or more consecutive years. Chronic bronchitis is usually a result of prolonged exposure to respiratory irritants, particularly tobacco smoke, air pollution, toxic fumes, and dust. The irritating agents produce a chronic inflammation that causes swelling and thickening of the lining of the bronchioles, along with enlargement of the mucous-producing glands. Repeated or prolonged inflammation eventually results in scarring and damage to the mucociliary lining of the respiratory tract. The small airways become distorted and begin to close prematurely when the patient exhales, causing air to be trapped within the lungs. Eventually the small airways are destroyed.

TAKE HOME POINTS

Chronic bronchitis is a result of exposure to respiratory irritants or a respiratory infection, such as a virus.

At-Risk Populations

Smoking and exposure to second-hand smoke are the two major causes of chronic bronchitis. COPD and associated respiratory disorders tend to run in some families, suggesting a genetic component in the development of this disorder.

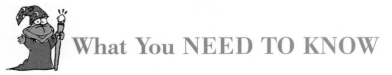

What You NEED TO KNOW

Clinical Manifestations

Patients with chronic bronchitis have a persistent, productive cough, particularly after a night's sleep. Frequently, the mucus is purulent because of a superimposed respiratory infection. Thick, sticky mucus that is associated with this disorder is a favorable breeding ground for respiratory infections. Recurrent infections cause further damage and scarring of the lungs. As the disease progresses, patients experience increased severe coughing, chest congestion, and shortness of breath. Patients with advanced disease can experience right-sided heart failure and chronic severe hypoxia.

Prognosis

The outcome of this disease depends on the presence of other concurrent health problems, such as heart disease, and the patient's access to and ability to comply with medical therapy. Few patients develop serious airway obstruction, but they may be disabled to the extent that they are unable to hold a job and have poor quality of life. In most cases, patients die from complications of this disease rather than the disease itself, particularly heart failure and respiratory infection.

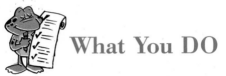

What You DO

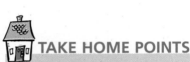

 See Chapters 6C and 7B in RWNSG: *Pharmacology*

Treatment

Medical therapy is directed toward slowing the progression of the disease and maintaining respiratory function. The single most important and effective intervention is to convince the patient who is still smoking to stop.

Inhaled bronchodilators are useful for patients with chronic bronchitis. Systemic and inhaled glucocorticoids are frequently used to reduce the inflammatory response. Glucocorticosteroids are discussed later in this section.

Continuous oxygen has also been shown to prolong life in patients with low arterial oxygen levels because it decreases the risk for development of pulmonary hypertension and right-sided heart failure. Patients with respiratory compromise also benefit from pulmonary rehabilitation, which will improve their level of fitness and exercise tolerance. Lung reduction surgery has been shown to improve respiratory function in some patients and is the subject of ongoing research.

Nursing Responsibilities

For the patient with chronic bronchitis, the nurse should:

Help the patient cope with this disease with extensive education and support. Provide the patient with comprehensive written and verbal information about medications, as well as the signs and symptoms of infection that require medical intervention.

- Instruct the patient in the proper use of metered dose inhalers (MDIs). Older or debilitated patients can have difficulty using an inhaler correctly and may require a spacer—a device that attaches to the inhaler that helps dispense the nebulized medicine.
- Teach patients the importance of avoiding potential sources of respiratory infection.
- Encourage patients to receive influenza shots annually, as well as vaccinations for pneumonia.

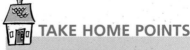

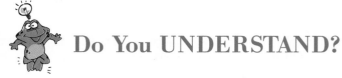

Do You UNDERSTAND?

DIRECTIONS: Indicate in the space provided whether each statement is *true* or *false*.

1. _____ Chronic bronchitis is characterized by thick, bloody sputum.
2. _____ Chronic bronchitis is primarily a disease of smokers.
3. _____ Patients with chronic bronchitis usually have a nonproductive cough.

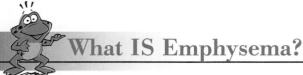

What IS Emphysema?

Pathogenesis

Emphysema is a chronic, progressive lung disease that is characterized by enlargement of distal air spaces in the lungs and destruction of the alveoli. Two types of emphysema have been identified. Centrilobular emphysema is strongly correlated with cigarette smoking. Panlobular emphysema tends to run in families.

Emphysema is a disease primarily of smokers. Irritating substances in cigarette smoke damage the epithelial lining of the alveoli, which causes a release of inflammatory mediators. Those who smoke have increased numbers of neutrophils and macrophages in their lungs. Smoking increases the availability and activity of elastase, an enzyme that is capable of digesting lung tissue. Smoking releases free radicals that inhibit the activity of protective agents in the lungs, contributing to further lung damage. Because of a genetic deficiency, some are unable to secrete a protein called alpha 1 antitrypsin, which minimizes the damage caused by elastase.

At-Risk Populations

People who began smoking at an early age or those who have a deficiency of alpha 1 antitrypsin are at the greatest risk for emphysema.

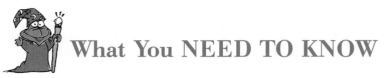

What You NEED TO KNOW

Clinical Manifestations

Gradually increasing breathlessness, particularly with exertion, is the hallmark of emphysema. Ultimately, the patient will be breathless at rest, with a prolonged expiratory phase of the respiratory cycle. Patients with emphysema tend to be chronically malnourished because eating increases their oxygen demands. Malnutrition causes loss of muscle mass, including the respiratory muscles, which leads to further decline in respiratory function. Patients are typically barrel-chested and breathe through pursed lips to open distal airways.

TAKE HOME POINTS

Emphysema is a chronic, progressive pulmonary disease that is caused by smoking.

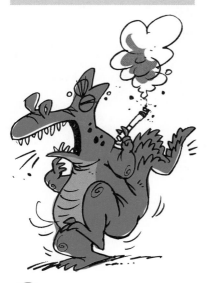

People with an alpha-1-antitrypsin deficiency usually develop severe emphysema in their 30s and 40s, particularly when they smoke.

Answers: 1. false; 2. true; 3. false.

Prognosis

Emphysema is a progressive, incurable disease. Most patients die of respiratory acidosis and coma, heart failure, or massive pneumothorax.

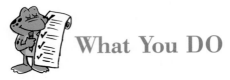

What You DO

Treatment

Therapy for emphysema focuses on maintaining respiratory function and preventing complications of the disease. Bronchodilators and glucocorticosteroids are the mainstay of treatment. Patients with emphysema benefit significantly from respiratory therapy treatments. Most individuals will require supplemental low-flow oxygen at some point in their illness.

See Chapters 6A, 6C, and 7B in RWNSG: *Pharmacology*

Nursing Responsibilities

For the patient with emphysema, the nurse should:

- Help the breathless patient minimize oxygen demands.
  1. Space out care and activities requiring exertion to provide adequate rest periods.
  2. Place frequently used items within convenient reach.
- Help the patient explore and develop strategies to maintain self-care ability, particularly after discharge from the hospital setting.
- Provide five to six nutrient-dense, high-calorie meals each day to help maintain nutritional status.
- Assist patients who are severely disabled and who require assistance with activities of daily living at home to find home care assistance. Placement in an extended care facility may be necessary when no other source of assistance is available.
- For additional nursing care measures, see the sections on asthma and bronchitis in this chapter.

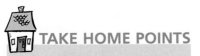

TAKE HOME POINTS

Emphysema is characterized by gradually increasing breathlessness with obstruction and reduction of exhaled air. Most emphysema patients eventually become oxygen dependent and require treatment with bronchodilators and steroids.

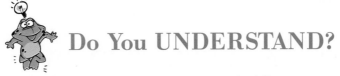

Do You UNDERSTAND?

DIRECTIONS: **Provide short answers to the following questions.**

1. Summarize the difference between asthma and emphysema.

2. List useful education topics for the patient with COPD.

Answers: 1. Asthma is characterized by hyperresponsiveness of the airways. Emphysema is characterized by destruction of the alveoli; 2. Smoking cessation, avoidance of respiratory infection, signs and symptoms of respiratory infection.

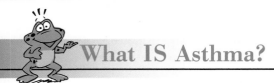

What IS Asthma?

Pathogenesis

Asthma is a respiratory disorder that has three main characteristics: recurring episodes of airway obstruction, hypersensitive ("twitchy") airways that narrow in response to certain stimuli, and inflammation of the airways. This hyperresponsiveness usually occurs after exposure to agents that would not bother a person without asthma. Inflammation of the bronchioles causes further hyperresponsiveness to other stimuli, ultimately resulting in episodes of airflow obstruction. Most people with asthma experience greater obstruction of airflow during the expiratory phase of breathing. Asthma attacks can range in severity from mild shortness of breath to respiratory failure and death. Various agents can trigger the inflammatory response associated with asthma, including dust, animal dander, and perfume.

Research indicates that respiratory viruses, gastroesophageal reflux disease, or chronic sinusitis triggers the inflammatory response. Other causes include extreme physical or emotional stress, cold or dry air, air pollutants (e.g., cigarette smoke, automobile emissions), and some foods (e.g., eggs, fermented alcohol). Forty percent of asthma is triggered by exercise.

Inflammation causes the production of cytokines within the lining of the bronchial tree. These substances prolong and amplify the inflammatory process within the airways. As a consequence of inflammation, collagen is deposited below the basement membrane of the bronchial lining, which causes thickening of the airway walls. In poorly controlled chronic asthma, overgrowth of glands and secretory cells that line the bronchial tree results, which causes further thickening of the airway walls and excess secretion of mucus. Some patients may have chronic asthma, with varying ranges of symptoms and respiratory compromise. With disease progression, the epithelial lining of the airways is lost, which causes increased airflow resistance and further hyperresponsiveness to stimuli. Hypersecretion of mucus and hyperresponsive airways cause blocked areas in the lungs with subsequent hypoxia and inadequate gas exchange.

Asthma attacks typically have two separate phases. The early phase occurs in reaction to the presence of a precipitating event or irritant. Mast cells in the bronchial lining release histamine, leading to contraction of the smooth muscles within the respiratory tree, swelling of the lining, and secretion of mucus. This phase tends to last approximately 2 hours. Without treatment, the inflammatory response will continue, which stimulates the release of other cytokines that support and prolong the inflammatory reaction. The late phase of asthma typically begins several hours after the triggering event and can evolve into severe respiratory compromise, unless the appropriate treatment is initiated.

Asthma that occurs in children is usually a result of allergies. In many cases, childhood asthma disappears when the person reaches adulthood. In adults, the cause of asthma is frequently unknown.

Certain drugs can cause asthmalike responses in susceptible individuals. These drugs include aspirin, nonsteroidal antiinflammatory agents, and propranolol.

Repeated asthma attacks can cause permanent changes in the pulmonary structure, with subsequent respiratory compromise and impairment.

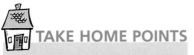

TAKE HOME POINTS

Asthma is frequently associated with allergies but may be of unknown origins.

Asthma can occur at any time in life, although it is generally more common in people under the age of 25. Many people with childhood asthma outgrow the condition as they reach adulthood.

Asthma is more common in African Americans than it is in Caucasians. Asthma appears to be most common in industrialized countries and appears to occur most frequently in socially and economically disadvantaged groups.

Status asthmaticus—a severe form of asthma that does not respond to normal treatment—is characterized by severe bronchospasm, mucous plugs, and increased airway resistance. Status asthmaticus is life threatening and requires immediate medical care.

Between 1979 and 1998 the age-adjusted death rate from asthma for African Americans is almost three times that of Caucasians. In the United States, approximately 5000 people die of asthma every year.

See Chapters 6C and 11 in RWNSG: *Pharmacology*

At-Risk Populations

The prevalence of asthma on a worldwide basis has increased by 30% in the last 20 years. The reason for this increase is unknown.

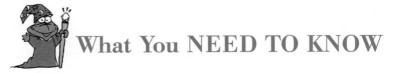

What You NEED TO KNOW

Clinical Manifestations

Breathlessness, severe cough, wheezing, and chest tightness are the hallmarks of asthma. Many patients also have thick, tenacious mucus that is difficult to clear from airways. A patient with mild asthma may be asymptomatic between attacks. Many people with more severe disease live in a chronic asthmatic state with varying degrees of respiratory compromise.

Prognosis

With appropriate treatment, most people with asthma live a normal life span.

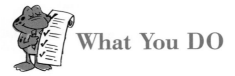

What You DO

Treatment

The goals of asthma management are to eliminate or control symptoms, maintain normal respiratory function, and minimize side effects and complications that are associated with both the disease and its therapy. Treatment is directed toward decreasing the inflammation and bronchospasm that are associated with this disease. Patients who work in farming, animal husbandry, mining, and steel production may need to seek other employment that minimizes their exposure to respiratory irritants.

Pharmacologic measures include oral and inhaled bronchodilators and anti-inflammatory drugs. Short- and long-acting beta-2 selective agonists are useful in treating symptoms and have a rapid effect, particularly when given via inhalers. Long-acting beta-2 agonists such as salmeterol are given on a routine twice-a-day schedule to prevent symptoms from occurring. The bronchodilating drug theophylline—a methylxanthine derivative—is also useful for some people with asthma, although it has a narrow therapeutic margin and may be poorly tolerated by some patients.

Glucocorticoids such as prednisone are highly effective in controlling inflammation. Eliminating or minimizing the chronic inflammation that is associated with severe asthma is important to prevent permanent structural damage to the lungs. Patients must be instructed that up to 1 year of steroid therapy may be required before an improvement in symptoms and pulmonary function is observed. For chronic use, these drugs have serious systemic effects that must be carefully considered when designing a plan of care. For some patients, side effects can be minimized and symptoms can be adequately controlled with the use of inhaled steroids.

See Chapter 7B in **RWNSG:** *Pharmacology*

Nursing Responsibilities

For the patient with asthma, the nurse should:

- Maintain and support adequate respiratory function for the patient. Carefully evaluate the patient's respiratory status and promptly report adverse changes to the patient's health care provider.
- Provide the patient with detailed information about asthma medications and signs and symptoms that require medical intervention.
- Teach medication-dependent patients to keep an extra supply available at all times and not to allow their prescriptions to run out.
- Instruct patients with exercise-induced asthma to use their medications before exertion is anticipated to improve exercise tolerance and minimize breathlessness.
- Evaluate the home and work environment of the person with asthma for possible asthma triggers and help the patient develop strategies to eliminate them.
- Advise patients who smoke to stop immediately. Provide assistance in the form of counseling, behavior modification, and referral to a smoking cessation support group. The patient should encourage friends and family not to smoke around them or in their home, because second-hand smoke frequently triggers an asthma attack.

Several strategies are available that can help the asthmatic patient in modifying the home environment. Carpets, curtains, and upholstered furniture frequently retain dust and residue from dust mites and insects. Whenever possible, carpets should be removed and replaced with rugs that can be easily laundered. Drapes should be replaced with blinds or shades. Down pillows should be replaced with hypoallergenic fiber pillows, and pillows and mattresses must be covered with impermeable, hypoallergenic material. All bedding, including blankets, must be laundered frequently in hot water. Ideally, a new home should be found for all pets, because animal dander and excrement can also be a source of allergy. When the patient is unwilling to comply with this restriction, all pets must be kept out of the patient's bedroom, and someone else in the household should assume responsibility for grooming the pet and cleaning up after it.

Patients who have no breath sounds, those who are using accessory muscles to breathe, and those who have tachypnea and tachycardia are in danger of respiratory arrest and require immediate emergency medical intervention.

Many patients with asthma, particularly older adults, have a decreased perception of breathlessness and may not seek medical help until they become desperately ill.

Parents of young children who are highly allergic (atopic), may need to modify the home environment.

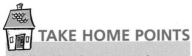
TAKE HOME POINTS

People with asthma may need to modify their home environment, lifestyle, and work setting to control their disease.

Do You UNDERSTAND?

DIRECTIONS: **In the space provided, write the letter(s) that correspond(s) to the word or phrase that answers each question. More than one answer may be chosen.**

_____ 1. Asthma can be caused by which of the following?
   a. Air pollution
   b. Food
   c. Warm moist air
   d. Animal dander

_____ 2. In what population does asthma typically occur?
   a. Under the age of 25
   b. Over the age of 50
   c. Of all ages

_____ 3. Drugs that are useful in the treatment of asthma include which of the following?
   a. Bronchodilators
   b. Diuretics
   c. Steroids

SECTION D

PULMONARY MALIGNANCIES

Cancer can affect nearly any tissue in the body. Cancer is classified and described according to the location in which it first appears (the primary site), the type of cell involved, the size of the tumor, whether the tumor has spread to other parts of the body (metastasized), and the way in which the cells appear under the microscope. This section will discuss lung cancer, the second most common type of cancer.

What IS Lung Cancer?

Pathogenesis

Two main types of lung cancer have been identified: small cell lung cancer (SCLC) and non–small cell lung cancer (NSCLC). The various types of lung cancer have different patterns of growth and respond differently to treatment.

SCLC grows rapidly and has, in many cases, already spread to other areas of the body by the time of diagnosis. SCLC usually responds well to chemotherapy or radiation, but the response is short-lived. SCLC has the poorest survival rates of all lung cancers.

Answers: 1. a, b, d; 2. a; 3. a, c.

NSCLC comprise 80% of lung cancers. The subcategories of NSCLC include squamous cell carcinoma, adenocarcinoma, and large cell carcinoma. Squamous cell cancers tend to originate in the central part of the chest and grow rapidly, but they are less likely to spread to other areas of the body. For this reason, squamous cell tumors have the greatest potential for cure of all the lung tumors, although overall survival rates remain poor. Adenocarcinomas tend to arise in the peripheral regions of the lungs, a location in which they frequently invade the lymphatics and then spread to other areas of the body, particularly the brain, bone, and liver (metastasize). Large cell tumors tend to behave in a manner similar to that of adenocarcinomas.

Prolonged exposure to respiratory irritants causes changes in the mucociliary lining of the lungs. Lung cancer is thought to be the result of repeated exposure to irritating substances, leading to inflammatory changes that eventually undergo malignant transformation. These substances are inhaled as part of the air. Most lung cancers originate in the epithelial lining of the lungs and bronchioles—the parts of the lungs that are exposed to ambient air and inhaled agents.

After cessation of smoking, 15 years may be required for lung tissue to return to normal. Research indicates that for women who smoke, a longer time may be required for their lungs to return to presmoking status.

At-Risk Populations

In most cases, carcinogenic agents in the tobacco combustion stream cause lung cancer. Smokers who use filtered, low-nicotine, low-tar cigarettes tend to inhale more deeply and, consequently, they have more tumors originating in the periphery of the lungs. Environmental agents that contribute to the development of lung cancer include silica, cadmium, chromium, and coal dust.

Occupations that entail exposure to respiratory irritants also convey an increased risk for lung cancer. These high-risk jobs include mining, some aspects of farming, and steel mills. The presence of multiple risk factors increases the overall risk for developing lung cancer. For example, miners who smoke have 20 times the risk of developing lung cancer when compared with a similar group of nonsmokers.

A small percentage of the population is genetically predisposed to the development of lung cancer. People who live in heavily industrialized areas with high levels of air pollution are also at risk for the disease.

What You NEED TO KNOW

Clinical Manifestations

Most lung cancers have metastasized by the time the disease is diagnosed. The signs and symptoms of the disease vary according to the size of the lung tumor, its location, and the number of other organs that are affected.

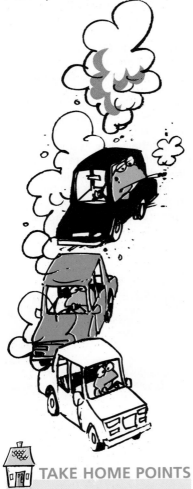

Lung cancer is the most commonly occurring fatal cancer in the United States and is now the leading cause of cancer deaths in both men and women. Over 90% of tumors arising in the lungs are malignant. The rising incidence of lung cancer over the last 70 years is directly linked to increased rates of tobacco use and air pollution.

TAKE HOME POINTS

Lung cancer is caused by prolonged exposure to respiratory irritants. Tobacco is responsible for 85% of all lung cancers.

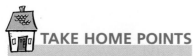

Patients with tumors in the central portion of the chest tend to present with coughing, shortness of breath, and persistent respiratory infections. Because many patients have a history of chronic lung disease, they may disregard the symptoms and fail to seek medical help. As the tumor progresses, the presenting symptoms become increasingly severe, and the patient may cough up blood (**hemoptysis**) and experience stridor and wheezing.

When the tumor is sufficiently large to compress the superior vena cava, the patient may have swelling of the face, neck, torso, arms, and hands (**superior vena cava syndrome**). Tumors that involve the thoracic nerves can cause pain in the shoulder that radiates down the arm. Patients who are hoarse and have trouble speaking or swallowing may have tumor involvement of the laryngeal nerve or compression of the esophagus. Tumors located in the peripheral area of the lungs may invade the pleura and chest wall, causing severe pain and difficulty breathing. Lung tumors can also invade and destroy bony tissue, causing pathologic fractures and subsequent pain.

Some tumors also have the ability to secrete substances that disrupt the electrolyte and metabolic balance of the body. Eleven percent of patients with SCLC will develop syndrome of inappropriate antidiuretic hormone (SIADH). Tumor cells create vasopressin, resulting in sodium loss and water retention. These patients experience decreased reflexes, confusion, lethargy, nausea, and vomiting. They may also be asymptomatic. Secretion of a substance that mimics the action of the parathyroid hormone, known as parathormone-related protein, can cause hypercalcemia and subsequent loss of appetite, as well as increased nausea, vomiting, constipation, and mental confusion.

Prognosis

The prognosis for lung cancer is poor for a variety of reasons. In most cases, the tumor is diagnosed when the disease has already spread to other parts of the body, substantially decreasing the likelihood of cure. Because most patients with this disease have a history of smoking, they tend to have other smoking-related problems, such as cardiovascular disease or respiratory compromise, which can disqualify them from aggressive but potentially curative therapies. Less than 10% of patients with SCLC are cured with standard therapy. Approximately 25% of patients with SCLC survive 2 years after diagnosis.

For patients with NSCLC, surgical excision of the tumor can be curative for some patients. The 5-year survival rate for patients with lung cancer that is diagnosed early is approximately 80%; however, most patients with lung cancer have metastatic disease at the time of diagnosis. For every eight patients diagnosed with lung cancer, only one will survive 5 years.

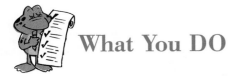

What You DO

Treatment

Currently, the three major medical therapies available for lung cancer are surgery, radiation therapy, and antineoplastic therapy. The overall status of the patient must be evaluated carefully before the start of treatment. Excision of the lung mass can offer prolonged survival and even a cure when the patient has a single lesion. Radiation therapy may be given in conjunction with surgery or antineoplastic therapy to control local disease. When tumor is obstructing airways or eroding mucosa, radiation therapy helps relieve breathlessness or hemoptysis. Radiation is also helpful in treating metastatic disease, particularly in bone or brain tissue.

Antineoplastic drugs are given to treat metastatic lung tumors that are too advanced to be treatable with surgery or radiation therapy. Drugs that are commonly used to treat lung cancer include cisplatin, carboplatin, ifosfamide, and Navelbine. Antineoplastic therapy offers limited benefit to most lung cancer patients, extending life expectancy only a few additional months in many cases.

> See Chapter 1D in **RWNSG:** *Pharmacology*

Nursing Responsibilities

Care of the patient with lung cancer is directed toward helping withstand the rigors of treatment or providing supportive and palliative care when active treatment is no longer an option. All patients and health care providers must understand the side effects of disease and treatment and be familiar with strategies to manage treatment and disease-related complications. The nurse should:

- Extensively monitor patients who are recovering from lung surgery to decrease the risk of further respiratory compromise.
- Take proactive measures, such as the use of incentive spirometers, respiratory therapy treatments, thoracentesis, oxygen therapy, diuretics, and steroids, when required.
- Remove respiratory irritants from the environment.
- Limit activity.
- Encourage diaphragmatic breathing.
- Keep a bedside fan blowing across the patient's face.
- Keep the ambient air cool and moist.
- Plan care around the patient's radiation therapy treatments to allow for rest periods. Radiation therapy can cause extreme fatigue, loss of appetite, difficulty eating and swallowing, and damage to skin and normal tissues within the radiation field.
- Position the patient upright to help relieve dyspnea.
- Monitor the patient who is receiving antineoplastic therapy for evidence of immunosuppression related to the effects of drugs on hematopoietic cells within the bone marrow. Anemia and thrombocytopenia are possible.
- Protect the patient who is undergoing antineoplastic therapy from infection.

- Manage pain. Encourage the patient to report his or her pain. Collaborate with other health care providers to establish a plan of care that controls pain and other distressing symptoms.
- Monitor patients for evidence of disabling depression or hopelessness, and prepare to intervene on their behalf. Patients and their caregivers frequently require intense emotional support. Some individuals can benefit from counseling from a social worker, chaplain, or psychiatrist. Further benefit can also be obtained by the judicious use of antidepressant drugs.
- Educate the public regarding the dangers of smoking, and motivate people who smoke to stop. Young people and nonsmokers must be targeted for educational programs before they actually start to smoke. Nurses must also be politically active and support public legislation that limits the sale and use of tobacco products.

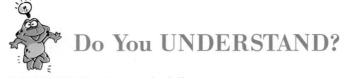

Do You UNDERSTAND?

DIRECTIONS: **Answer the following questions.**

1. What type of lung cancer has the greatest potential for cure?

2. What are three environmental agents that contribute to the development of lung cancer?

3. What are two side effects associated with radiation therapy?

Answers: 1. squamous cell carcinoma; 2. radon, asbestos, chromium; 3. fatigue, skin damage.

7 Endocrine System

SECTION A
PITUITARY DISORDERS

The pituitary gland and hypothalamus, as parts of the central nervous system, are responsible for many endocrine functions. The pituitary gland, known as the *master gland* of the endocrine system, is located at the base of the brain and is attached to the hypothalamus. The pituitary gland is divided into the anterior and posterior lobes.

The anterior lobe of the pituitary gland secretes six important hormones: human growth hormone (HGH), thyroid-stimulating hormone (TSH), adrenocorticotropic hormone (ACTH), prolactin, follicle-stimulating hormone (FSH), and luteinizing hormone (LH). These hormones are responsible for regulation of growth, development, and proper functioning of other endocrine glands. Additionally, these hormones are vital for the growth, maturation, and reproduction of the individual.

The posterior lobe stores and secretes two hormones: oxytocin and antidiuretic hormone (vasopressin). Antidiuretic hormone is responsible for reducing urine formation. Oxytocin acts as a powerful stimulant to the uterus, particularly toward the end of pregnancy.

Hormones are chemical messengers that are transported in body fluids. A single hormone can exert a variety of effects in different tissues, or several hormones can regulate a single body function. Water-soluble hormones combine with receptors on the surface of the cell membrane to exert their effects. Fat-soluble hormones permeate the cell membrane to combine with receptors found in the nucleus of the cell. Every cell contains approximately 2000 to 100,000 hormone receptor sites.

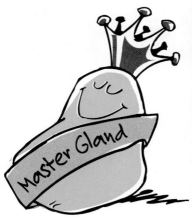

The oxytocin hormone causes milk to be expressed from the breasts during suckling.

Anterior Pituitary Disorders

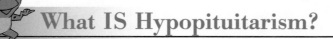

What IS Hypopituitarism?

Pathogenesis

Hypopituitarism results from a decrease in or a cessation of hormonal secretion by the anterior lobe of the pituitary gland. Any disorder that leads to obstruction or constriction (**vasospasm**) of the artery supplying blood to the pituitary gland leads to tissue death (**necrosis**) and loss of pituitary hormones. After tissue death, the pituitary gland swells, which further interrupts the blood supply. Causes of the reduction in blood supply fall into nine categories, known as the "nine I's" of hypopituitarism:

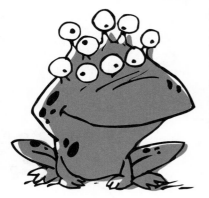

1. **I**nvasive (most common)—pituitary tumors, central nervous system tumors, carotid aneurysm
2. **I**nfarction—postpartum necrosis, pituitary stroke, malformation of pituitary blood vessels
3. **I**nfiltrative—sarcoidosis, hemochromatosis
4. **I**njury—head trauma, child abuse
5. **I**mmunologic—white blood cell invasion of pituitary gland, sickle cell disease, diabetes mellitus
6. **I**atrogenic—surgery, radiation therapy
7. **I**nfectious—fungal infections, tuberculosis, syphilis
8. **I**diopathic—familial
9. **I**solated—deficiency of anterior pituitary hormones

At-Risk Populations

Patients who are at risk for hypopituitarism include those who have any of the "nine I's." Patients who are most at risk for hypopituitarism are those who have pituitary or central nervous system tumors or those who have a weakness in the carotid artery (**aneurysm**).

The risk of hypopituitarism is increased during pregnancy because of the pituitary gland's increased size and large blood supply.

What You NEED TO KNOW

Clinical Manifestations

The signs and symptoms of hypopituitarism vary depending on the hormones affected. When all of the hormones are absent, the patient experiences signs and symptoms of dwarfism from growth hormone deficiency, cortisol deficiency from the lack of ACTH, thyroid hormone deficiency from the lack of TSH, diabetes insipidus from the lack of ADH, and gonadal failure and loss of secondary sex characteristics from the absence of FSH and LH.

Hypopituitarism in postpartum women results in loss of breast milk because of the absence of prolactin.

Prognosis

Patients with ACTH deficiency must be on drug therapy for life to compensate for the lack of cortisol.

ACTH deficiency is potentially life threatening because cortisol is required to sustain life.

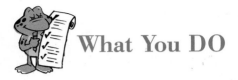

What You DO

Treatment

The treatment of hypopituitarism involves removal of the cause and replacement of hormones. Medications used to replace the hormones include growth hormone to treat HGH deficiency, glucocorticosteroids for correcting ACTH deficiency, thyroid hormones to treat thyroid hormone deficiency (hypothyroidism), and sex hormones to correct the decreased functional activity of the gonads (hypogonadism).

See Chapters 7A and 7B in RWNSG: *Pharmacology*

Nursing Responsibilities

The nursing responsibilities for the patient with hypopituitarism are directed toward the problems that result from deficiency at the target organ (e.g., thyroid, adrenal glands, gonads). The nurse should:

- Encourage the patient to verbalize concerns about body image and self-concept.
- Teach the patient and family about the prescribed medication therapy and the importance of continued follow-up and adherence to therapy.
- Monitor laboratory test results to ensure medication therapy is at a safe level.

Do You UNDERSTAND?

DIRECTIONS: **Indicate in the space provided whether the site of secretion for each hormone is the anterior pituitary (A) or the posterior pituitary (P).**

_____ 1. Growth hormone
_____ 2. Prolactin
_____ 3. Antidiuretic hormone
_____ 4. Thyroid-stimulating hormone
_____ 5. Follicle-stimulating hormone
_____ 6. Adrenocorticotropic hormone
_____ 7. Oxytocin
_____ 8. Luteinizing hormone

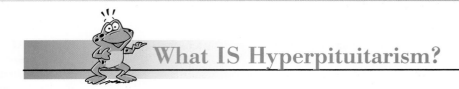

What IS Hyperpituitarism?

Pathogenesis

Increased activity of the pituitary gland, particularly, secretion of HGH and prolactin, causes hyperpituitarism. The disorders that result from the increased secretion of HGH include acromegaly and gigantism, as well as abnormal milk secretion (galactorrhea).

The most common cause of acromegaly is continuous hormonal secretion, a primary HGH-secreting pituitary tumor (adenoma). An unpredictable secretion pattern develops with the excess levels, which stimulates growth. In the adult, the growth of long bones has ceased and HGH can no longer stimulate long bone growth. Rather, connective tissue and the bony matrix multiply, which results in the enlargement of facial features and long bones (acromegaly).

Oversecretion of HGH in children and adolescents leads to increased proportional growth (gigantism). Secretion of HGH is also increased during exercise, hypoglycemia, stress, and nervous-system stimulation.

The metabolic effect of HGH on the renal tubules contributes to high levels of phosphates in the blood. Carbohydrate intolerance and an increased metabolic rate are present. Blood glucose levels elevate, followed by insulin resistance. Diabetes mellitus develops when the pancreas cannot secrete sufficient insulin to offset the effects of HGH.

At-Risk Populations

Patients who are most at risk for hyperpituitarism are those who have a pituitary adenoma. Approximately one third of patients with HGH abnormalities have glucose intolerance and one half of these patients develop diabetes mellitus. Of all pituitary adenomas, 30% secrete sufficient prolactin to cause galactorrhea, and approximately 25% of those secrete both HGH and prolactin.

What You NEED TO KNOW

Clinical Manifestations

In adults whose bone growth has stopped, a gradual enlargement and coarsening of facial features, hands, and feet is observed. Early signs include increased metabolism and strength and excessive sweating. The patient experiences joint pain, weakness, visual disturbances, and signs and symptoms of diabetes mellitus. Female patients with excessive prolactin levels develop abnormal milk secretion

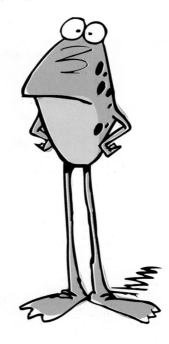

Acromegaly, an uncommon disorder, appears more frequently in women than it does in men and is diagnosed most frequently between ages 40 and 60.

in the nonlactating breast, cessation of menses (amenorrhea), and vaginal dryness. Male patients with excessive prolactin levels experience a loss of interest in sex and an inability to obtain and sustain an erection. Depression, anxiety, headaches, and vision loss occur in both genders.

Prognosis

Without treatment, hyperpituitarism, specifically acromegaly, is a slow progressive disease associated with decreased life expectancy.

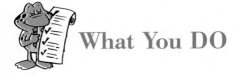

What You DO

Treatment

Treatment of patients with acromegaly or excessive prolactin secretion consists of radiation or surgical removal of the pituitary gland (hypophysectomy). Adjunctive drug therapy with a dopamine receptor agonist (e.g., bromocriptine) can be used for patients with excessive prolactin. The use of bromocriptine can reduce prolactin levels in 90% of patients. Octreotide, a growth hormone analog, is effective in reducing HGH levels in 60% to 80% of patients.

Gigantism can be corrected only through early diagnosis in childhood and surgical removal of a portion of the pituitary gland or through radiation therapy.

Nursing Responsibilities

Nursing care of the patient with hyperpituitarism is most frequently related to perioperative care. The nurse should:

- Assess the patient's expectations involving the surgery, educational needs related to diagnosis and treatment regimen, and the available support system.
- Obtain baseline vital signs.
- Perform perioperative neurologic assessments that include pupil equality and reactivity to light; handgrip; level of consciousness; orientation to time, place, and situation; appropriate response to stimuli; and visual acuity and visual fields.
- 🍎 Teach the patient and family about the diagnosis, surgical intervention, and medication therapy that are required after surgery.
- 🍎 Instruct the patient to avoid sneezing, coughing, and bending over from the waist to avoid disrupting the surgical site.
- Support changes in patient's self-image and self-concept.
- Administer glucocorticoids as ordered preoperatively to help the patient tolerate the stress of surgery and the absence of cortisol.

In children, overproduction of HGH stimulates growth of long bones and results in an unusually tall adult. When the abnormality is extreme, the child can reach a height of 8 feet or more, although the body proportions are usually normal. An underproduction of HGH, conversely, causes dwarfism.

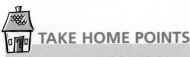
See Chapters 2A and 7A in RWNSG: *Pharmacology*

TAKE HOME POINTS

Patients who have had their pituitary gland completely removed or destroyed with radiation therapy must take hormone replacements, particularly cortisone, for the remainder of their lives.

Lack of cortisone can be life threatening.

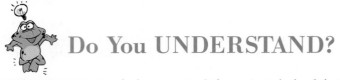

Do You UNDERSTAND?

DIRECTIONS: **Match the terms in Column A with the definitions in Column B.**

Column A

_____ 1. Hyperpituitarism

_____ 2. Adenoma

_____ 3. Prolactin

_____ 4. Growth hormone

_____ 5. Hypophysectomy

Column B

a. A benign tumor in which the cells form a recognizable glandular structure or in which the cells are derived from glandular epithelium

b. Surgical removal of a portion or all of the pituitary gland; indicated when there is a tumor of the gland

c. The anterior pituitary hormone controls general growth of the skeleton and influences metabolism

d. An anterior pituitary hormone that promotes the growth of breast tissue and stimulates and sustains milk production during the postpartum period

e. A condition from pathologically increased activity of the pituitary gland, especially growth hormone or prolactin

---

Posterior Pituitary Disorders

What IS Syndrome of Inappropriate Antidiuretic Hormone?

Pathogenesis

Syndrome of inappropriate antidiuretic hormone (SIADH) is the secretion of excessive amounts of antidiuretic hormone (ADH) from the posterior pituitary gland and other areas outside the pituitary gland. The most common cause of excessive production of ADH is carcinoma. The carcinoma produces an additional source of ADH. Tumors that are associated with SIADH include carcinoma of the tongue, lung, duodenum, pancreas, and connective tissues, as well as leukemia, lymphoma, and Hodgkin's diseases. A transient SIADH can follow pituitary surgery or the use of certain drugs (e.g., barbiturates, general anesthetics, vincristine, nicotine, morphine, diuretics, synthetic hormones). These drugs serve either to simulate ADH release or to enhance the physiologic effects of ADH.

Answers: 1. e; 2. a; 3. d; 4. c; 5. b.

ADH is normally released in response to elevated serum concentrations and a decrease in extracellular fluid volume. ADH increases the kidney's permeability to water thus promoting reabsorption and a decrease in urine output. In SIADH, ADH is not inhibited by the low concentration of solutes in the extracellular fluid.

Continual release of ADH causes water retention from renal tubules and collecting ducts. Extracellular fluid volume increases with a dilution of serum sodium. Hyponatremia suppresses renin and aldosterone secretions. The result of hyponatremia is a suppression of renin and aldosterone, causing a decrease in the reabsorption of sodium by the renal tubules.

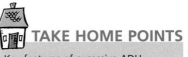

TAKE HOME POINTS

Key features of excessive ADH include water retention, low serum sodium levels, and dilute urine.

At-Risk Populations

Patients who are at risk for SIADH include those with a history of carcinoma of the lung, duodenum, brain, bladder, pancreas, or prostate. Patients with an infection of the brain, brain trauma, or infectious processes of the lungs are also at risk. Patients who are taking certain drugs (e.g., morphine, diuretics, barbiturates, nicotine) that serve either to stimulate ADH release or to enhance its effects can also be predisposed to SIADH.

No single, specific population of patients is more susceptible to this disorder than are other groups.

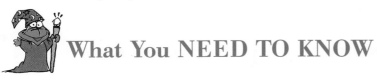

What You NEED TO KNOW

Clinical Manifestations

The signs and symptoms of SIADH are related to the onset and severity of low serum sodium levels. A rapid decrease in serum sodium level from 140 to 130 mEq/L produces thirst, impaired taste, anorexia, dyspnea-on-exertion, fatigue, and dulled mentation. Severe gastrointestinal symptoms appear with a drop in serum sodium from 130 to 120 mEq/L.

A serum sodium level below 115 mEq/L produces confusion, lethargy, muscle twitching, seizures, coma, and, occasionally, irreversible neurologic damage.

Prognosis

The prognosis of SIADH depends on the cause and sodium level. Resolution of SIADH usually occurs within 3 days. The prognosis is poor for patients who have carcinoma of the lung. Seizures and coma can contribute to chronic brain dysfunction.

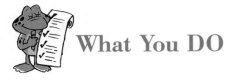

What You DO

Treatment

Treatment for SIADH includes identifying and treating the underlying cause. SIADH ordinarily resolves with the correction of hyponatremia. No drug is available that suppresses sources of ADH coming from outside the posterior pituitary gland. Demeclocycline (Declomycin) inhibits the action of pituitary-secreted ADH, although the mechanism is unknown. Hypertonic intravenous fluids can be used to correct low serum sodium levels, along with a fluid restriction of 600 to 800 ml per day. Diuretics are given to correct low plasma osmolality.

Nursing Responsibilities

For the patient with SIADH, the nurse should:

- Identify patients who are at risk for SIADH.
- Monitor the results of serum and urine tests.
- Assess for signs and symptoms of hyponatremia through evaluation of neurologic status.
- Monitor fluid restriction to avoid exceeding daily fluid-restriction requirements.
- Obtain weight readings at same time daily, on same scale, and in same type of clothing and accurately record intake and output.
- Administer medication therapy as ordered.
- Use strategies appropriate to reduce the patient's risk of injury secondary to altered neurologic status.
- Teach age-appropriate and culturally appropriate patient and family information regarding the disorder.

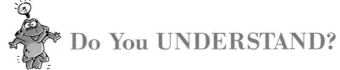

Do You UNDERSTAND?

DIRECTIONS: **Unscramble the italicized letters to form terms associated with SIADH.**

1. _____ *(noedhraiydt)*
2. _____ *(dutecnaiirti)*
3. _____ *(mecllyoecenidc)*

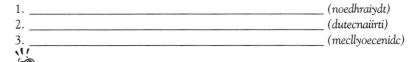

What IS Diabetes Insipidus?

Diabetes insipidus results in a deficiency of ADH. Two types of this disorder have been classified. In neurogenic diabetes insipidus, ADH is either missing or present at a low level. ADH synthesis or release is affected from a malfunction of the posterior pituitary gland. Injury to the brain, tumors, neurosurgical operations, infections, or bleeding can affect the brain's ability to release ADH.

In nephrogenic diabetes insipidus, ADH is produced normally, but the distal tubules and collecting ducts cannot respond to the hormone's signal to reabsorb water. This form of the disorder can be acquired or inherited by male children.

Pathogenesis

The hypothalamus normally produces ADH and is stored in the posterior pituitary gland. ADH is released into the bloodstream when needed to cause the kid-

http://www.cc.nih.gov/ccc/ patient_education/pepubs/ di/pdf

ney tubules to reabsorb water. Water that cannot be reabsorbed is passed out of the body in the form of urine. Decreased secretion of ADH causes less water to be reabsorbed and more urine to be produced. The result is diabetes insipidus with elimination of large volumes of dilute urine.

At-Risk Populations

Patients who are at risk for diabetes insipidus include those with head injuries, patients who have had neurosurgery or pituitary tumors, or those who have had inflammation or infection of brain tissue. Drugs that inhibit ADH release (e.g., ethanol, glucocorticosteroids, adrenergics, phenytoin, opioid antagonists, lithium) can also increase the patient's risk of developing diabetes insipidus.

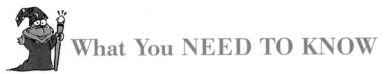

What You NEED TO KNOW

Clinical Manifestations

Although the two forms of diabetes insipidus are different in cause, the signs and symptoms are similar. Changes in mentation, insomnia, excessive continued thirst (polydipsia), weight loss, urinary frequency with a urinary output of 4 to 18 liters per day, and nighttime voiding (nocturia) are common. The skin and mucus membranes are cool.

Prognosis

The prognosis for the patient with diabetes insipidus is excellent as long as the prescribed medications are taken.

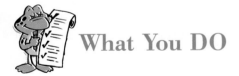

What You DO

Treatment

Treatment of the patient with either type of diabetes insipidus includes identifying and treating the underlying cause of the disorder. Fluid intake is balanced with urinary output. ADH is replaced using intravenous, subcutaneous, or intranasal desmopressin (DDAVP) or intramuscular Pitressin. Surgical removal of the posterior pituitary gland may be required in some patients.

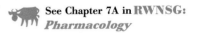
See Chapter 7A in RWNSG:
Pharmacology

Nursing Responsibilities

For patients with either type of diabetes insipidus, the nurse should:
- Know which patients are at risk for the disorder.
- Monitor for excessive urination or thirst.
- Obtain weights at same time daily, on same scale, and in same type of clothing; accurately monitor intake and output.

- Monitor urine-specific gravity and osmolality.
- Administer desmopressin, pitressin, or diuretic as prescribed
🍎 Provide age-appropriate and culturally appropriate patient and family information regarding the disorder and the importance of adherence to medication therapy.

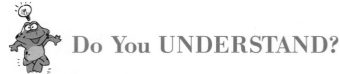

Do You UNDERSTAND?

DIRECTIONS: Indicate in the space provided whether the statement is *true* or *false*. If false, then correct the statement in the margin space to the left to make it true.

_____ 1. Excessive urination is known as polydipsia.

_____ 2. Patients who have diabetes insipidus are seldom thirsty.

_____ 3. Patients should be taught to call the health care provider when they are unable to balance their fluid intake with fluid output.

_____ 4. Patients need not call their health care provider when they cannot balance their fluid intake and output.

_____ 5. The lack or deficiency of ADH causes diabetes insipidus.

SECTION B

THYROID AND PARATHYROID DISORDERS

Thyroid abnormalities are of three types: enlargement of the thyroid, known as a goiter; hypofunction, known as hypothyroidism; and hyperfunction, known as hyperthyroidism. Hypothyroidism and hyperthyroidism represent disorders of thyroid hormone secretion.

What IS Hypothyroidism

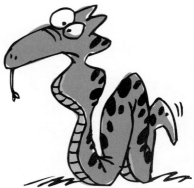

Pathogenesis

In hypothyroidism, the production of thyroid hormones is inadequate, which results in a decrease in the basal metabolic rate. The thyroid gland may enlarge in an attempt to compensate for the inadequacy, and a goiter is formed.

Congenital defects of thyroid function, defective hormone synthesis, iodine deficiency, antithyroid drugs, or chronic autoimmune Hashimoto's disease can cause primary hypothyroidism. Surgery or radiation therapy for hyperthyroidism can also contribute to a hypothyroidism state. Secondary hypothyroidism occurs when TSH levels are increased as a result of insufficient stimulation of a normal

Answers: 1. false, excessive urination is known as polyuria; 2. false, patients are usually very thirsty; the medical term for this thirst is polydipsia; 3. true; 4. false, patients should call their health care provider to avoid dehydration; 5. true.

thyroid gland. Peripheral resistance to thyroid hormones can also cause secondary hypothyroidism. Tertiary hypothyroidism develops when the hypothalamus fails to produce thyroid-releasing hormone (TRH) and thus no stimulation of the pituitary to secrete TSH is present. This form of hypothyroidism can be a result of a tumor or another destructive lesion in the hypothalamus.

A goiter is an enlargement of the thyroid gland. A deficiency of iodine that develops most frequently in the autumn and winter is a primary cause of endemic goiter. Sporadic goiter is related to genetic defects that result in faulty iodine metabolism, to the ingestion of large amounts of nutritional goitrogens, and to the ingestion of medical goitrogens.

At-Risk Populations

Hypothyroidism affects more women than it does men by a ratio of 4:1.

The ingestion of large amounts of foods that inhibit thyroxine production (goitrogens) such as rutabagas, cabbage, soybeans, peanuts, peaches, peas, strawberries, spinach, and radishes contribute to goiter formation. Patients who take lithium, cobalt, aminosalicylic acid, phenylbutazone, tolbutamide, and iodine in large doses are also at risk.

The highest incidence of hypothyroidism occurs in women between 30 and 65 years of age.

People living in the Midwest, Northwest, and Great Lakes regions in which the soil and water are deficient in iodine are at greater risk for developing goiter.

Endemic goiter most frequently affects adolescents who have decreased thyroid hormones during periods of growth spurts, pregnant women, and nursing mothers who are living in iodine-deficient regions.

What You NEED TO KNOW

Hypothyroidism

SIGNS AND SYMPTOMS	ASSOCIATED PATHOPHYSIOLOGY
Respiratory distress and dysphagia	Goiter formation
Hypoxia and mental status changes, forgetfulness, depression	Decreased cerebral blood flow
Reduced stroke volume and heart rate	Reduced cardiac output
Increased systolic blood pressure	Increased peripheral vascular resistance
Reduced urinary output, increase in total body water, low serum sodium levels	Reduced renal blood flow
Anemia	Reduced production of erythropoietin and red blood cells
Decreased appetite, weight gain, constipation; increased cholesterol and triglyceride levels with subsequent development of atherosclerosis and heart disease; decreased absorption of glucose	General slowing of gastrointestinal function; abnormalities in lipid metabolism; increased sensitivity to exogenous insulin

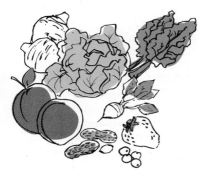

Continued

Hypothyroidism—cont'd

SIGNS AND SYMPTOMS	ASSOCIATED PATHOPHYSIOLOGY
Sensitivity to cold; reduced inability to sweat; dry flaky skin; brittle head and body hair; nails are slow growing	Decreased metabolic rate and basal body temperature; reduced secretions from sweat and sebaceous glands
Delayed skeletal and soft tissue growth; delayed wound healing	Decreased protein metabolism

Clinical Manifestations

Hypothyroidism in its severe form (myxedema) is characterized by physical and mental sluggishness, obesity, hair loss, enlargement of the tongue, and thickening of the skin. Myxedematous changes in respiratory muscles lead to hypoventilation and carbon dioxide retention. Pleural effusions associated with dyspnea are possible, although patients can be asymptomatic. Complicating factors to myxedema coma include hyponatremia, hypercalcemia, secondary adrenal insufficiency, hypoglycemia, and water intoxication. Myxedema can also be brought on by the stress of surgery, infection, or noncompliance with thyroid replacement hormone therapy.

Hypothyroidism is diagnosed based not only on signs and symptoms, but also on thyroid function tests. The serum TSH is elevated in an attempt to compensate for low levels of thyroid hormones. Thyroxine (T_4) and triiodothyronine (T_3) levels are low as is the free thyroxine concentration (fT_4), which is the metabolically active form of T_4. The radioactive iodide uptake is decreased. TRH levels are elevated.

Prognosis

Most patients with hypothyroidism have a good prognosis with treatment.

Severe hypothyroidism in children is known as cretinism.

Unrecognized and undiagnosed hypothyroidism can progress to myxedema coma, which has a mortality rate approaching 100%.

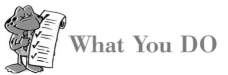

What You DO

Treatment

The primary treatment for hypothyroidism is life-long hormonal replacement therapy. The patient is encouraged to use iodized salt to ensure sufficient iodine intake. Levothyroxine sodium (Synthroid and Levoxyl) is the primary drug used. After therapy is started, patients will notice an improvement in their signs and symptoms within 2 to 3 weeks. Levothyroxine sodium and corticosteroids are administered intravenously to patients with myxedema coma.

Patients with cardiac disease must be started on low doses of thyroid hormone to reduce the risk of heart failure or myocardial infarction. These complications of therapy develop as a result of increasing metabolism, myocardial oxygen requirements, and, consequently, the workload on the heart.

See Chapter 7B in **RWNSG:** *Pharmacology*

Nursing Responsibilities

For the patient with hypothyroidism, the nurse should:

- Assess the patient for manifestations of hypothyroidism and response to therapy (e.g., mental status, quality of skin and hair, subnormal temperature, bradycardia, respiratory rate, blood pressure, worsening heart failure, weight gain or loss).
- Provide instructions for adhering to a low-calorie diet until the patient's weight stabilizes within an ideal range. Weight gain develops when the patient's appetite improves with the start of therapy, but energy levels have not yet improved.
- Encourage activity as tolerated to reduce constipation.
- Advise the patient to drink six to eight glasses of water daily and eat high-fiber foods. A stool softener may be needed if diet and exercise are ineffective. Reassure the patient that energy levels will return to normal after hormone therapy is begun.
- Teach the patient and family the importance of life-long drug therapy, about the disease and the importance of monitoring thyroid hormone levels, the benefits and adverse effects of hormone replacement therapy, and when to contact the health care provider for assistance.
- Maintain a patent airway, administering oxygen, and intravenous fluids for the patient with myxedema coma.
- Monitor intake, output, and daily weights.
- Provide the patient with a comfortable, warm environment. Supply extra clothing and warm blankets when necessary.
- Administer no more than $1/2$ to $1/3$ of the usual dose when the patient requires a sedative or opioid analgesic. Reassess the patient for manifestations of respiratory depression or a decreased level of consciousness after medication administration.
- Monitor the sacrum, coccyx, elbows, scapula, and other pressure points for evidence of redness or tissue breakdown. The edematous tissues are prone to decubitus ulcers formation. Turn the patient on a regular schedule. Use a pressure-reduction mattress.
- Advise the patient to take the medication at the same time every day to maintain blood levels. Taking the drug in the morning will help prevent insomnia.

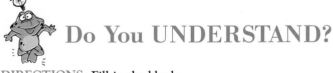

Do You UNDERSTAND?

DIRECTIONS: Fill in the blanks.

1. The primary food source of iodine is _____.
2. List five foods that can precipitate development of goiter:

   _____
   _____
   _____
   _____
   _____

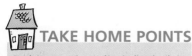

TAKE HOME POINTS

Explain to patients that iodized salt is a prevention for goiter.

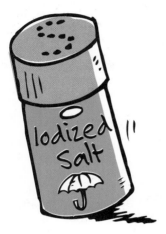

 Examine package labeling carefully because the medication order may be written in micrograms or milligrams.

 TAKE HOME POINTS

Do not administer thyroid hormone replacement medications if the patient has had a heart attack, thyrotoxicosis, or untreated adrenal insufficiency.

Use the medications cautiously in patients who have angina pectoris and other cardiovascular disorders, renal insufficiency or failure, or poor circulation.

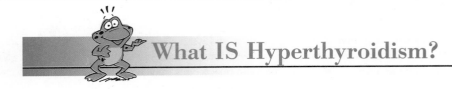

What IS Hyperthyroidism?

Pathogenesis

Excessive thyroid hormone secretion (hyperthyroidism) can cause various thyroid disorders. Graves' disease, the most common hypersecretion condition, is an autoimmune disorder mediated by the IgG antibody that binds to and activates TSH receptors on the surface of thyroid cells. Excessive stimulation of the sympathetic nervous system can also cause hyperthyroidism. In either case, a loss of the normal regulatory controls of thyroid hormone secretion is present. Because the activity of thyroid hormones on the body is stimulation, hypermetabolism results with increased sympathetic nervous system activity.

Overtreatment of hypothyroidism in its clinical state (thyrotoxicosis) with thyroid hormones can result in hyperthyroidism. Hyperthyroidism can also result from single or multiple functioning thyroid cancer (thyroid adenoma).

At-Risk Populations

Hyperthyroidism is predominantly a disorder of women. Graves' disease tends to occur in twins. Patients who are at risk also include those who have been overtreated for hypothyroidism. Patients also at risk for hyperthyroidism include those who have a history of posterior pituitary disease, hypothalamic disease, or those who use amiodarone to treat atrial fibrillation.

 Hyperthyroidism affects women four times as frequently as it does men, particularly young women age 20 to 40 years.

What You NEED TO KNOW

Clinical Manifestations

The signs and symptoms of hyperthyroidism vary from mild to severe. Excessive amounts of thyroid hormones stimulate the cardiovascular system and increase the number of beta-adrenergic receptors. This increase leads to tachycardia and increased cardiac output, stroke volume, peripheral blood flow, and adrenergic responsiveness.

The metabolic rate increases significantly, leading to a negative nitrogen balance, lipid depletion, and nutritional deficiency. Weight loss occurs despite a ravenous appetite. The patient will also experience loose bowel movements, heat intolerance, profuse sweating, tachycardia, and a lack of coordination. The skin becomes warm, smooth, and moist. The hair appears thin and soft.

The patient's emotions are volatile because of the turbulent activity within the body. Moods can be cyclic, ranging from mild euphoria to extreme hyperactivity, delirium, fatigue, and depression. As a consequence of the chaotic emotional state, interpersonal relationships can deteriorate. The patient may appear extremely agitated and irritable with a resting tremor of the hand.

A thyroid crisis (thyroid storm) is an acute exacerbation of hyperthyroidism. A thyroid storm is a medical emergency that leads to life-threatening cardiac, hepatic, or renal failure.

The patient with Graves' disease also exhibits an enlarged thyroid and abnormal protrusion of the eyes (exophthalmia). Exophthalmos appears to be an autoimmune problem of the tissues behind the eye. The patient has protruding eyes and a fixed stare resulting from the accumulation of fluids in the fat pads and muscles that lie behind the eyes. Because the eyes are surrounded by bone, edema forces the eyes forward out of their sockets, producing the typical appearance of hyperthyroidism.

Hyperthyroidism alters the metabolism of hypothalamic, pituitary, and gonadal hormones. It is diagnosed based on thyroid function tests. The serum TSH is decreased in primary hyperthyroidism and elevated when excessive TSH secretion is the cause. T_4 and T_3 levels are elevated, as is fT_4. The radioactive iodide uptake is increased. TRH levels are decreased.

Prognosis

With treatment, the prognosis for hyperthyroidism is good. Inadequate treatment of hyperthyroidism, stressors (e.g., stroke, surgery, infection, pulmonary embolism, myocardial infarction, diabetic ketoacidosis), and preeclampsia can precipitate a thyroid storm. The patient may have marked tachycardia, vomiting, and stupor. Other findings include a combination of irritability and restlessness, double vision (diplopia), tremor and weakness, cough with shortness of breath, angina, and extremity edema. A high fever can develop insidiously, rising rapidly to a lethal level. Without treatment, the patient will experience vascular collapse, hypotension, coma, and death.

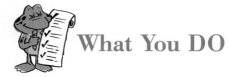

What You DO

Treatment

The treatment for hyperthyroidism includes antithyroid medications, radioactive iodine therapy, iodine therapy, dietary therapy, and surgery.

Radioactive iodine therapy (^{131}I) is used primarily for middle-age and older patients. The rationale for this therapy is simple: the thyroid gland is unable to distinguish between regular iodine atoms and radioiodine atoms, thus the thyroid gland picks up the radioiodine and concentrates it precisely as it would regular iodine. As a result, the cells that concentrate ^{131}I to make T_4 are destroyed by the irradiation, and thyroid hormone secretion diminishes. In most patients, hypermetabolic symptoms diminish within 6 to 12 weeks. A few patients may require a second dose. Because of the delay in drug activity, concurrent treatment with beta-adrenergic blockers may be desirable. The beta-adrenergic blocking medications used most frequently are propranolol and reserpine.

Iodine therapy reduces the vascularity of the thyroid gland before surgery and is prescribed to treat a thyroid storm. Iodine preparations such as potassium iodide act temporarily to prevent the release of thyroid hormones into the

When hyperthyroidism alters hypothalamic, pituitary, and gonadal metabolism before puberty, sexual development is delayed. After puberty, hyperthyroidism results in decreased libido in both men and women. Women note menstrual irregularities and decreased fertility.

American Thyroid Association
http://www.thyroid.org/patient/brochur3.htm.

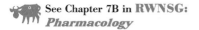
See Chapter 7B in **RWNSG:** *Pharmacology*

Antithyroid medications such as propylthiouracil (PTU) and methimazole are used for children, young adults, pregnant women, and patients who are not candidates for radioactive iodine therapy or surgery.

circulation by increasing the amount of hormone stored within the gland. When surgery is warranted, a partial thyroidectomy is most frequently used thus decreasing its size and capacity for hormone production.

Nursing Responsibilities

For the patient with hyperthyroidism, the nurse should:

- Provide education regarding the signs and symptoms of hyperthyroidism for persons at risk.
- Instruct the patient about the importance of a well-balanced, high-calorie diet, while discouraging foods that increase peristalsis and thus result in diarrhea (highly seasoned, bulky, or fibrous foods).
- Advise the patient to notify the health care provider when a weight loss of more than 2 kg (4.4 lb) occurs.
- Assign a hospitalized patient with hyperthyroidism to a private room to promote rest and prevent being disturbed by others through restlessness and hyperactivity.
- Inform the patient of the use of artificial tears and eye patches as needed to prevent irritation if exophthalmos develops.
- Teach the patient to stay in a cool environment, primarily because heat intolerance is common. Use lightweight linens and encourage the wearing of light, loose clothing.
- Monitor the patient who has had a thyroidectomy for weakness and hoarseness of the voice as a result of trauma or damage to the laryngeal nerve, hypocalcemia, and tetany; respiratory obstruction as a result of edema of the glottis; laryngeal nerve damage; or tracheal compression from hemorrhage.
- Maintain intake and output record for 2 to 3 days while watching for difficulty swallowing.
- Assess for signs of a thyroid storm (e.g., elevated temperature, extreme restlessness, agitation, tachycardia). Report temperature elevations over 100° F (37.7° C).
- Teach the patient to support the head and neck when sitting up in bed to prevent stress on the suture line. Be certain to check the patient's neck for bleeding at the front, sides, and back of the neck because blood tends to drain posteriorly.
- Emphasize the importance of routine follow-up laboratory testing.

Inadvertent removal of the parathyroid glands can cause postoperative hypoparathyroidism manifesting as hypocalcemia.

What IS Hypoparathyroidism?

Pathogenesis

Hypoparathyroidism is the result of inadequate circulating parathyroid hormone (PTH). By stimulating bone resorption, renal tubular reabsorption of calcium, and activation of vitamin D, PTH helps regulate calcium and phosphate levels.

Hypoparathyroidism is characterized by hypocalcemia, resulting from a lack of PTH to maintain serum calcium levels. PTH resistance at the cellular level can also occur. This resistance is the result of a genetic defect from hypocalcemia, in spite of normal or high PTH levels and is frequently associated with hypothyroidism and hypogonadism. The most common cause of hypoparathyroidism is iatrogenic; that is, accidental removal of the parathyroid glands or damage to the vascular supply of the glands during neck surgery.

At-Risk Populations

All forms of hypoparathyroidism are rare, but the disorder affects all ages with both genders equally at risk. Hypomagnesemia, as observed in alcoholism or malabsorption, impairs PTH secretion and its action on bone and kidneys thus increasing the risk of hypocalcemia. Other risk factors include neck trauma or surgery and carcinoma of the head and neck.

Most patients with congenital hypoparathyroidism have no family history of the disease. The pattern of inheritance is as varied as are the kinds of genetic abnormalities that cause the disease. Children in some families are at a 50% risk for contracting the disease (dominant gene defect); others are at a risk of 25% or less (recessive gene defect).

Hypocalcemia is fairly common in the older adult and can be a result of multiple abnormalities, not hypoparathyroidism alone.

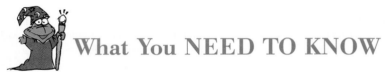

What You NEED TO KNOW

Clinical Manifestations

The signs and symptoms of hypoparathyroidism are those of hypocalcemia. Sudden decreases in calcium concentration result in neuromuscular irritability (tetany). Tetany is characterized by tingling of the lips, fingertips, and, occasionally, the feet and increased muscle tension, leading to paresthesias and stiffness. Patients are usually anxious and apprehensive. Painful tonic spasms of smooth and skeletal muscles of the extremities and face, as well as dysphagia, a constricted feeling in the throat, laryngospasms, and hyperactive deep tendon reflexes are also present. Accessory muscle spasm and laryngeal spasm-induced airway obstruction can compromise respiratory function. Other signs include irritability of the facial nerve when tapped (Chvostek's sign) and carpopedal spasm within 2 minutes of inflating a blood pressure cuff over systolic pressure (Trousseau's sign). The serum total and ionized calcium level is decreased (less than 8.5 mg/dl) and the serum phosphorous level is increased (greater than 5.4 mg/dl).

See Chapter 7A in **RWNSG:**
Fluids & Electrolytes

Prognosis

Death can result from respiratory obstruction secondary to tetany and laryngospasm if treatment is not begun rapidly for patients with hypoparathyroidism. Patients with chronic hypoparathyroidism will develop calcifications of the eye and basal ganglia if treatment is delayed.

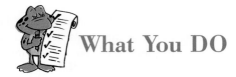

What You DO

Treatment

Vitamin D and calcium supplements are the primary treatments for hypoparathyroidism, regardless of the cause. The only exception is the point at which the inactivity of PTH is a result of hypomagnesemia, which is readily treated with magnesium supplementation. Currently, a replacement form of PTH is unavailable. Oral vitamin D (ergocalciferol [vitamin D_2], calcitriol, 1,25-dihydroxycholecalciferol [Rocaltrol], dihydrotachysterol [Hytakerol]) increases intestinal absorption of calcium from the diet. Along with calcium supplements (e.g., calcium carbonate, calcium lactate, calcium gluconate), vitamin D helps maintain normal blood calcium levels.

Life-long treatment may be required for patients with a chronic form of the disease. For some patients, a thiazide diuretic can be used to increase phosphate excretion and decrease calcium excretion.

See Chapters 7B, 9B, and 12 in RWNSG: *Pharmacology*

An acute attack of hypoparathyroidism is life threatening and requires immediate attention to airway maintenance and intravenous calcium gluconate given slowly until tetany ceases. When the patient is awake, breathing into a paper bag can help raise serum ionized calcium levels.

Nursing Responsibilities

The primary objectives of treatment are to treat tetany when present and prevent long-term complications by maintaining normal serum calcium levels. As such, for the patient with hypoparathyroidism, the nurse should:

- Identify patients at risk for hypoparathyroidism and periodically assessing for presence of Chvostek's and Trousseau's signs.
- Maintain a patent airway, and administer intravenous calcium as needed for tetany. Monitor electrocardiogram while administering calcium.
- Provide for seizure precautions during tetany.
- Provide careful and detailed teaching about life-long maintenance therapy with oral calcium preparations and the signs and symptoms of overtreatment (hypercalcemia), as well as undertreatment (hypocalcemia).
- Teach the patient about the importance of a high-calcium, low-phosphate diet and of avoiding foods containing oxalic acid (e.g., spinach, rhubarb), phytic acid (e.g., bran, whole grains), and phosphorus. These food substances reduce calcium absorption. Milk and cheese contain high levels of phosphorus and should also be avoided.
- Encourage the patient to keep appointments for follow-up and periodic laboratory testing of serum calcium and phosphorous levels (three to four times per year and as needed).
- Encourage the use of skin softeners for scaly skin.
- Use stool softeners, adequate fluids, and fresh fruits to prevent constipation associated with calcium supplements.

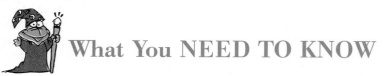

What IS Hyperparathyroidism?

Pathogenesis

The primary disease of parathyroid glands is overactivity (hyperparathyroidism). One or more of the parathyroid glands behaves inappropriately by making excess hormone, regardless of the level of calcium. In other words, the parathyroid glands continue to make large amounts of parathyroid hormone, even when the calcium level is normal, and they should not be making the hormone at all.

Primary hyperparathyroidism is a result of either glandular hyperplasia of all four glands or adenoma of only one gland. The result is an unregulated increase of PTH production and release and a subsequent rise in serum calcium levels. Secondary hyperparathyroidism occurs when the glands are hyperplastic from malfunction of another organ system. This condition is usually found in patients with chronic renal failure but can also occur with vitamin D deficiency, osteogenesis imperfecta, Paget's disease, multiple myeloma, and carcinoma with bone metastasis.

At-Risk Populations

Hyperparathyroidism is rare in children. Male and female adults over age 50 are most at risk, with women more frequently involved than men. Hyperparathyroidism is not related to age in patients with renal failure. The disorder occurs more frequently in temperate climates and in persons exposed to therapeutic low levels of radiation. Medications associated with hyperparathyroidism include thiazide diuretics, furosemide, excessive amounts of vitamins A and D, and exogenous calcium intake. Long periods of immobilization predispose a patient to hypercalcemia.

What You NEED TO KNOW

Clinical Manifestations

Some patients with hyperparathyroidism can be entirely asymptomatic. In patients with the severe form, bones can give up calcium to the extent that they become brittle and break (osteoporosis and osteopenia). This problem is even more of a concern in older patients. Bones can also have small hemorrhages within their center, which will cause bone pain.

Because the major function of the kidney is to filter and clean the blood, constant exposure of the kidney to high levels of calcium causes a collection of calcium within the renal tubules, which leads to kidney stones.

TAKE HOME POINTS

Because hyperparathyroidism was first described in 1925, the symptoms have become known as "painful bones, renal stones, abdominal groans, and psychic moans."

In extreme cases, the entire kidney can become calcified, taking on the characteristics of bone because of deposition of excess calcium within the tissues. Not only is this condition painful because of the presence of kidney stones, in severe cases, it can also cause kidney failure.

High levels of calcium in the blood can be dangerous to a number of cells, including the lining of the stomach and the pancreas. The cells of both of these organs become inflamed and painful (ulcers and acute pancreatitis).

Mental fatigue, somnolence, apathy, anxiety, depression, and psychosis are possible. Changes in the mental status observed in the older adult can be misinterpreted as senile dementia.

Diagnosis of hyperparathyroidism is made when the serum calcium level is greater than 10.2 mg/dl on three successive measurements. Elevated PTH levels and low serum phosphate levels (less than 2.5 mg/dl) are also noted.

Prognosis

The prognosis of the patient with hyperparathyroidism depends primarily on the duration and severity of the disease. The cure rate for primary hyperparathyroidism after surgical removal of the glands is greater than 95%. Secondary hyperparathyroidism carries a poor prognosis because of the primary disease state of chronic renal failure.

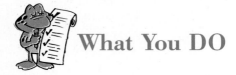 **What You DO**

Treatment

Surgical removal of the parathyroid glands is the only proven curative therapy for hyperparathyroidism. Antihypercalcemic drugs such as plicamycin (Mithracin) and gallium nitrate (Ganite) lower serum calcium levels within 48 hours, the use of which is limited to patients with hyperparathyroidism caused by parathyroid carcinoma. Biphosphonates such as etidronate (Didronel), pamidronate (Aredia), and calcitonin (Cibacalcin) inhibit osteoclastic bone resorption and helps normalize serum calcium levels. Estrogen or progestin therapy can reduce serum and urinary calcium levels in postmenopausal women and may retard demineralization of the skeleton. Oral phosphates can be used in patients with normal kidney function and low serum phosphate levels to inhibit the calcium-absorbing effects of vitamin D in the intestine. Glucocorticoids can be used to reduce hypercalcemia by decreasing the gastrointestinal absorption of calcium. Diuretics can be given to increase the urinary elimination of calcium. Administration of furosemide (Lasix) can be helpful in well-hydrated patients to promote sodium loss and decrease renal tubular reabsorption of calcium.

See Chapters 1A, 7B, 9B, 10B, and 12 in RWNSG: *Pharmacology*

Nursing Responsibilities

The treatment of hyperparathyroidism is directed at lowering severely elevated serum calcium levels, increasing calcium excretion, and increasing the bone resorption of calcium. Thus for the patient with hyperparathyroidism, the nurse should:

• Ensure that serum calcium levels are lowered by hydration (a minimum of 3000 ml per day) and that the calcium in the urine is eliminated with the administration of furosemide.

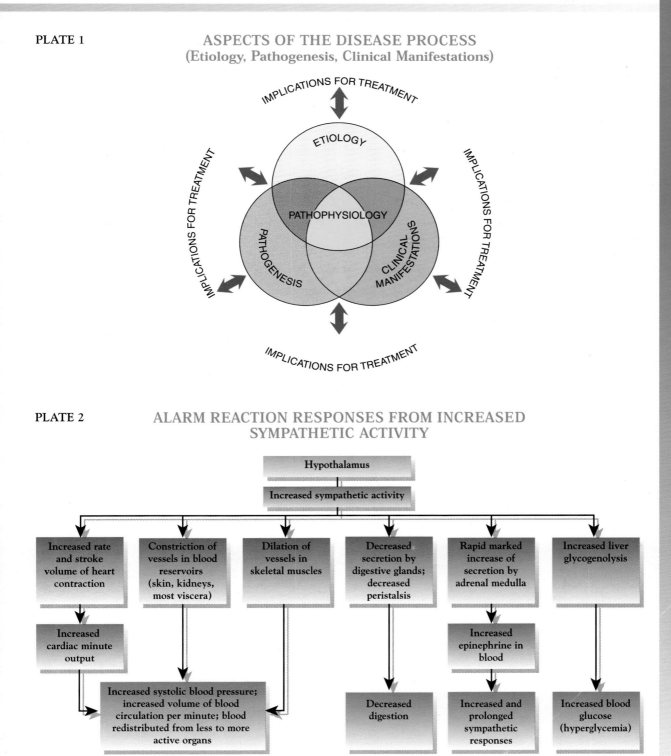

PLATE 1

ASPECTS OF THE DISEASE PROCESS
(Etiology, Pathogenesis, Clinical Manifestations)

IMPLICATIONS FOR TREATMENT

IMPLICATIONS FOR TREATMENT

IMPLICATIONS FOR TREATMENT

IMPLICATIONS FOR TREATMENT

ETIOLOGY

PATHOPHYSIOLOGY

PATHOGENESIS

CLINICAL MANIFESTATIONS

PLATE 2

ALARM REACTION RESPONSES FROM INCREASED SYMPATHETIC ACTIVITY

Hypothalamus

Increased sympathetic activity

Increased rate and stroke volume of heart contraction

Constriction of vessels in blood reservoirs (skin, kidneys, most viscera)

Dilation of vessels in skeletal muscles

Decreased secretion by digestive glands; decreased peristalsis

Rapid marked increase of secretion by adrenal medulla

Increased liver glycogenolysis

Increased cardiac minute output

Increased systolic blood pressure; increased volume of blood circulation per minute; blood redistributed from less to more active organs

Decreased digestion

Increased epinephrine in blood

Increased and prolonged sympathetic responses

Increased blood glucose (hyperglycemia)

PLATE 3

EFFECTS OF EXCESSIVE STRESS ON TARGET ORGANS AND ORGAN SYSTEMS

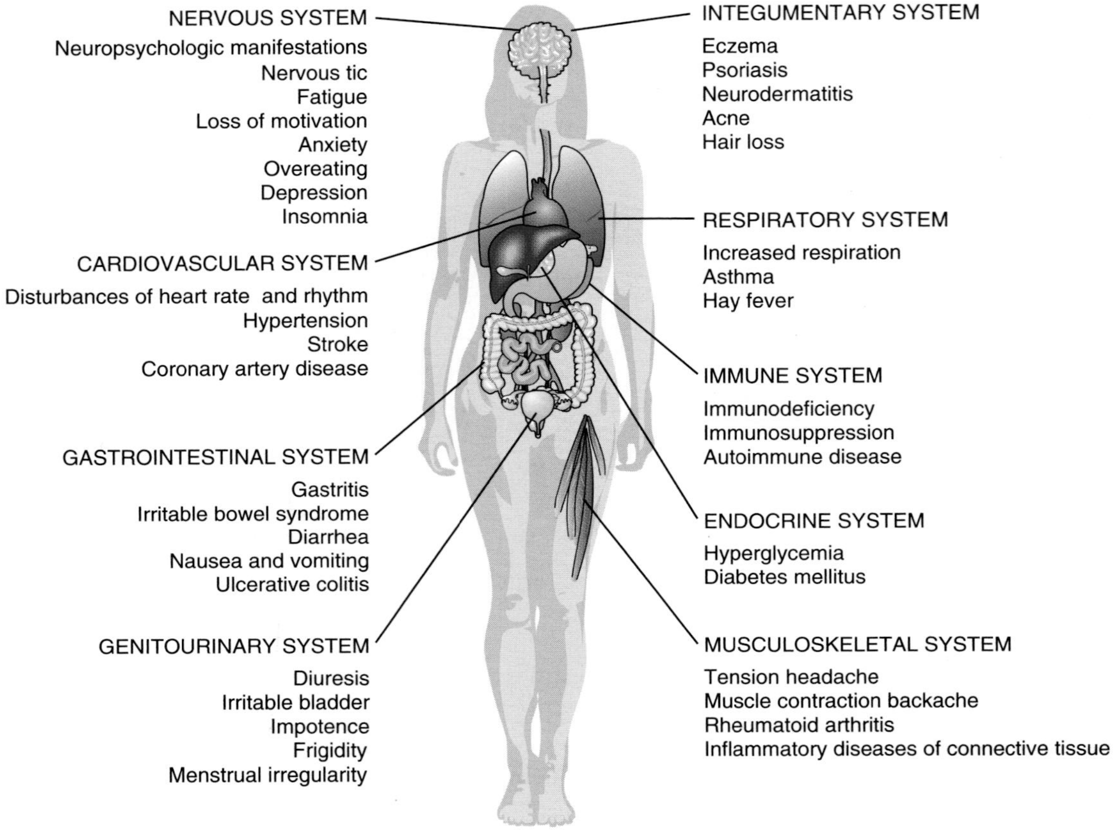

NERVOUS SYSTEM

Neuropsychologic manifestations
Nervous tic
Fatigue
Loss of motivation
Anxiety
Overeating
Depression
Insomnia

CARDIOVASCULAR SYSTEM

Disturbances of heart rate and rhythm
Hypertension
Stroke
Coronary artery disease

GASTROINTESTINAL SYSTEM

Gastritis
Irritable bowel syndrome
Diarrhea
Nausea and vomiting
Ulcerative colitis

GENITOURINARY SYSTEM

Diuresis
Irritable bladder
Impotence
Frigidity
Menstrual irregularity

INTEGUMENTARY SYSTEM

Eczema
Psoriasis
Neurodermatitis
Acne
Hair loss

RESPIRATORY SYSTEM

Increased respiration
Asthma
Hay fever

IMMUNE SYSTEM

Immunodeficiency
Immunosuppression
Autoimmune disease

ENDOCRINE SYSTEM

Hyperglycemia
Diabetes mellitus

MUSCULOSKELETAL SYSTEM

Tension headache
Muscle contraction backache
Rheumatoid arthritis
Inflammatory diseases of connective tissue

PLATE 4

THEORETICAL STEPS IN THE DEVELOPMENT OF CANCER

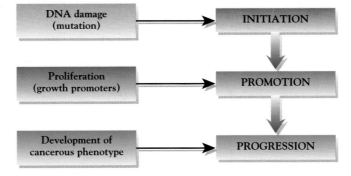

DNA damage (mutation) → INITIATION

Proliferation (growth promoters) → PROMOTION

Development of cancerous phenotype → PROGRESSION

PLATE 5   INTEGRATED FUNCTION OF IMMUNE COMPONENTS

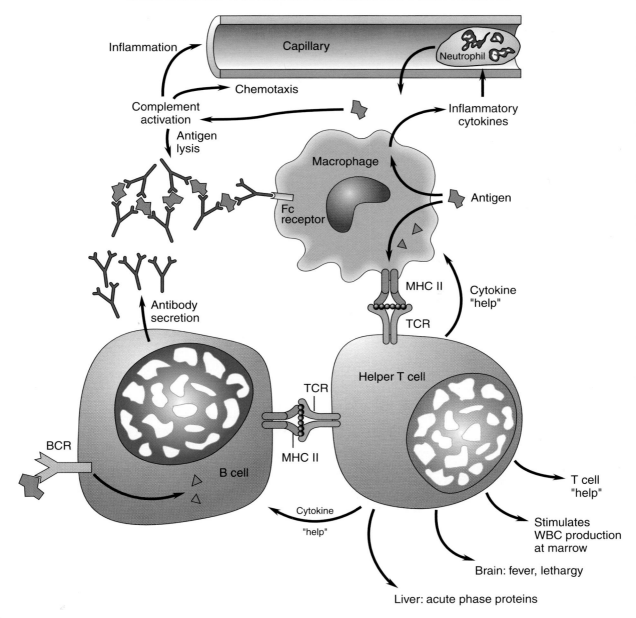

PLATE 6

RENIN-ANGIOTENSIN-ALDOSTERONE SYSTEM

PLATE 7

CONDUCTION SYSTEM OF THE HEART

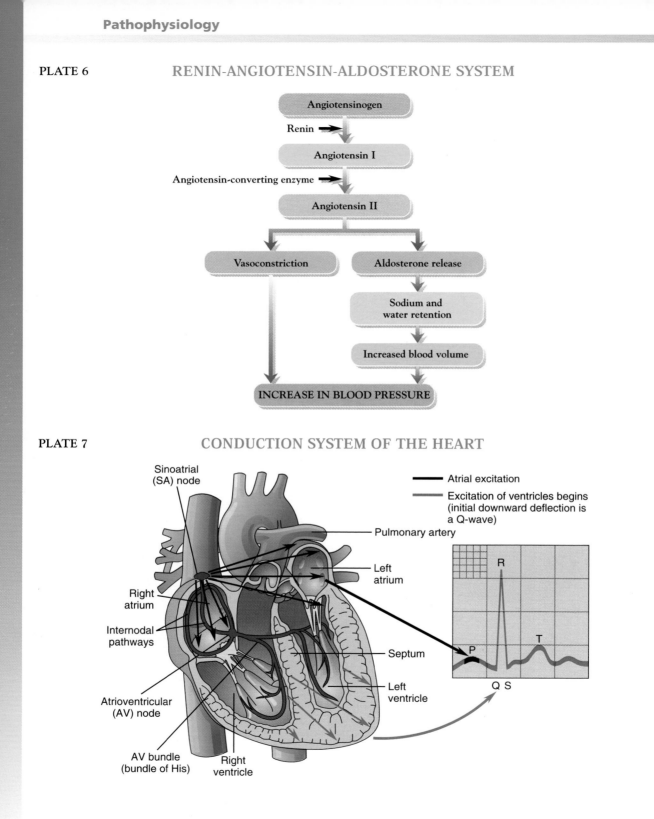

PLATE 8   SUMMARY OF EVENTS AFTER MYOCARDIAL INFARCTION

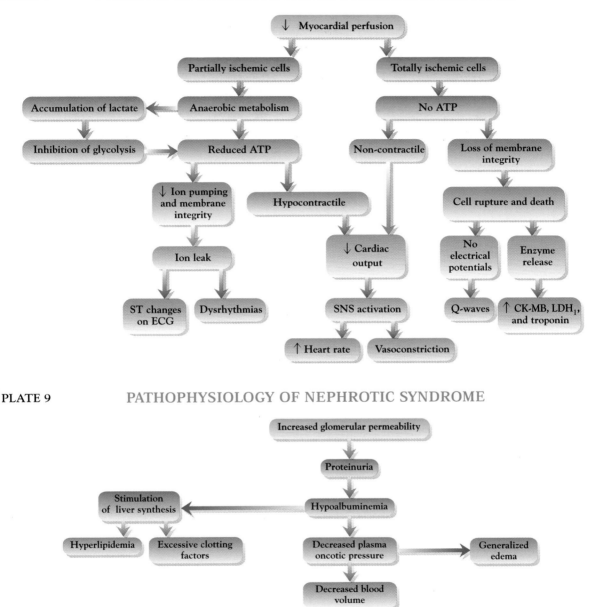

PLATE 9   PATHOPHYSIOLOGY OF NEPHROTIC SYNDROME

PLATE 10

PATHOGENESIS OF ACUTE PANCREATITIS

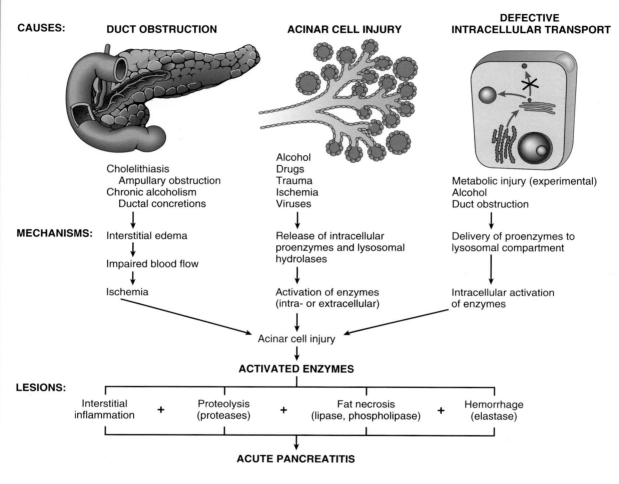

CAUSES:

DUCT OBSTRUCTION	ACINAR CELL INJURY	DEFECTIVE INTRACELLULAR TRANSPORT

Cholelithiasis
  Ampullary obstruction
Chronic alcoholism
  Ductal concretions
	Alcohol
	Drugs
	Trauma
	Ischemia
	Viruses
		Metabolic injury (experimental)
		Alcohol
		Duct obstruction

MECHANISMS:

Interstitial edema → Impaired blood flow → Ischemia

Release of intracellular proenzymes and lysosomal hydrolases → Activation of enzymes (intra- or extracellular)

Delivery of proenzymes to lysosomal compartment → Intracellular activation of enzymes

Acinar cell injury

ACTIVATED ENZYMES

LESIONS:

Interstitial inflammation + Proteolysis (proteases) + Fat necrosis (lipase, phospholipase) + Hemorrhage (elastase)

ACUTE PANCREATITIS

PLATE 11

NEGATIVE-FEEDBACK LOOP

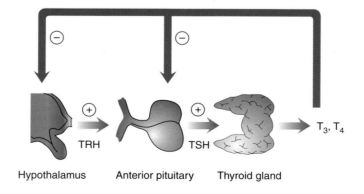

$\ominus$ $\ominus$

$\oplus$ TRH $\oplus$ TSH T_3, T_4

Hypothalamus   Anterior pituitary   Thyroid gland

PLATE 12
SYNDROME OF INAPPROPRIATE ANTIDIURETIC HORMONE (SIADH)

PLATE 13
CUSHING'S SYNDROME CLINICAL MANIFESTATIONS

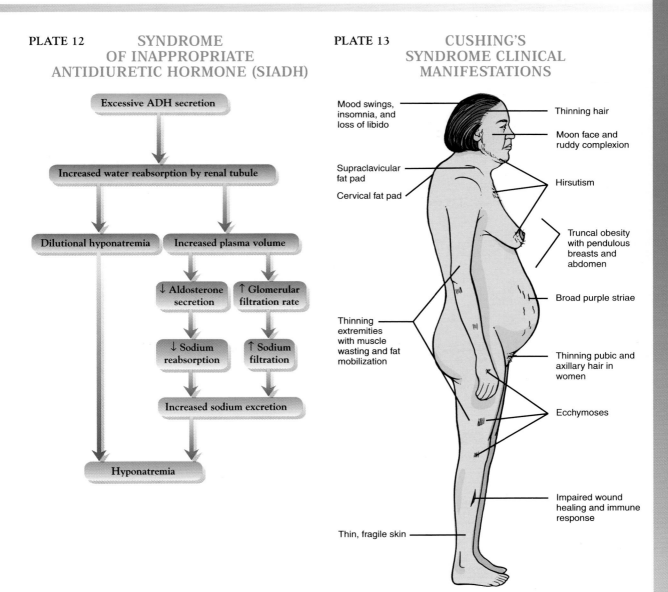

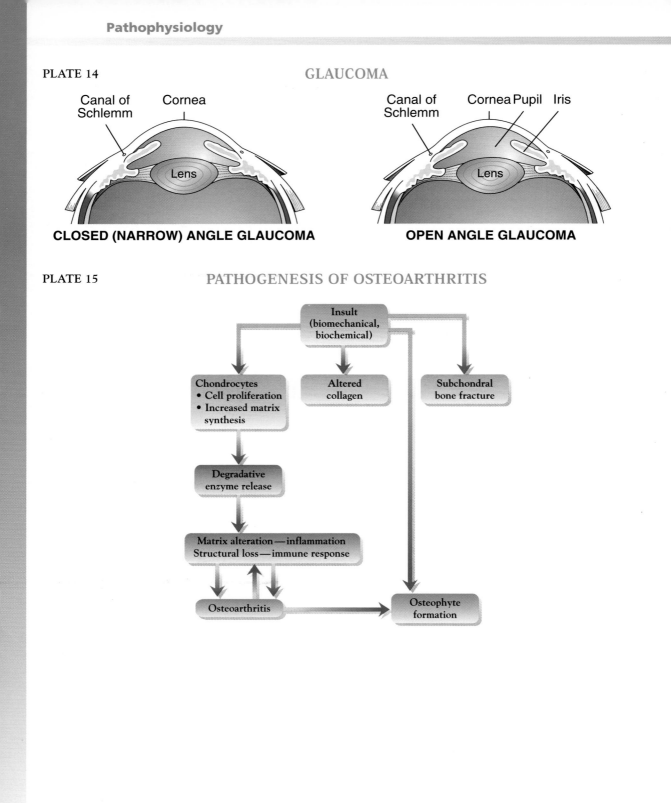

PLATE 14

GLAUCOMA

Canal of Schlemm — Cornea

Lens

CLOSED (NARROW) ANGLE GLAUCOMA

Canal of Schlemm — Cornea — Pupil — Iris

Lens

OPEN ANGLE GLAUCOMA

PLATE 15

PATHOGENESIS OF OSTEOARTHRITIS

Insult
(biomechanical,
biochemical)

Chondrocytes
• Cell proliferation
• Increased matrix synthesis

Altered collagen

Subchondral bone fracture

Degradative enzyme release

Matrix alteration — inflammation
Structural loss — immune response

Osteoarthritis

Osteophyte formation

- Administer antiresorption medications as prescribed and monitor for adverse effects.
- Teach the patient about the importance of adherence to medication therapy and the importance of periodic laboratory testing to be certain that the hyperparathyroid state does not redevelop.
- Instruct the patient about the importance of a diet low in calcium and vitamin D. Cranberry and prune juice make urine more acidic thus helping to prevent renal stones. Calcium is more soluble in acid urine.
- Instruct the patient to use stool softeners, drink adequate fluids, and eat fresh fruits to prevent constipation associated with hypercalcemia.
- Strain the urine for the patient who has developed kidney stones.
- Teach about and monitor the patient's environment for safety.
- Postoperatively monitor for signs and symptoms of transient tetany, laryngeal nerve damage, bleeding, and infection.
- Encourage ambulation as soon as possible after surgery because weight-bearing speeds the recalcification process.

SECTION C
ADRENAL DISORDERS

The adrenal gland is a small triangular endocrine gland located on the top of each kidney and is composed of two parts: the center of the gland (medulla) and the outer portion of the gland (cortex). The adrenal cortex secretes more than 30 different steroids. These steroids are divided into three major groups: the glucocorticoids, the mineralocorticoids, and the androgens. The glucocorticoids received their name because they raise blood glucose levels (gluco), are produced by the adrenal cortex (corti), and are made from cholesterol, which is a steroid (oid). The mineralocorticoids, as their name implies, involve the concentration of minerals (electrolytes) in the fluid between the cells. Androgens are any steroid hormones that promote male characteristics, such as beard growth and the deepening of the voice at puberty. Many androgens are converted to estrogens elsewhere in the body.

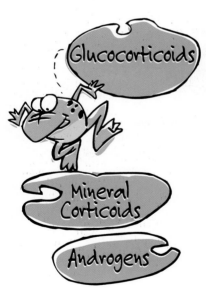

The primary glucocorticoid is cortisol (hydrocortisone), which is responsible for more than 95% percent of all glucocorticoid activity. The most important job of cortisol is to help the body respond to stress. Additionally, cortisol helps maintain blood pressure and cardiovascular function, helps slow the immune system's inflammatory response, helps to balance the effects of insulin in breaking down sugar for energy, and regulates the metabolism of carbohydrates, proteins, and fats.

Disorders of the adrenal gland are organized into two groups: those affecting the medulla and those affecting the cortex. The disorders can be further divided into two other additional groups: those that are caused by too much activity (hyperfunction) and those that are caused by too little activity (hypofunction).

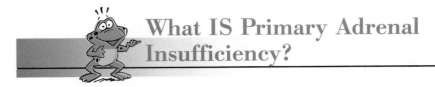

What IS Primary Adrenal Insufficiency?

Pathogenesis

Primary adrenal insufficiency is a chronic autoimmune disorder (Addison's disease) that can occur as either a primary or a secondary deficit in the production of glucocorticoids and mineralocorticoids. Primary adrenal insufficiency is a result of an autoimmune inflammation of the adrenal gland as a consequence of tuberculosis, fungal infections, or nonsecreting tumors of the adrenal cortex. Basically, some factor causes the adrenal glands to produce insufficient cortisol, and, occasionally, the hormone aldosterone. Infiltration of the adrenal cortex by a type of white blood cell (lymphocyte) is the characteristic feature. Gradual, continued destruction of the adrenal gland leads to inadequate amounts of mineralocorticoids, as well as glucocorticoids and androgens. The autoimmune process accounts for 75% of primary adrenal insufficiency.

A lack of ACTH from the anterior pituitary gland causes secondary adrenal insufficiency. Hypofunction of the pituitary gland, surgical removal, and certain tumors of the gland eventually result in a decrease or total absence of ACTH, the hormone that triggers the release of other hormones from the adrenal cortex.

At-Risk Populations

This potentially life-threatening autoimmune disorder affects persons of all ages and occurs equally in both genders and all races. Individuals who are at risk for primary adrenal insufficiency include those with a history of other endocrine disorders. Persons taking glucocorticoids for more than 3 weeks who suddenly stop therapy and those taking glucocorticoids more frequently than once every other day are at risk. Surgical removal of the adrenal glands also increases the risk. Tuberculosis is the cause in approximately 20% of the cases. Other causes include metastatic carcinomas of the lung, breast, or gastrointestinal tract.

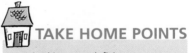

TAKE HOME POINTS

Acquired immunodeficiency syndrome (AIDS) is becoming a more common cause of adrenal insufficiency than are autoimmune processes and tuberculosis.

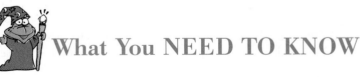

What You NEED TO KNOW

Clinical Manifestations

Symptoms are slow and progressive such that they are frequently unnoticed until a stressor appears, such as illness or accident. The development of signs and symptoms appears with the loss of over 90% of both adrenal cortices. A profound drop in blood sugar occurs (hypoglycemia), in addition to orthostatic hypotension, cardiac irregularities (arrhythmias), sodium loss with potassium retention, and, when acute, volume depletion. Mental confusion, mood swings, loss of consciousness, and shock, when the condition is acute, also occurs. Muscle pain and weakness, fatigue, and sudden penetrating pain in the back, abdomen, or legs are also present, when an acute deficiency exists. An unusual darkening (bronzing) of skin folds, pressure areas, the areolae, fingers and toes, and sun-exposed body parts also appears.

 Without treatment, acute adrenal insufficiency is fatal.

Prognosis

The patient with primary adrenal insufficiency can lead a fairly normal life with hormonal replacement therapy. Hormonal replacement therapy usually brings about a rapid recovery.

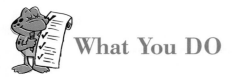 # What You DO

Treatment

The treatment of primary adrenal insufficiency focuses on replacing hormones, using exogenous glucocorticoids (dexamethasone) and mineralocorticoids. Intravenous feedings of glucose are used to prevent a severe drop in blood glucose levels when fasting is required for diagnostic studies or surgery.

See Chapter 7B in **RWNSG:** *Pharmacology*

The treatment goal for acute adrenal insufficiency is to prevent the morbidity and mortality associated with the crisis. After the cause of the crisis has been determined, the low blood pressure and electrolyte imbalance are quickly corrected. An isotonic intravenous solution will usually correct the volume depletion, salt depletion, and hypotension. Low blood sugar is corrected with glucose. The patient also receives oxygen, drugs to raise blood pressure (vasopressors) or volume expanders, and hydrocortisone.

Nursing Responsibilities

For the patient with adrenal insufficiency, the nurse should:
- Monitor vital signs, including orthostatic blood pressure readings and electrocardiogram tracings, when indicated.
- Provide for adequate rest periods.
- Monitor for signs and symptoms of hypoglycemia and infection.
- Obtain daily weights at same time, on same scale, and in same type of clothing; accurately record intake and output.
- Assess for manifestations of sodium and potassium imbalance; check bony prominences for pressure areas and the apical-radial pulse.
- Implement safety measures to prevent falls and injury.
- Administer hormonal replacement therapy as ordered.
- Provide age-appropriate and culturally appropriate patient and family teaching regarding disorder and stress reduction strategies.

Symptoms of acute adrenal insufficiency (Addisonian crisis) can occur when the patient has been under stress without appropriate hormonal replacement. Stressors include pregnancy, surgery, infection, dehydration, anorexia, fever, and emotional upheaval.

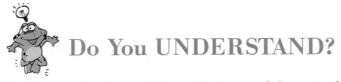

Do You UNDERSTAND?

Ms. McMahon has Addison's disease. She is worried about going home from the hospital because she is too tired to clean her house. Most of the time she is too tired to cook dinner.

DIRECTIONS: **Place a check next to the priority nursing intervention for Ms. McMahon.**

_____ 1. Encourage Ms. McMahon to consume a diet that is high in sodium, potassium, and fats.
_____ 2. Help her break her house cleaning and dinner preparation into small manageable tasks that can be separated by rest periods.
_____ 3. Teach stress-reduction strategies to Ms. McMahon.
_____ 4. Arrange for a housekeeper to help Ms. McMahon.

What IS Cushing's Syndrome?

Pathogenesis

National Institute of Diabetes and Diseases of the Kidney: Cushing's Disease
www.niddk.nih.gov/health/endo/pubs/cushings/cushings.htm

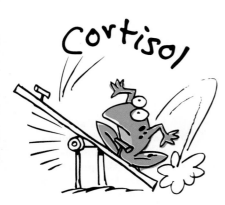

Cushing's syndrome is a group of symptoms resulting from prolonged exposure of the body's tissues to high levels of the glucocorticoid hormone cortisol for long periods (hypercortisolism). Approximately 85% of patients with Cushing's syndrome have a tumor of the pituitary gland that causes excessive secretion of ACTH. Many people experience iatrogenic Cushing's because they take high-dose, long-term glucocorticoid hormones, such as prednisone for asthma, rheumatoid arthritis, lupus, or other inflammatory diseases.

The signs and symptoms of Cushing's syndrome are the result of the action of cortisol. Normally, the production of cortisol follows a precise chain of events. First, the hypothalamus sends corticotropin-releasing hormone (CRH) to the pituitary gland. CRH causes the pituitary gland to secrete ACTH, a hormone that stimulates the adrenal glands. When the adrenal glands receive the ACTH, they respond by releasing cortisol into the bloodstream.

When the amount of cortisol in the blood is adequate, less CRH and ACTH are released. This mechanism ensures that the amount of cortisol released is precisely balanced to meet the body's daily needs. However, when "something goes wrong" with the adrenal glands or their regulating switches in the pituitary gland or the hypothalamus, cortisol production can go awry.

At-Risk Populations

Cushing's syndrome affects mostly adults ages 20 to 50 years. Patients at risk for Cushing's syndrome include those with a history of a cortisol-secreting adrenal tumor, adrenal hyperplasia, or those who are receiving glucocorticoid drugs (steroids).

Answer: 2.

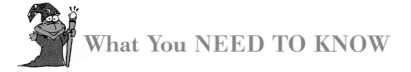

What You NEED TO KNOW

Clinical Manifestations

The signs and symptoms of Cushing's syndrome vary but most people have hypertension, arrhythmias, low serum potassium levels, sodium and fluid retention, and elevated blood glucose levels (hyperglycemia). The upper body becomes obese with a rounded face and increased fat around the neck. The arms and legs are thin because of loss of muscle mass. Generalized weakness and osteoporosis are present. Men become impotent with decreased fertility and loss of sex drive. Women develop excessive hair growth on the face, neck, chests, abdomen, and thighs. Menstrual periods can become irregular or stop. The skin is thin with bruising from even minor injuries. Purplish-pink stretch marks (atropic striae) appear on the abdomen, thighs, buttocks, arms, and breasts.

Prognosis

Cushing's syndrome causes many other serious health problems. Without treatment, approximately 50% of patients who have Cushing's die within 5 years of the onset of the disease. The major causes of death include overwhelming infection, suicide, complications from generalized hardening of the arteries (arteriosclerosis), and hypertension.

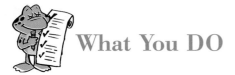

What You DO

Treatment

Treatment of Cushing's syndrome is complex and depends on the specific reason for cortisol excess. Therefore differentiation among pituitary, adrenal, and ectopic causes of the excess cortisol secretion is essential for effective treatment. Generally, treatment includes removal of the adrenal gland or the causative tumor, radiation therapy, and antineoplastic therapy.

Cortisol-inhibiting drugs such as aminoglutethimide (Cytadren) and mitotane (Lysodren) inhibit glucocorticoid synthesis without destroying the adrenal cortex. ACTH-reducing drugs such as somatostatin may be used when the cause of the disorder is a pituitary tumor. When the cause of excess cortisol is long-term use of glucocorticoid hormones to treat another disorder, the dosage is reduced to the lowest dose that controls that disorder. After control is established, the daily dose of glucocorticoid may be doubled and given on alternate days to reduce the side effects.

See Chapter 7B in RWNSG: *Pharmacology*

Nursing Responsibilities

For the patient with Cushing's syndrome, the nurse should:

- Support patient and family during diagnostic phase of the disease.
- Take measures to prevent injury and infection.
- Keep the bed in lowest position and raising the side rails for protection.
- Assist the patient to ambulate to reduce risk of falls.
- Promote periods of mental and physical rest.
- Provide good skin care to reduce the likelihood of skin breakdown.
- Assess the patient closely for manifestations of severe hypertension (e.g., elevated blood pressure, headache, failing vision, irritability, dyspnea).
- Obtain daily weights at same time, on same scale, and in same type of clothing and monitoring vital signs at frequent intervals.
- Obtain daily blood sugar readings via fingerstick to monitor for hyperglycemia.
- Assist in the collection of 24-hour urine specimen for free cortisol.
- Encourage a diet low in calories, carbohydrates, and sodium but with ample protein and potassium.
- Help the patient and family acquire effecting coping mechanisms.
- Anticipate mood swings and provide reassurance that physical appearance and moods will most likely return to normal after the disorder is treated.
- Administer medications as prescribed and monitor for adverse effects.
- Provide age-appropriate and culturally appropriate patient and family teaching regarding the disorder.

For patients who have had their adrenal glands removed (**adrenalectomy**), **teach that lifelong glucocorticoid replacement is essential to life.**

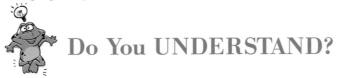

Do You UNDERSTAND?

Mr. Rodriquez is a 26-year-old elementary school teacher who is seeking the advice of his health care provider because of changes in his appearance over the last year. Mr. Rodriquez comes to the office today complaining of weight gain, particularly through his mid-section, easy bruising, and edema of his feet, lower legs, and hands; he has been having increasing problems sleeping (insomnia). Blood pressure is 150/110; he has 2+ edema of lower extremities, striae on the abdomen, birdlike extremities with thin, friable skin, and severe acne on the face and neck.

DIRECTIONS: **Place a check next to four of the seven treatments listed below that are most appropriate for Mr. Rodriquez.**

_____ 1. Use of cortisol-inhibiting drugs
_____ 2. Removal of the causative tumor
_____ 3. Radiation therapy
_____ 4. Intravenous fluids low in sodium and potassium and high in glucose
_____ 5. Antineoplastic therapy
_____ 6. Brushing teeth twice daily
_____ 7. Driving only during daylight hours

Answers: 1, 2, 3, and 6.

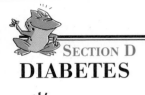

SECTION D
DIABETES

What IS Type 1 Diabetes Mellitus?

Pathogenesis

Type 1 diabetes mellitus is a disorder resulting from absolute insulin deficiency and is characterized by chronic hyperglycemia and the presence of disturbances in the metabolism of carbohydrates, fats, and proteins. In the past, type 1 diabetes was known by several names, such as insulin-dependent diabetes mellitus (IDDM), juvenile-onset diabetes, brittle diabetes, or ketosis-prone diabetes.

Type 1 diabetes results from the destruction of the pancreatic beta cells of the islet of Langerhans. The damage results from a cell-mediated autoimmune mechanism, genetic susceptibility, or environmental factors. Environmental factors include viruses or exposure to a toxic agent.

In 85% to 90% of cases, autoantibodies to the islet cells are present, which damage the pancreas. The autoantibodies can be present for years before insulin secretion is affected and symptoms appear.

Viruses such as those that cause mumps, Coxsackie, and cytomegaloviruses are associated with the development of type 1 diabetes. Drugs and chemicals such as alloxan, streptozocin, pentamidine, and Vacor (a rat poison) are environmental influences.

The lack of insulin production affects the metabolism of carbohydrates, fats, and proteins. Without insulin, glucose cannot enter adipose and muscle tissues, leading to elevated blood glucose levels (hyperglycemia). High blood glucose levels cause osmotic fluid loss from the cells, resulting in intracellular dehydration. The dehydration stimulates the hypothalamus and subsequent thirst (polydipsia). When the amount of glucose filtered by the glomeruli and reabsorbed by the renal tubules is exceeded, glucose spills into the urine (glycosuria) resulting in large amounts of osmotic fluid loss. In the absence of insulin, glucose cannot be transported into cells; thus the cells are depleted of carbohydrates, fats, and protein stores, resulting in cellular starvation and an increase in hunger (polyphagia). As fats and proteins are used for energy, body tissue is lost. Osmotic diuresis (polyuria) causes fluid to be lost, resulting in weight loss. Fatigue is a result of the metabolic changes.

Hyperglycemia, along with the presence of the autoantibodies, indicates that the islet cells of the pancreas have been damaged to the extent that the secretion of insulin by these cells is severely inadequate or nonexistent. The destruction of 80% to 90% of the beta cells occurs before hyperglycemia is observed. Beta cell destruction causes an imbalance of the hormones produced by the islets of Langerhans. When beta cells cannot produce insulin and blood glucose levels are

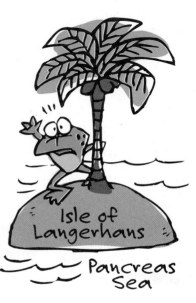

Isle of Langerhans

Pancreas Sea

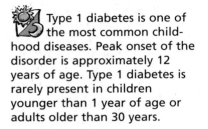

Type I diabetes is more prevalent in Caucasians than it is in other ethnic groups.

Type 1 diabetes is one of the most common childhood diseases. Peak onset of the disorder is approximately 12 years of age. Type 1 diabetes is rarely present in children younger than 1 year of age or adults older than 30 years.

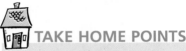

TAKE HOME POINTS

Kussmaul respirations and "fruity" (acetone odor) breath are the first presenting symptoms of ketoacidosis.

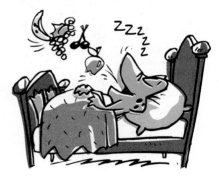

elevated, the alpha cells overproduce glucagon. Because no insulin is present to oppose the production of glucose, the overproduction of glucagon stimulates the new production of glucose from glycogen (glycogenolysis) and the production of glucose from amino acids and glycerol in the liver (gluconeogenesis).

At-Risk Populations

From 5% to 10% of all cases of diabetes are type 1. Genetic predisposition increases the risk of developing type 1 diabetes. Approximately 10% of diagnosed individuals have a parent or sibling with type 1 diabetes. Type 1 diabetes occurs in 40% of individuals who had congenital rubella.

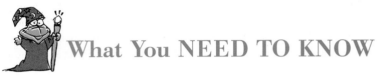

What You NEED TO KNOW

Clinical Manifestations

Classic symptoms of diabetes mellitus are polydipsia, polyphagia, and polyuria. Other clinical manifestations are fluctuations in blood glucose levels, weight loss, and fatigue. Individuals with type 1 diabetes are also prone to ketoacidosis.

The increased metabolism of fat and protein results in the increase of circulating ketones. Excess ketones decrease blood pH, causing a decrease in the bicarbonate concentration, which results in metabolic ketoacidosis. To compensate for metabolic acidosis, the lungs blow off acetone through Kussmaul respirations, giving the breath a sweet, "fruity" odor. Hypokalemia occurs in response to the metabolic acidosis. Hypovolemia can result in decreased, normal, or elevated sodium, magnesium, and phosphorus levels, depending on the extent of fluid loss. The hematocrit, hemoglobin, white blood count, serum creatinine, blood urea nitrogen (BUN), and serum osmolality are increased during ketoacidosis because of hypovolemia.

Prognosis

Acute or chronic complications of diabetes result in morbidity and mortality. Over 15% of patients with type 1 diabetes die by the age of 40. Most complications are the result of chronic hyperglycemia and metabolic alterations. Microvascular, macrovascular, and neuropathic insults are responsible for many of the serious complications. Periodontal disease occurs in 30% of persons with diabetes who are 19 years or older. Diabetes is the leading cause of new blindness in patients between the ages of 20 and 74 and is also the leading cause of end-stage renal failure.

The leading cause of diabetic-related deaths is heart disease.

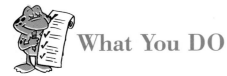

What You DO

Treatment

The treatment goal is to maintain near normal blood glucose levels (euglycemic), avoid hypoglycemia (blood glucose of 45 to 60 mg/dl) or hyperglycemia (fasting blood glucose over 126 mg/dl), and to avoid complications. The treatment plan is individualized and specific, considering the patient's lifestyle, age, and activity level. Treatment includes strict dietary adherence, planned exercise, and daily self–blood-glucose monitoring (SBGM).

Periodic measurement of glycosylated hemoglobin (Hgb A1c) should be monitored to evaluate the effectiveness of the treatment plan and, if any adjustments are required, to maintain normal blood glucose levels.

Nursing Responsibilities

For the patient with type 1 diabetes, the nursing responsibilities are primarily supportive. The nurse should:

- Provide information to the newly diagnosed patient and family about the disorder and prevention, as well as the ways to reduce the risk of complications.
- Stress the importance of adherence to the treatment plan, including the technique for insulin administration, SBGM, dietary and exercise regimes, proper foot care, and ways to recognize signs and symptoms of hypoglycemia and hyperglycemia.
- Provide instruction of the management of diabetes during illness and any needed adjustments to dosage or diet.
- Assess the patient's psychosocial resources and provide information on support groups and community resources that are available for patients with diabetes, such as the American Diabetes Association.
- Instruct the patient to wear Medic-Alert identification.
- Encourage the patient to have annual eye and foot examinations during each visit.
- Periodically assess Hgb A1c levels to evaluate the effectiveness of the treatment plan and encourage patients to see their health care provider every 3 months.

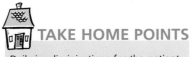

See Chapter 7C in RWNSG:
Pharmacology

National Diabetes Data Group of the National Institute of Diabetes and Digestive and Kidney Diseases: Diabetes in America
http//www.niddk.nih.gov/health/diabetes/diabetes.htm#stats.

Do You UNDERSTAND?

DIRECTIONS: Fill in the blanks.

1. Type 1 diabetes results from an _____ insulin deficiency.
2. The peak onset of type 1 diabetes is approximately _____ years of age.
3. A metabolic complication of hyperglycemia that those with type 1 diabetes are prone to is _____.

Answers: 1. absolute; 2. 12; 3. ketoacidosis.

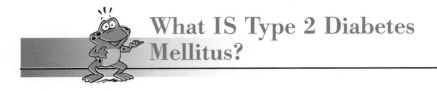

What IS Type 2 Diabetes Mellitus?

Pathogenesis

Type 2 diabetes is characterized by a relative insulin deficit, the development of insulin resistance in peripheral tissues and excessive glucose production by the liver. The result is similar to type 1 diabetes (hyperglycemia). In the past, type 2 diabetes was called other names, such as non–insulin-dependent diabetes mellitus (NIDDM), adult-onset diabetes, maturity-onset diabetes, or ketosis resistant diabetes. Because of its insidious nature, approximately 50% of all cases of type 2 diabetes have actually been diagnosed.

Type 2 diabetes most commonly results from obesity, increasing age, physical inactivity, and genetic predisposition.

Insulin resistance is associated with decreased number of insulin receptors, decreased action of glucose transporters, and increased production of glucagon. Obesity and inactivity increase insulin resistance. The insulin resistance is initially compensated for by increased insulin production. However, because the beta cells are unable to produce sufficient insulin, decreased numbers and abnormal function of beta cells result. The increased insulin resistance, decreased production of insulin, and increased production of glucagon result in hyperglycemia.

At-Risk Populations

Approximately 90% to 95% of all diagnosed cases of diabetes mellitus in the United States are type 2. Major risk factors include a family history of diabetes, age over 40, obesity, hypertension, and a history of gestational diabetes.

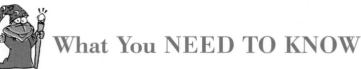

What You NEED TO KNOW

Clinical Manifestations

Type 2 diabetes is an insidious disease. Initially, the patient usually has no symptoms. The patient frequently reports nonspecific symptoms, such as itching (pruritus), recurrent infections, visual changes, fatigue, and burning or prickling sensation (paresthesias). From 60% to 80% of patients with type 2 diabetes are obese. The classic symptoms of polydipsia, polyuria, and polyphagia may be present, as well as fluctuations in blood glucose levels.

 An increased risk of developing diabetes exists after the age of 40.

The risk of developing type 2 diabetes is high in the older adult and non-Caucasian populations. Type 2 diabetes is more common in the African-American, Hispanic-American, and Native-American populations and is more prevalent in women than it is in men.

The life-threatening complication common in type 2 diabetes is hyperglycemic hyperosmolar nonketotic (HHNK) coma. HHNK is characterized by severe dehydration and hyperglycemia with little or no ketosis. The production of ketone bodies, which results from lipolysis, is suppressed by the presence of endogenous insulin, thus no ketosis is present, as it is in type 1 diabetes.

Prognosis

The mortality of patients with type 2 diabetes is twice that of persons without diabetes. Life expectancy is reduced by 5% to 10% among middle-age populations. Early detection and treatment reduces the microvascular, macrovascular, and neuropathic changes that are responsible for the retinopathy, renal, cardiovascular, and peripheral vascular complications of diabetes mellitus.

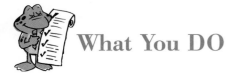

What You DO

Treatment

Similar to type 1 diabetes, the treatment goals for type 2 diabetes is to maintain euglycemia, correct related metabolic disorders, and avoid complications.

Drug therapy for type 2 diabetes includes the use of antidiabetic drugs such as sulfonylureas, biguanides, alpha glucosidase inhibitors, meglitinides, and thiazolidinediones. Treatment includes using a single antidiabetic agent (*monotherapy*), combination therapy using two drugs, or insulin therapy. Insulin therapy is used when oral agents fail to maintain a near normal blood glucose level.

Nursing Responsibilities

The nursing responsibilities for patients diagnosed with type 2 diabetes are similar to those for type 1, primarily, being supportive and educating the patient and family in medical and nutritional therapy, using oral antidiabetic agents or insulin when necessary, and preventing complications.

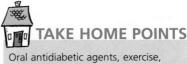

TAKE HOME POINTS

Oral antidiabetic agents, exercise, and diet therapy are basic treatments for type 2 diabetes.

See Chapter 7C in **RWNSG:** *Pharmacology*

Do You UNDERSTAND?

DIRECTIONS: Fill in the blanks.

1. Type 2 diabetes accounts for _____ to _____ of all diagnosed cases of diabetes in the United States.

2. The three basic pathologic changes causing type 2 diabetes are
   _____,
   _____, and
   _____.

3. Type 2 diabetes is most prevalent in the ethnic or cultural groups of
   _____,
   _____, and
   _____ populations.

Answer: 1. 90%, 95%; 2. insulin resistance, insulin production deficiency, excessive glucose production by the liver; 3. African American, Hispanic American, native American.

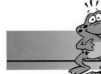

What IS Gestational Diabetes Mellitus?

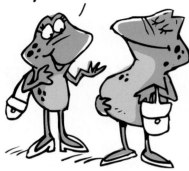

When are you due?

Pathogenesis

The onset or first recognition of gestational diabetes (GDM) occurs during pregnancy. The cause of GDM is similar to that of type 2 diabetes: tissue resistance and deficiency in insulin production.

During normal pregnancy, tissue resistance to insulin is present. Weight gain and the presence of placental hormones can cause this insulin resistance. Pregnant women require two to three times as much insulin than do women who are not pregnant. The deficiency in insulin production and increased tissue resistance causes glucose intolerance.

At-Risk Populations

Women at the highest risk for GDM are those who are obese, have a first-degree relative with diabetes, have a previous history of GDM, or have had infants whose birth weights exceeded 9 pounds.

GDM affects approximately 4% of all pregnancies.

What You NEED TO KNOW

TAKE HOME POINTS

During pregnancy, a deterioration of glucose tolerance is present, particularly during the third trimester during which insulin needs increase significantly.

Clinical Manifestations

The signs and symptoms of gestational diabetes are similar to those of type 2 diabetes. The classic symptoms of polydipsia, polyuria, and polyphagia may be present, as well as fluctuations in blood glucose levels and fatigue. Complications of GDM are infants of high birth weight (over 4000 grams) and neonatal hypoglycemia.

Prognosis

The woman should be reclassified approximately 6 weeks after delivery, according to the American Diabetes Association's diagnostic criteria, as having diabetes, impaired fasting glucose, impaired glucose tolerance, or normoglycemic. A woman with GDM has an increased risk of developing glucose intolerance or type 2 diabetes later in life. GDM will reoccur in future pregnancies in as many as 90% of women.

Women of Hispanic-American, Native American, Asian-American, African-American, and Pacific Islander ethnic or racial groups are at risk for the development of GDM.

Women who are over 40 years of age are also at risk for GDM.

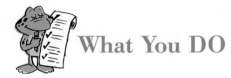

What You DO

Treatment

Similar to type 1 and type 2 diabetes, the goal is to maintain blood sugar levels in the normal range and to prevent hypoglycemia, hyperglycemia, and complications. Treatment of GDM includes blood glucose and urine ketone monitoring, exercise, and dietary counseling. The safe use of oral hypoglycemic agents has not been determined; therefore if hyperglycemia continues, insulin therapy should be used.

Nursing Responsibilities

The nursing responsibilities for patients diagnosed with GDM are similar to those for patients with type 1 diabetes, primarily, being supportive and educating the patient and family involving medical and diet therapy, in the use of insulin when necessary, and in the prevention of complications.

Women with high-risk characteristics should have their glucose tested initially and, when negative for GDM, they should be retested again at 24 to 28 weeks gestation. Women with an average risk should be glucose tested between 24 and 28 weeks gestation.

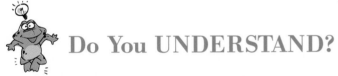

Do You UNDERSTAND?

DIRECTIONS: **Answer the following questions.**
1. How does GDM differ from type 1 diabetes?

2. Do all women who have GDM develop type 2 diabetes?

 When GDM is not treated during pregnancy, stillbirth of the infant and metabolic abnormalities can occur. An increased rate of cesarean delivery and chronic hypertension, as well as the development of diabetes later in life, are maternal complications related to GDM.

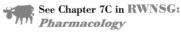 **See Chapter 7C in** RWNSG: *Pharmacology*

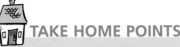 **TAKE HOME POINTS**

Recognition and treatment of GDM early in pregnancy can reduce complications in both the mother and infant.

A risk assessment for GDM should be completed at the first prenatal visit.

Answers: 1. Type 1 diabetes results from an absolute insulin deficiency, whereas GDM and type 2 diabetes both result from insulin resistance and a deficiency in insulin production; 2. No, but they are at a higher risk for type 2 diabetes than are women who have not had GDM.

8 Gastrointestinal System

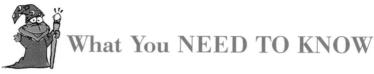

SECTION A
DISORDERS OF THE ESOPHAGUS

What IS Gastroesophageal Reflux Disorder?

Pathogenesis

Normally, contents of the stomach are prevented from entering the esophagus because of the structural location and pressures within the lower esophageal sphincter (LES). Gastroesophageal reflux disorder (GERD) is one in which the LES is relaxed or ineffective, permitting upward movement of gastric secretions from the stomach into the lower portion of the esophagus.

At-Risk Populations

Patients who are at risk for GERD include those who have hiatal hernias, delayed gastric emptying, and inappropriate relaxation of the LES. Additionally, people who smoke, consume alcohol, eat irritating foods, or take medications that irritate the gastrointestinal (GI) tract are at risk for developing GERD.

What You NEED TO KNOW

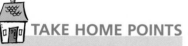

TAKE HOME POINTS

A strong relationship exists between GERD and asthma. Approximately 89% of asthmatics have GERD.

Clinical Manifestations

The pain of GERD is described as a burning sensation running up and down the esophagus. The pain is usually more severe when the patient is lying down. In some situations, the pain may radiate to the jaw, neck, or back. Common symptoms of GERD include a bitter or sour liquid entering the esophagus or mouth (eructation), a feeling of a lump in the throat, and difficulty swallowing (dysphagia). The pain of GERD may mimic that of a myocardial infarction (MI).

Prognosis

The prognosis of GERD depends on early identification and treatment. When the underlying cause is not treated, the patient continues to have symptoms. Fifty percent of patients have chronic symptoms but with no real progression of the illness. Patients with chronic GERD develop alterations of the distal esophageal mucosa, changing from the usual stratified squamous epithelium to a columnar epithelium (Barrett's esophagus). This mucosal change is associated with esophageal ulcers, strictures, hemorrhage, and increased risk of adenocarcinoma. Five percent of patients progress to these severe stages of GERD and may require surgery.

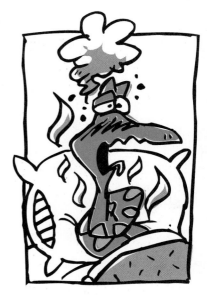

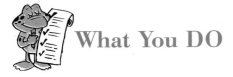

What You DO

Treatment

Treatment of the patient with GERD includes weight reduction and avoidance of foods and medications that increase acid secretion and decrease LES pressure. A high-protein, low-fat diet with small, frequent meals should be encouraged. Tobacco products should be avoided. The head of the patient's bed should be elevated on 4- to 6-inch blocks to facilitate gastric emptying. The patient should avoid eating for at least 2 to 3 hours before going to bed thus avoiding a full stomach at bedtime. Fluids should be taken between meals to decrease gastric distention. The patient should avoid lifting, straining, and bending. Tight-fitting clothing around the abdomen should also be avoided.

Medications frequently used in the treatment of GERD include antacids, as well as cytoprotective agents, histamine 2 antagonists, proton pump inhibitors, and medications that increase LES pressure. Surgical intervention using antireflux procedures is sometimes required. A Nissen fundoplication, Hill posterior gastropexy, and Belsey Mark IV repair may be used to relieve symptoms. These surgical procedures strengthen the LES thus preventing acid reflux. Either an open surgical approach or a laparoscopic approach may be used.

Nursing Responsibilities

For the patient with GERD, the nurse should:
- Provide patient and family teaching regarding nutrition and medication management while assessing the effects of medications administered.
- Maintain intravenous (IV) fluids when required.
- Promote comfort and managing the patient's pain (see Chapter 14).
- Maintain nasogastric tube patency and monitor the amount and color of drainage.
- Keep the head of patient's bed elevated.

🏠 **TAKE HOME POINTS**

Heartburn is the hallmark symptom of GERD. Try this pneumonic exercise to help you remember gastro-esophageal reflux disease:
- **G**astric secretions
- **E**ructation
- **R**elaxed LES
- **D**ysphagia

 See Chapter 8A in RWNSG: *Pharmacology*

🏠 **TAKE HOME POINTS**

The patient with symptoms of GERD but who has not been diagnosed with GERD is treated as though an MI has occurred until an accurate diagnosis is made. An electrocardiogram will rule out an MI.

- Monitor respiratory status and facilitate deep breathing and coughing while splinting the incision.
- Monitor the incision for drainage and redness and maintaining a closed-chest drainage system, when needed.
- Provide discharge instructions regarding diet, medications, and symptom management.

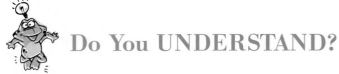

Do You UNDERSTAND?

DIRECTIONS: Complete the following crossword puzzle.

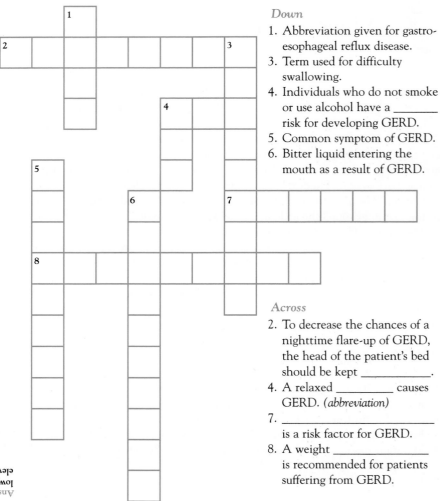

Down

1. Abbreviation given for gastro-esophageal reflux disease.
3. Term used for difficulty swallowing.
4. Individuals who do not smoke or use alcohol have a _____ risk for developing GERD.
5. Common symptom of GERD.
6. Bitter liquid entering the mouth as a result of GERD.

Across

2. To decrease the chances of a nighttime flare-up of GERD, the head of the patient's bed should be kept _____.
4. A relaxed _____ causes GERD. (*abbreviation*)
7. _____ is a risk factor for GERD.
8. A weight _____ is recommended for patients suffering from GERD.

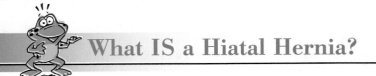

What IS a Hiatal Hernia?

Pathogenesis

A hiatal hernia is an extension of part of the stomach through the diaphragm into the thoracic cavity. The actual cause of a hiatal hernia is unknown. Muscle weakness of the esophageal junction with the stomach and increased intraabdominal pressure contribute to the development of hiatal hernias.

Two major types of hiatal hernias have been identified: sliding hernias and rolling hernias. A sliding hiatal hernia involves extension of the LES and the upper portion of the stomach through the diaphragm and is the most common type of hiatal hernia. In a rolling hernia, the LES stays below the level of the diaphragm, but the upper portion of the stomach protrudes through the diaphragm.

At-Risk Populations

Women are affected more frequently than are men. Any factor that increases intraabdominal pressure (e.g., pregnancy, obesity, ascites, straining at stool) increases the risk for hiatal hernia. Research studies have refuted a close association between hiatal hernia and GERD.

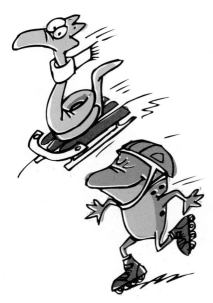

Advancing age is a risk factor for hiatal hernia. Of those over the age of 60, 60% may have hiatal hernias.

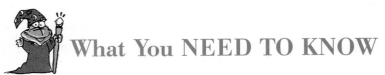

What You NEED TO KNOW

Clinical Manifestations

The signs and symptoms vary, depending on the type of hernia. With a sliding hiatal hernia, heartburn related to reflux is common. However, the patient with a rolling hernia frequently complains of a feeling of fullness and pain that is frequently compared with anginal pain. In both cases, symptoms are worse when the patient is in a reclining position.

Prognosis

The prognosis for a patient with a hiatal hernia depends on the severity of the problem. A herniated gastric pouch can cause difficulty swallowing and can be the site of gastritis and ulceration, the latter of which causes chronic blood loss.

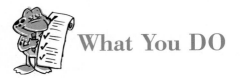

What You DO

Treatment

Treatment of the patient with a hiatal hernia is the same as that for the patient with GERD. Patients are advised to lose weight. Treatment includes small, frequent meals of high-protein, low-fat foods, although eating is avoided within 2 to 3 hours of bedtime. The head of the bed is elevated on 4- to 6-inch blocks to facilitate gastric emptying. Patients should avoid alcohol, tobacco, and constrictive clothing around the abdomen.

Medications frequently used in the treatment of hiatal hernias include the nonsystemic antacids, H2 antagonists, and proton pump inhibitors. The surgical management of hiatal hernia is similar to that of the patient with GERD.

See Chapter 8A in RWNSG:
Pharmacology

Nursing Responsibilities

For the patient with a hiatal hernia, the nurse should:
- Provide patient and family teaching regarding nutrition and medication management.
- Assess the effects of medications administered.
- Maintain IV fluids for the patient who has had surgery.
- Promote comfort and manage the patient's pain.
- Monitor nasogastric tube for patency, amount, and color of drainage.
- Keep the head of the bed elevated.
- Monitor respiratory status, encourage deep breathing and coughing (despite any postoperative discomfort), and splint the incision.
- Monitor the incision for drainage and redness.
- Maintain closed-chest drainage when a thoracic approach was used for the surgery.
- Discharge education regarding diet, medications, and symptom management.

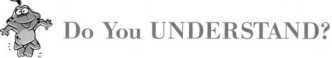

Do You UNDERSTAND?

DIRECTIONS: **Fill in the blanks.**

1. Muscle weakness and increased _____ pressure contributes to the formation of hiatal hernias.
2. In a hiatal hernia, part of the stomach extends through the diaphragm and into the _____ cavity.
3. The major symptom observed with a sliding hiatal hernia is _____.
4. One medication that is frequently used for treatment of hiatal hernias is _____.
5. The most common type of hiatal hernia is termed a _____ hernia.
6. _____, _____, and _____ can increase abdominal pressure and predispose the individual to the development of a hiatal hernia.
7. In a _____ hiatal hernia, the LES stays below the diaphragm, but the upper portion of the stomach protrudes through the diaphragm.

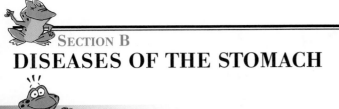

SECTION B
DISEASES OF THE STOMACH

What IS a Stress Ulcer?

Pathogenesis

Stress ulcers are gastric ulcerations that occur as a result of excessive stress. In burn patients, stress ulcerations are also known as Curling's ulcers. Curling's ulcers develop within 72 hours of the patient's injury. Stress ulcerations that occur in patients with severe head injuries are known as Cushing's ulcers.

Excessive physical or psychologic stress can lead to the development of stress ulcers. Severe injury or illness causes a decreased gastric blood flow (related to sympathetic nervous system stimulation) as the body shunts blood to vital organs. This activity produces ischemia of gastric tissues, which leads to a loss of the normal protective functions of the stomach lining. Multiple erosions of the gastric lining occur, which can lead to GI bleeding.

At-Risk Populations

Individuals who are at risk for stress ulcers include those with a major illness or severe injury, such as burns, shock, sepsis, head injuries, and spinal cord injury. Most people with burns over 35% or more of their body will develop stress ulcers. Other patients at risk include those receiving large doses of medications, particularly corticosteroids and NSAIDs.

See Chapters 7B and 11 in RWNSG: *Pharmacology*

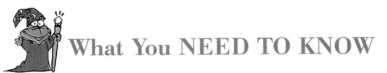

What You NEED TO KNOW

Clinical Manifestations

The clinical manifestations of a stress ulcer include painless upper GI tract bleeding until complications such as hemorrhage develop. Bleeding may present as blood in the stools (melena) or as bloody sputum (hematemesis).

Prognosis

Because a stress ulcer is a complication of a preexisting condition, the prognosis depends on the predisposing cause. Early recognition and treatment contribute to a positive outcome.

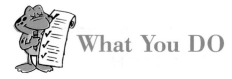

What You DO

Treatment

The treatment of the patient with a stress ulcer includes nasogastric intubation with suction when hemorrhage occurs. Endoscopic procedures may be needed to treat the bleeding. Medications used in the treatment of stress ulcers include histamine 2 antagonists, proton-pump inhibitors, mucosal protectants, and noncalcium-containing antacids. IV fluids may be started to maintain and improve fluid and electrolyte balance. For severe hemorrhage or perforation, surgical procedures may be required.

See Chapters 8A and 8B in RWNSG: *Pharmacology*

Nursing Responsibilities

For the patient with a stress ulcer, the nurse should:

- Identify patients who are at risk for the disorder while assessing for early signs and symptoms.
- Monitor stools for hidden or occult blood and vital signs for evidence of hemorrhage or shock.
- Palpate the abdomen. A boardlike or rigid finding may indicate perforation of the viscera.

Do You UNDERSTAND?

Juan, a 55-year-old trauma victim, has been hospitalized for 3 days. The health care provider has noticed symptoms of a developing stress ulcer.

DIRECTIONS: **Provide answers for the following questions.**

1. What is a stress ulcer?

2. What occurs physiologically in a trauma situation that causes a stress ulcer to develop?

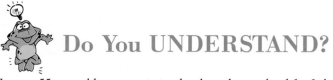

Answers: 1. A gastric ulcer that develops as a result of excessive physical or psychological stress; 2. A reduced blood flow to the GI tract is present as the body moves blood to more vital organs; this activity results in ischemia of gastric tissues, which, in turn, leads to a loss in the normal protective functions of the stomach lining, and ulcers form.

3. What factors might place John Smith at increased risk for developing a stress ulcer?

4. What symptoms might you assess if John develops a stress ulcer?

5. What measures might be taken to prevent the development of a stress ulcer?

What IS Peptic Ulcer Disease?

Pathogenesis

Peptic ulcer disease (PUD) is a chronic inflammation from altered gastric secretions that produces erosions in the lining of the esophagus, stomach, or duodenum. Several factors are involved in the development of PUD. Chronic inflammation, altered acid and pepsinogen secretion, damage to the protective mucosal barrier by irritating substances, and infection from *Helicobacter pylori* (*H. pylori*) bacteria have all been implicated.

An *H. pylori* infection is the most significant factor in the development of PUD and is associated with more than 90% of all duodenal peptic ulcers and 70% of all gastric ulcers. This organism releases mucolytic enzymes and toxins that breakdown the mucosal lining, which produces cellular injury and inflammation. This process alters gastric secretions and sustains inflammation, resulting in ulcerative lesions. In addition to *H. pylori*, two different mechanisms for the disease have been proposed as contributing to the development of ulcerations.

The tight, nonpermeable junctions between epithelial cells and the slightly alkaline layer of mucus that coats the surface of the gastric epithelium normally prevent the flow of hydrochloric acid from the lumen of the stomach. When gastric ulcers form, numerous injurious substances (e.g., aspirin, NSAIDs, glucocorticoids, caffeine, alcohol, phenylbutazone, adrenocorticotropin hormone) interrupt this diffusion barrier. These substances stimulate acid production and cause local mucosal damage or suppress mucus secretion. The epithelial cell membranes degenerate with massive backward diffusion of acid into the gastric epithelial wall.

Answers: 3. The patient was in a traumatic accident that placed significant physical and psychological stress on his body; 4. Most stress ulcers are painless until GI bleeding occurs; hematemesis or melena can occur; 5. Prophylactic administration of histamine 2 antagonists, proton-pump inhibitors, mucosal protectants, and noncalcium-containing antacids.

The pathogenesis of duodenal ulcer formation appears to be different. Vagus nerve activity is increased in patients with duodenal ulcers, particularly at night or when the patient is fasting. The vagus nerve stimulates the antrum cells in the pylorus to release gastrin. The gastrin travels through the circulation to act on the gastric parietal cells. The parietal cells stimulate the release of hydrochloric acid.

At-Risk Populations

Individuals with *H. pylori* infection are at high risk for developing PUD. Other individuals who are at risk include those who abuse alcohol, smoke, use NSAID medications on a chronic basis, and those who have type O blood. The incidence of PUD is increased in individuals with Crohn's disease, Zollinger-Ellison syndrome, and hepatic or biliary disease.

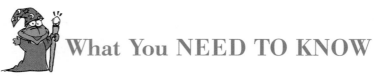

What You NEED TO KNOW

Clinical Manifestations

The signs and symptoms of PUD include pain localized to the epigastric region. Gastric ulcer pain occurs in the upper epigastrium and is localized to the left of midline. The pain of gastric ulcers is variable and frequently described as aching, gnawing, burning, and cramplike, occurring from 1 to 3 hours after eating. The condition is made worse with eating but relieved with vomiting. Antacids fail to relieve the pain. Patients with duodenal ulcers have pain on an empty stomach and at night. Ingesting food or antacids frequently relieves the discomfort.

Patients with ulcers bleed when the ulcer erodes through a blood vessel. Massive bleeding can develop or the bleeding can be occult from slow oozing. Approximately 25% of patients with gastric ulcers experience bleeding. Steady pain near the midline of the back can indicate perforation of the ulcer. The patient may also complain of nausea, eructation, constipation, or diarrhea, and may show evidence of blood in the stools.

Prognosis

The pain of both gastric and duodenal ulcers tends to recur daily for a time, and then it and all signs and symptoms disappear for months or years, to be followed eventually by another episode of pain. Reoccurrence of the disease is likely if risk factors are not reduced.

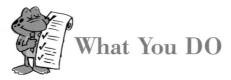

What You DO

Treatment

The treatment of PUD includes H2 antagonists, proton pump inhibitors, mucosal protectants, and stress modification strategies. Additionally, antibiotics (e.g.,

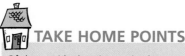

Gastric ulcerations are likely to occur during the fifth and sixth decades of life. Duodenal ulcerations commonly occur during the fourth and fifth decades in men. In women, the occurrence is approximately 10 years later in life. Men are more likely to develop both gastric and duodenal ulcers than are women.

TAKE HOME POINTS

Of those with chronic gastric ulcer disease, 10% are at risk for gastric malignancy. Early treatment and preventive health measures are vital to prevent future disease.

clarithromycin, tetracycline, metronidazole, amoxicillin) in combination with the medications mentioned now play a crucial role in the treatment and prevention of further disease.

Surgical intervention may be required in some cases. The surgical interventions include a vagotomy, pyloroplasty, antrectomy, subtotal gastrectomy, and total gastrectomy. A vagotomy is the partial or complete severance of the vagal nerve to reduce the acid-secreting stimulus to gastric cells. A pyloroplasty is a widening of the exit of the stomach to prevent stasis of stomach contents. This procedure is usually performed in connection with a vagotomy. An antrectomy is the removal of the antrum of the stomach. This portion of the stomach contains the cells that secrete gastrin. A subtotal gastrectomy (i.e., partial removal of the stomach) may be performed using a Billroth I or a Billroth II technique. A Billroth I procedure removes the distal portion of the stomach, including the antrum with anastomosis to the duodenum. The Billroth II procedure removes the distal portion of the stomach, including the antrum and the duodenum with anastomosis to the jejunum. Removal of the stomach with anastomosis of the esophagus to the jejunum is known as a total gastrectomy and is a typical surgery for gastric cancer.

See Chapters 1A, 8A, and 8B in RWNSG: *Pharmacology*

Nursing Responsibilities

For the patient with PUD, the nurse should:

- Provide health teaching for patient and family regarding the disease, treatment regimen, and importance of proper completion of antibiotic regimen to help ensure eradication of the bacterium.
- Promote comfort, adequate hydration, and nutrition.
- Monitor drug therapy for effectiveness and adverse effects.
- Monitor for signs and symptoms of complications, such as perforation (assess abdomen for pain, tenderness, and rigidity and monitor vital signs), hemorrhage (assess vital signs, symptoms of shock, emesis of coffee-ground material), upper GI bleeding or for blood in the stool, and obstruction (monitor for nocturnal pain, assess type and amount of emesis).
- Assess for postoperative complications, such as the following:
  1. *Dumping syndrome*. Occurs after a gastrectomy when food rapidly enters the jejunum. Symptoms include distention, feelings of fullness, cramping, nausea, and rumbling and gurgling in the bowel (borborygmi). To slow gastric emptying, the nurse should advise an increased fat and protein diet with avoidance of sugars. Patients should drink liquids between meals and rest after meals.
  2. *Anemia*. Loss of absorbing surface in the intestine predisposes the patient to anemia. Assess lab data for signs of anemia. Administer vitamin B12 and iron as appropriate.
- Promote postoperative wound healing.

See Chapter 12 in RWNSG: *Pharmacology*

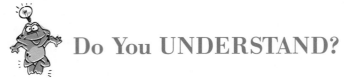

Do You UNDERSTAND?

DIRECTIONS: **Provide answers for the following questions.**

1. What are three factors that predispose an individual to the development of gastric ulcers?

2. What factor has been identified as the most significant in the development of gastric ulcers?

3. What clinical manifestations are observed in the patient with a gastric ulcer?

4. What is the difference between the Billroth I and Billroth II surgical procedures for treatment of gastric ulcer disease?

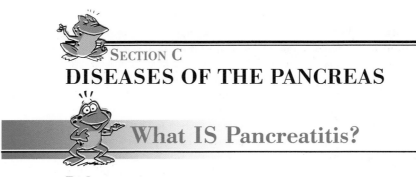

Section C

DISEASES OF THE PANCREAS

What IS Pancreatitis?

Pathogenesis

Pancreatitis is an inflammation of the pancreas that results in a release of pancreatic enzymes. This process can lead to autodigestion of the pancreas by its own enzymes. Pancreatitis can be acute or chronic. Although the process is unclear, the causative factors activate enzymes in the pancreas rather than in the intestine, leading to autodigestion of the pancreas and surrounding tissues. The enzyme activity can be triggered by reflux of bile from the duodenum into the pancreatic duct or by pancreatic duct obstruction. After pancreatic inflammation begins, a vicious cycle continues the process of further tissue damage and enzyme activation. As the process continues, destruction of the pancreas itself occurs. Severity of the disease varies from edema and pain to hemorrhage and necrosis of the pancreas.

Answers: 1. chronic inflammation, altered acid and pepsinogen secretion, and damage to the protective mucosal barrier from irritating substances (e.g., alcohol, caffeine, smoking, medications); 2. Infection with H. pylori; 3. pain described as gnawing, aching, and burning is localized in the epigastric region left of midline; the symptoms can be made worse by eating; hematemesis, weight loss, and nausea; 4. Billroth I or removal of the distal portion of the stomach, including the antrum with anastomosis to the duodenum; Billroth II or removal of the distal portion of the stomach, including the antrum and the duodenum with anastomosis to the jejunum.

At-Risk Populations

Ninety percent of acute pancreatitis is related to excessive alcohol intake or biliary disease. Other known causes of pancreatitis are pancreatic trauma, infection, drug reactions, and gastrointestinal surgery. Additionally, patients who are obese, those who have had pancreatic trauma or surgery, or those who have any condition that blocks the pancreatic ducts have an increased risk of developing pancreatitis. Other individuals at risk for pancreatitis include those who have hyperlipidemia, hypercalcemia, or pancreatic ischemia. Pancreatic ischemia occurs during periods of hypotension, cardiopulmonary bypass, and vasculitis. Visceral atheroembolism also raises the risk of developing pancreatitis.

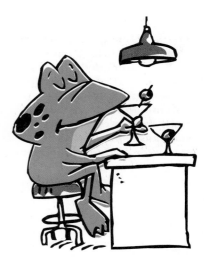

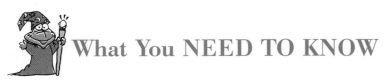

What You NEED TO KNOW

Clinical Manifestations

The primary symptom of pancreatitis is pain. The pain is sudden in onset, constant, and severe, located in the midepigastrium. The pain can also radiate to the back and is accompanied by nausea and vomiting, abdominal distension, and decreased bowel sounds. Jaundice may become apparent. When the pancreatitis is related to gallstones, the stools can be pale, bulky, and foul smelling (steatorrhea) as a consequence of decreased fat digestion. In patients with alcohol-related pancreatitis, the pain frequently begins 12 to 48 hours after an episode of drinking.

A low-grade fever, hypotension, tachycardia, and decreased breath sounds with increased crackles can also be present. The decreased breath sounds and crackles are related to irritation of the pleura from pancreatic enzyme action. Laboratory values are altered, with elevations in serum and urinary amylase, serum lipase, leukocytosis, hyperglycemia, hyperlipidemia, and hypocalcemia.

Other clinical manifestations include subcutaneous fat necrosis and alterations in consciousness, such as belligerence, confusion, psychosis, and coma. Transient hypoglycemia is evident in 50% of patients, most likely because of damage to the islets of Langerhans. Because all endocrine functions of the pancreas are disrupted, the patient can develop diabetes secondary to tissue damage.

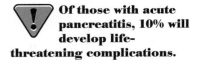

Middle-age men have the highest incidence of pancreatitis.

Of those with acute pancreatitis, 10% will develop life-threatening complications.

Prognosis

Acute pancreatitis usually resolves when the cause has been eliminated. Patients with severe pancreatitis can experience circulatory complications, such as hypotension, pallor, cool and clammy skin, hypovolemia, hypoperfusion, and obtundation. One third of the patients develop a left pleural effusion or an elevation of the left side of the diaphragm.

Premature return to oral intake has been associated with the development of pancreatic abscess and worsening inflammation. Morphine is contraindicated because it can cause spasm of the sphincter of Oddi, which can then cause ongoing pancreatic injury.

See Chapters 1A, 2A, 8A, and 8B in **RWNSG:** *Pharmacology*

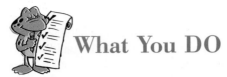 # What You DO

Treatment

The primary treatment goal for the patient with pancreatitis is to decrease pancreatic enzyme function thus resting the GI tract. Withholding food and fluids, inserting a nasogastric tube, and giving pain medication accomplish this goal. Oral intake is resumed after abdominal pain and tenderness have subsided.

IV fluids help maintain or improve fluid and electrolyte balance. IV lines can also be used to administer pain medications. Patients with moderate to severe pancreatitis will need total parenteral nutrition (TPN) and lipids to support nutritional status. Pancreatic enzymes, such as pancrelipase, are also used for patients who have pancreatitis or for those who have had pancreatic surgery. H2 receptor antagonists, anticholinergics, and antacids may be used. Antibiotics may be used prophylactically, particularly in patients with more severe pancreatitis.

Peritoneal dialysis may be required to rid the peritoneum of potentially toxic compounds that are commonly found in the exudate (e.g., histamine, vasoactive kinins, elastase, prostaglandins, phospholipase A, trypsin, chymotrypsin). These toxins can contribute to the hypotension, respiratory failure, hepatic failure, and altered vascular permeability that are present in pancreatitis. Peritoneal dialysis is usually reserved for patients who show a worsening state, despite other medical interventions.

In severe cases of pancreatitis, surgery may be necessary to drain the pancreatic duct and remove injured and necrotic tissue. A Roux–en–Y procedure connects (anastomoses) the pancreatic duct to the proximal jejunum. A subtotal pancreatectomy (removal of a portion of the pancreas) or a Whipple's procedure (removal of the distal third of the stomach, duodenum, common bile duct, gallbladder, and the head of the pancreas) may be required in advanced disease states.

Nursing Responsibilities

For the patient with pancreatitis, the nurse should:
- Maintain nasogastric (NG) tube patency and vital signs while monitoring for evidence of hemorrhage, shock, and infection.
- Administer IV fluids to prevent fluid and electrolyte imbalance, monitoring vital signs, weight, and lab values, such as glucose, calcium, chloride, sodium, and potassium.
- Administer pancreatic enzyme medications as ordered.
- Monitor respiratory status.

🍎 Provide health education regarding restriction of alcohol intake, dietary restrictions, preventive measures, and follow-up care.

P— Pain control with Demerol (morphine causes contraction of the sphincter of Oddi)

A—Antacids to neutralize acidity

N—NPO and use of NG to rest GI tract and decrease pancreatic activity

C—Calcium replacement, check for tetany with possible hypocalcemia

R—Rest and replacement fluids

E— Electrolyte replacement

A—Antibiotics for acute pancreatitis

S— Surgery, usually Roux-en-Y procedure

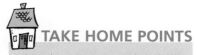

TAKE HOME POINTS

Advise the patient to avoid alcohol, reduce dietary intake of fats, and avoid ingestion of drugs known to cause pancreatitis.

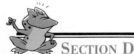

Do You UNDERSTAND?

DIRECTIONS: Fill in the blanks.

1. Inflammation of the pancreas results in the release of
_____ that lead to _____
of the pancreas itself.
2. _____ have the
highest incidence of pancreatitis.
3. The primary clinical manifestation of pancreatitis is _____.
4. When the pancreatitis is related to gallstones, the stools can be pale, bulky, and foul smelling as a consequence of decreased fat digestion. This type of stool is referred to as _____.
5. The primary goal of treatment for the patient with pancreatitis is to decrease _____ _____ _____
thus resting the GI tract.

SECTION D
DISEASES OF THE INTESTINES

Inflammatory bowel disease (IBD) includes two chronic disorders: Crohn's disease and ulcerative colitis. Both diseases are autoimmune disorders characterized by periods when symptoms are worse (exacerbations) and periods when the diseases are less problematic. The recurrent diseases affect predominantly younger people. Treatment is symptomatic, and responses are frequently unpredictable.

What IS Crohn's Disease?

Pathogenesis

Crohn's disease is a chronic, recurring inflammation of the small intestine, usually occurring in the terminal ileum. Although the cause is unknown, Crohn's disease is believed to be a genetic disorder related in some way to an abnormal immune response to an unidentified etiologic agent. Extensive research continues the attempt to identify the cause of the disease. Possible causes include infection, autoimmune reaction, food allergies, and hereditary factors.

Crohn's disease is considered as another manifestation of irritable bowel syndrome. Rectal involvement is common (up to 95% of cases). Chronic, extensive inflammation develops in segments throughout the bowel, concentrating primarily in the distal ileum. Inflammation results in ulcerations involving the entire thickness of the intestinal wall. Multiple abscesses develop and leave ulcerations, which bleed and cause increased peristalsis and diarrhea. As the disease progresses, the bowel mucosa thickens and shortens, decreasing the surface area for absorption of water and nutrients.

At-Risk Populations

Stressful events frequently precipitate exacerbations.

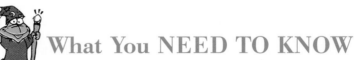

What You NEED TO KNOW

Clinical Manifestations

The signs and symptoms of Crohn's disease include diarrhea up to 20 times a day. Steatorrhea is common. The stools are pale, bulky, greasy, and foul smelling. The stools are also the color and consistency of oatmeal. Rectal bleeding is not typically present in Crohn's disease. A cramping (colicky) abdominal pain is common. Systemic symptoms such as fever, malaise, anorexia, dehydration, and weight loss are also noted. Anemia and extraintestinal manifestations include arthritis, finger clubbing, and a transient, inflammatory, nonulcerating nodular rash that is common over the shins (erythema nodosum). In some cases, strictures, internal fistulas, and anorectal fissures can form.

Prognosis

The segmental nature of Crohn's disease results in reoccurrence in the majority of patients postoperatively in a different area of the intestine.

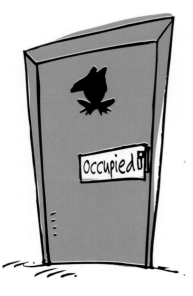

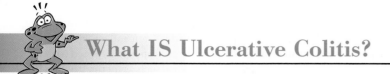

What IS Ulcerative Colitis?

Pathogenesis

Ulcerative colitis is an inflammation and ulceration of the mucosa and submucosa of the entire length of the colon. The cause of ulcerative colitis is unknown. Extensive research continues the attempt to identify the cause. Infection, autoimmune reactions, food allergies, and hereditary factors have been identified as possible causes of the disorder.

Ulcerative colitis is one of the manifestations of inflammatory bowel disease. Usually beginning in the rectum, ulcerative colitis moves up the colon in a continuous pattern. Inflammation causes edema and an increase of blood (hyperemia) of the bowel mucosa. Multiple abscesses develop leaving ulcerations, which bleed and cause increased peristalsis and diarrhea. As the disease progresses, the bowel mucosa thickens and shortens, decreasing the surface area available for absorption of water and nutrients.

At-Risk Populations

Stressful events frequently precipitate exacerbations.

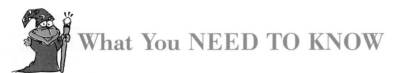

What You NEED TO KNOW

Clinical Manifestations

The signs and symptoms of ulcerative colitis include bloody diarrhea, occasionally up to 20 times a day. Abdominal pain can be cramplike in nature. The patient may develop systemic symptoms such as fever, malaise, and anorexia; they may also experience weight loss, anemia, and dehydration.

Prognosis

Ulcerative colitis progresses with periods of exacerbations and remissions but can be cured with surgery. Those who have had the disease more than 20 years have an increased incidence of cancer of the colon.

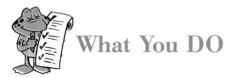

What You DO

Crohn's Disease Treatment

The treatment for Crohn's disease is symptomatic with the goals of good nutrition and prevention of a secondary infection. Antibiotics such as sulfasalazine and mesalamine—a combination of sulfapyridine and 5-aminosalicyclic acid—

The highest incidence of ulcerative colitis is among females ages 10 to 40.

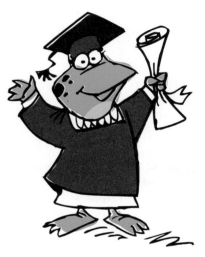

Ulcerative colitis is more prevalent in urban, upper middle-class, and higher educated populations.

A genetic predisposition to inflammatory bowel disease may be present because ulcerative colitis and Crohn's disease are observed frequently in Caucasians and Jews.

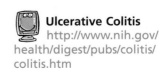

Ulcerative Colitis
http://www.nih.gov/
health/digest/pubs/colitis/
colitis.htm

See Chapters 1A, 2B, 7A, 8B, and 8C in **RWNSG:** *Pharmacology*

are the mainstay of treatment because of their antimicrobial and antiinflammatory effects. Corticosteroids are also used for their antiinflammatory effect. Immunosuppressive drugs such as azathioprine or cyclosporine are used to reduce the immune response. Anticholinergic medications, such as methantheline bromide and propantheline, help slow gastric motility.

Providing the patient a low-residue diet maintains nutritional balance. Ordering the patient to receive nothing by mouth (NPO) and providing TPN may be necessary during acute exacerbations. TPN provides total bowel rest and decreases gastric stimulation. Stress reduction techniques are helpful in reducing the anxiety and symptoms associated with Crohn's disease.

Surgical intervention is used only to treat complications. The length of the small bowel is protected, when possible, to preserve the patient's ability to absorb nutrients.

Ulcerative Colitis Treatment

The treatment of ulcerative colitis varies somewhat with the severity of the disorder. Stress-reduction strategies are used regardless of the severity of the disease. Sulfasalazine and mesalamine is the mainstay of treatment because of their antimicrobial and antiinflammatory effects. Corticosteroids are also used for their antiinflammatory effect. Immunosuppressive drugs such as azathioprine and cyclosporine may be used to reduce the immune response associated with the disorder. Anticholinergic medications such as methantheline bromide and propantheline slow gastric motility. Nutritional balance is maintained with a low-residue diet. During acute exacerbations, the patient is NPO and provided TPN.

See Chapters 1A, 2B, 7A, 8B, and 8C in **RWNSG:** *Pharmacology*

Four surgical procedures are used to treat chronic ulcerative colitis that fails to respond to drug therapy. A J-pouch (ileal pouch–anal anastomosis) prevents the need for an ostomy and preserves the rectal sphincter muscle. The colon is removed and the ileum attached to a reservoir created in the anal canal. This surgical procedure is frequently preferred for patients with ulcerative colitis.

The entire colon and rectum may be removed and the anus closed. The terminal ileum is brought out through the abdominal wall and a permanent ileostomy is formed (total proctocolectomy with ileostomy). This procedure is the most extreme measure. An ileorectal anastomosis attaches the ileum to the rectum while removing the remainder of the colon, representing an early alternative to total proctocolectomy.

A procedure known as a continent ileostomy (Kock's pouch) creates a reservoir constructed from a loop of the ileum. Stool is stored in the ileum until it is drained through a nipple valve. This procedure is rarely performed as a first choice.

Nursing Responsibilities

For patients with ulcerative colitis or Crohn's disease, the nurse should:
- Provide health teaching regarding medication therapy, diet, and stress-management strategies.
- Provide information about community resource support groups to help the patient cope with changes in body image and self-esteem.

Gastrointestinal System CHAPTER 8 237

- Monitor the effectiveness and adverse effects of drug therapy.
- Monitor intake, output, and daily weights.
- Monitor the number and consistency of stools while teaching the patient about nutritional needs. Small, frequent meals that are low in residue and high in protein, carbohydrates, and calories are recommended after surgery, along with supplemental fat-soluble vitamins and vitamin B12.
- Administer antidiarrheal medications as needed.
- Encourage the patient to verbalize fears regarding changes in sexuality. The patient with an ileostomy has no physiologic reasons for sexual dysfunction; however, psychological changes can occur.

In addition, for the patient with ulcerative colitis, the nurse should:
- Educate the patient about the implications of a proposed surgical procedure.
- Involve an enterostomal therapist and recommend a preoperative visit from a member of the ostomy association early in the treatment.
- Provide postoperative care and pain management as necessary.
- Help the patient manipulate ostomy equipment or supplies that will be needed postoperatively while monitoring skin for breakdown.

 Inflammatory bowel disease affects young people with many issues related to body image. Nurses advocate for both physical and psychosocial needs.

 TAKE HOME POINTS

Inflammatory bowel disease takes a person away from family and friends and focuses attention on the disease process. Educate the patient to help them maintain a more normal lifestyle.

Do You UNDERSTAND?

DIRECTIONS: Indicate in the space provided whether the statement is *true* or *false*. If false, then correct the statement in the margin space to the right to make it true.

_____ 1. Crohn's disease is a chronic, inflammatory disease that usually affects the terminal ileum.

_____ 2. Occult blood in the feces is a common finding in patients with Crohn's disease.

_____ 3. An expected outcome of Crohn's disease is increased absorption of the fat-soluble vitamins.

_____ 4. Rectal involvement is rare in Crohn's disease.

_____ 5. Steatorrhea is absent in Crohn's disease.

_____ 6. The lesions of Crohn's disease typically develop in several discontinuous segments of the bowel.

_____ 7. Anticholinergic medications are given to the patient with Crohn's disease to relieve abdominal cramping and help control diarrhea.

_____ 8. Sulfasalazine is the most commonly prescribed drug used in the treatment of Crohn's disease.

_____ 9. Vitamin D deficiency predisposes the patient with Crohn's disease to bleeding disorders.

_____ 10. TNP provides total bowel rest and decreases gastric stimulation for the patient with Crohn's disease.

Answers: 1. true; 2. true; 3. false; an expected outcome of Crohn's disease is decreased absorption of the fat-soluble vitamins; 4. false; rectal involvement is common in Crohn's disease; up to 95% of patients have rectal involvement; 5. true; 6. true; 7. true; 8. true; 9. false; vitamin K deficiency predisposes the patient with Crohn's disease to bleeding disorders; 10. true.

You are caring for a 21-year-old female college student who was admitted to your unit with severe abdominal pain. She states she has had 25 episodes of bloody diarrhea today and has lost 15 pounds in the last 2 weeks. She has not been able to eat and feels extremely weak and tired.

11. What indicators would you assess to indicate a positive outcome in treatment for the patient?

12. What nursing interventions would you initiate to detect or prevent complications?

What IS Diverticular Disease?

Pathogenesis

Saclike outpouchings of mucosa through the muscle layers of the colon wall (diverticula) develop most frequently in the sigmoid colon but can occur anywhere in the GI tract. Diverticulosis occurs when the large intestine, usually the descending and sigmoid portions, tries to move highly compacted fecal material. To accomplish this task, the longitudinal and circular muscles of those areas enlarge. The resulting increase in force on the nonmuscular tissues of the large intestine is similar to squeezing clay between the fingers as you clamp down on the soft clay. The clay between the fingers represents the diverticula, the outpouchings of soft tissue between the muscle fibers. Hypertrophy and contraction of the colonic muscles increase the pressure and can add to the degree of herniation.

Diverticulitis develops when small amounts of undigested foods (e.g., nuts, seeds) or stool (fecaliths) become trapped. The area becomes irritated, and infection and inflammation result. The inflamed area may bleed as it becomes congested with blood. Diverticulitis can lead to perforation of the colon when the trapped mass in the diverticulum erodes through the colon wall. Chronic diverticulitis can result in scarring and narrowing of the lumen of the colon, potentially leading to colon obstruction. Extension of the inflammation to adjacent organs can lead to fistulas of the bladder or vagina.

At-Risk Populations

Diverticular disease is common in men and women over age 45 and in obese individuals. This disorder is present in approximately one-third of the population over the age of 60 who do not have adequate cellulose in their diets. The incidence appears to be increasing, particularly for persons who live in developing countries in which much of the diet consists of refined foods and little residue. Cellulose is commonly called fiber or roughage. Many older adults have lost their teeth or simply prefer a soft diet. As a result, these people do not have adequate cellulose to prevent diverticular disease.

Answers: 11. the patient will experience a decrease in the number of stools; increase intake to meet metabolic needs; provide relief from abdominal pain and effective coping with the disease; 12. administering antidiarrheal medications as ordered and needed; monitoring the skin for breakdown, keeping it clean and dry; monitoring intake, output, and daily weights; consuming small, frequent easily digestible meals; monitoring IV fluids and TPN as indicated; assessing frequently the patient's pain level; administering pain medication as needed and assessing the adequacy of pain management; and educating the patient and family about disease and course of treatment.

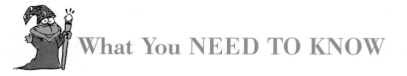

What You NEED TO KNOW

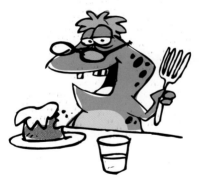

Clinical Manifestations

The signs and symptoms of diverticular disease can be vague or even absent in some patients. A change in bowel habits (constipation, diarrhea, or both), distention, cramping pain of the lower abdomen, or the development of gas (flatulence) may be observed. When diverticula become inflamed or abscesses form, the patient develops fever, increased white blood cell count (leukocytosis), and tenderness of the left lower quadrant. Assessment reveals alterations in bowel habits (constipation, diarrhea, or both), increased flatus, anorexia, and low-grade fever. Bleeding of arterial blood (bright, bright red) from the rectum is a serious sign of diverticular disease.

Diverticular disease is common in the United States, the United Kingdom, Australia, and France.

Prognosis

Habitual consumption of low-residue diet reduces fecal bulk thus reducing the diameter of the colon. Pressure within the narrow lumen of the colon can thus increase sufficiently to rupture the diverticula. However, severe complications, such as hemorrhage, peritonitis, bowel obstruction, and fistula formation, are rare.

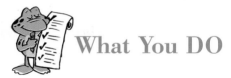

What You DO

Treatment

Diverticular disease is frequently discovered during diagnostic tests for other problems. Direct observation of the lesions is possible through examination of the rectal colon (sigmoidoscopy). A barium enema can reveal muscle hypertrophy, but the barium can become trapped in the outpouchings and form hard masses.

Asymptomatic diverticular disease requires no specific treatment other than dietary modification. Mild disease is treated with a high-fiber diet and the use of bran and bulk laxatives.

Diverticulitis is treated conservatively by allowing the colon to rest. The patient is made NPO, an NG tube is inserted, and IV fluids administered until pain, inflammation, and fever subside. When the acute episode has quieted, the patient can take in oral fluids and slowly advance the diet as tolerated.

A colon resection may be needed if the patient develops complications such as hemorrhage, obstruction, abscesses, or perforation. With abscess or obstruction, a colon resection with temporary colostomy may be performed until the patient's condition improves. A colostomy permits evaluation of the colon by creating an artificial opening (stoma) in the large intestine and bringing it to the surface of the abdomen. For some patients, the temporary colostomy allows the colon to rest and heal.

See Chapters 8C and 12 in
RWNSG: *Pharmacology*

Nursing Responsibilities

For the patient with diverticular disease, nursing responsibilities are aimed at controlling inflammation. The nurse should:

- 🍎 Teach the patient to consume a high-fiber diet, bulk laxatives, and at least eight glasses of water every day to help prevent constipation.
- Encourage the obese patient to lose weight.
- 🍎 Advise the patient to notify the health care provider of any change in bowel pattern (constipation or diarrhea) or character (presence of blood or mucus), or when fever, abdominal pain, or urinary symptoms develop.
- 🍎 Teach the patients with acute diverticulitis to rest the colon by remaining NPO until the pain, fever, and inflammation subside.
- Administer IV fluids and antibiotics as prescribed.
- Insert and maintain patency of an NG tube in some cases to rest the bowel.
- Provide postoperative care as needed for the patient who has had a colon resection with colostomy.
- 🍎 Teach patients with chronic diverticulitis about the importance of avoiding indigestible fiber foods such as nuts, corn, popcorn, tomatoes, cucumbers, or strawberries to help prevent further inflammation.

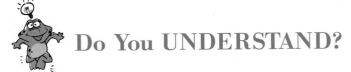

Do You UNDERSTAND?

DIRECTIONS: **Provide answers to the following questions.**

1. Diverticula is defined as what?

2. When does diverticulitis develop?

3. At what age is diverticular disease found most frequently in patients? It is also becoming more common in what other age group?

4. What is the most common treatment for mild diverticular disease?

5. When surgery is required for the patient with diverticulitis, what is the procedure most commonly performed?

Answers: 1. saclike outpouchings of mucosa through the muscle layers of the colon wall; 2. undigested foods, such as nuts and seeds, block the diverticula; 3. 60 years of age, young; 4. the amount of fiber in the diet is increased and bran and bulk laxatives are consumed; 5. colon resection with temporary colostomy.

What IS Gluten-Sensitive Enteropathy?

Pathogenesis

Patients with gluten-sensitive enteropathy (celiac sprue) are unable to digest and use sugars, starches, and fats. Intolerance to gluten—a protein found in wheat, barley, rye, malt, and possibly oats—triggers an autoimmune response in genetically predisposed individuals. Autoimmune responses damage the villa of the small intestines, resulting in flattening of the surface of the intestine with a loss of surface area and decreased absorption. The damaged surface cells have a decreased ability to stimulate pancreatic sections, which leads to further impaired digestion and absorption of nutrients.

Destruction of mucosal cells causes inflammation and the secretion of water and electrolytes, which leads to watery diarrhea. The loss of potassium leads to muscle weakness. The malabsorption of calcium and magnesium can cause seizures or tetany. Unabsorbed fatty acids combine with calcium, and secondary hyperparathyroidism increases phosphorus excretion, resulting in bone reabsorption. Fat malabsorption in the jejunum leads to steatorrhea. Malabsorption of vitamin K leads to a deficiency of prothrombin in the blood. The absorption of B12, iron, and folic acid also occurs, leading to anemia.

At-Risk Populations

Seventy percent of persons diagnosed with this disease are female. A strong genetic influence has been identified.

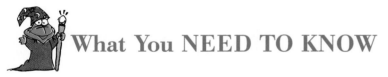

What You NEED TO KNOW

Clinical Manifestations

The signs and symptoms of this disorder include steatorrhea; three to five such movements occur daily. Malnutrition, anemia, weight loss, abdominal distention, and a symmetric skin rash (dermatitis herpetiformis) are also present. Low serum magnesium and calcium levels cause irritability, tremor, seizures, tetany, bone pain, osteomalacia, and dental deformities. Rickets and clubbing of the fingers are likely when vitamin D deficiency is prolonged.

Prognosis

The prognosis for the patient with gluten-sensitive enteropathy is good, as long as a gluten-free diet is maintained. Dietary management can prevent acute episodes of the disease. The incidence of non-Hodgkin's lymphoma is greatly increased in patients who fail to respond to gluten-free diets.

Gluten-sensitive enteropathy affects primarily infants and children.

Gluten-sensitive enteropathy occurs largely in Caucasians and has been documented in persons from India and Pakistan. In native African, Japanese, and Chinese populations, gluten-sensitive enteropathy is nearly nonexistent. The incidence has been estimated to be 1 in 1000 in Europe, South America, and North Africa; however, it is diagnosed infrequently in the United States.

As early as 3 to 4 months of age, growth failure, anorexia, and constipation can begin. In older children, constipation is observed occasionally despite steatorrhea. Vomiting and cramplike abdominal pain are prominent in infants but are unusual in older children. In older children, delayed puberty and infertility can develop.

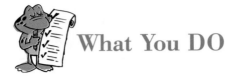

What You DO

Treatment

The treatment for gluten-sensitive enteropathy includes life-long, permanent attention to a gluten-free diet. A gluten-free diet means avoiding cereal grains such as wheat, rye, barley, oats, and malt. Milk-sugar (lactose) intolerance is presumed, thus these products are also excluded from the diet.

Corticosteroids may be used in acute episodes along with antidiarrheal and anticholinergic medications.

See Chapters 7A, 8C, and 12 in RWNSG: *Pharmacology*

Nursing Responsibilities

For the patient with gluten-sensitive enteropathy, the nurse should:
- Monitor nutritional adequacy while the patient adheres to a gluten-free diet.
- Monitor daily weights and periodic evaluations of growth status.
- Monitor of laboratory values for anemia and vitamin deficiency.
- Monitor the frequency and consistency of stools while maintaining fluid and electrolyte balance.
- Provide health teaching for the patient or caregiver regarding gluten-free diets, the disease process, and medications.

Infants are routinely given vitamin D, iron, and folic acid supplements to treat deficiencies.

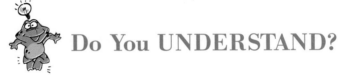

Do You UNDERSTAND?

DIRECTIONS: **For each of the following nursing diagnoses for gluten-sensitive enteropathy, identify the appropriate outcome statement and interventions.**

1. Altered nutrition, less than body requirements related to inability to use gluten.
   a. Evaluation and outcome statement: _____
   _____
   b. Interventions: _____
   _____

2. Diarrhea related to intestinal response to gluten in the diet.
   a. Evaluation and outcome statement: _____
   _____
   b. Interventions: _____
   _____

3. Fluid volume deficit related to losses via excessive diarrhea.
   a. Evaluation and outcome statement: _____
   _____
   b. Interventions: _____
   _____

Answers: 1. a, the patient will experience no further weight loss; the patient will meet metabolic needs through adequate nutritional intake; b, maintain gluten-free diet high in calories, protein and vitamins; monitor daily weights, intake, and output; 2. a, the patient will experience a normal number and consistency of stools; b, monitor frequency and consistency of stools; maintain gluten-free diet; administer antidiarrheal medications as ordered and needed; maintain good skin care to perianal area; 3. a, the patient will obtain and maintain a normal fluid and electrolyte balance; b, monitor intake and output; assess for symptoms of dehydration; monitor laboratory values for electrolyte imbalance.

4. Knowledge deficit related to dietary restrictions.
   a. Evaluation and outcome statement: _____

   _____

   b. Interventions: _____

   _____

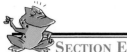

SECTION E
DISEASES OF THE LIVER AND GALLBLADDER

The liver is responsible for over 1300 functions within the body. Included among these functions are the storing and filtering of blood, production of bile (bile is then stored in the gallbladder), conversion of sugars to glycogen, and the synthesis and breakdown of fats. The liver also temporarily stores fatty acids. As the chief supplier of glucose for the body, the liver is occasionally called on to convert glucose from protein and fats. This conversion may also work in reverse. The liver cells can convert excess sugar into fat and send it for storage in other parts of the body. The liver is also responsible for the synthesis of serum proteins, such as steroids, globulins, and albumin (which helps regulate blood volume), as well as fibrinogen and prothrombin (essential clotting factors). In addition to these functions, the liver stores many essential vitamins until they are needed by other parts of the body.

The liver protects the body by disposing of depleted blood cells, filtering, and destroying bacteria. One of the most important protective functions of the liver is the detoxification of medications, alcohol, and environmental poisons by the endoplasmic reticulum. Kupffer cells are an important part of the mononuclear phagocyte system (known previously as the reticuloendothelial system). The liver also helps maintain the balance of sex hormones in the body. Finally, the liver monitors the proteins that pass through the digestive system. The body cannot use some of the amino acids that pass through the digestive tract. The liver rejects and neutralizes these acids and sends them to the kidneys for disposal. When the liver is affected by disease, any or all of the these functions are affected.

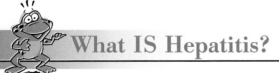

What IS Hepatitis?

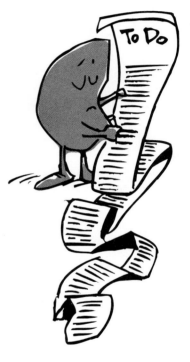

Pathogenesis

Hepatitis is an inflammation of the liver. Several different causes of hepatitis have been identified, including viral, bacterial, and toxic substances. Viral hepatitis is the most common. The pathogenesis of viral hepatitis is similar regardless of the cause. Liver cells are damaged, become inflamed, and die (**necrosed**) as a result of the body's immune response to the illness. The degree of impair-

Answers: 4. a, the patient will develop a working understanding of their disease and treatment; **b,** provide health education to patient and family concerning the nature of disease; establish dietary restrictions and allowances; monitor for complications and effects of noncompliance with diet; maintain medications and other treatments.

ment depends on the amount of cellular damage and the subsequent inflammatory process. The endoplasmic reticulum (responsible for the synthesis of protein and steroids and the detoxification of drugs and poisons) is the first to be affected. Liver functions that depend on the endoplasmic reticulum and Kupffer cells are altered. The degree of impairment depends on the amount of damage. The disease may manifest acutely and, without treatment, may become chronic.

At-Risk Populations

Hepatitis occurs worldwide. The incubation period ranges from 2 weeks to 6 months, depending on the specific type of hepatitis (A, B, C, D, E). Patients who abuse alcohol or who are exposed to hepatotoxic substances are at risk for developing hepatitis. Other persons at risk include those with poor sanitation and those exposed to infected individuals or blood. Hepatitis can also be transmitted via feces, contaminated shellfish, sexual contact, and contaminated water.

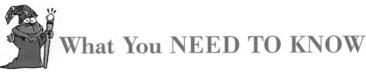 What You NEED TO KNOW

Clinical Manifestations

The greatest danger for developing hepatitis is during the incubation period and early appearance of symptoms (prodromal period), during which the patient is likely unaware of the illness. As the disease progresses and jaundice appears, the patient becomes less infectious, and danger of transmission is decreased.

Most symptoms of viral hepatitis are mild. The low-grade fever results from the release of pyrogens in the inflammatory process. Reduced energy metabolism by the liver causes fatigue and malaise. Impaired excretion of conjugated bilirubin and the build-up of urobilin in the blood cause jaundice (noted first in the sclera), clay-colored stools, increased serum bilirubin levels, and dark urine. The dark urine and clay-colored stools appear before the onset of jaundice. Itchy skin (pruritus) results from the accumulation of bile salts in the skin. Stretching of the liver capsule produces right upper quadrant pain. Changes in the stomach or bowel produce anorexia, nausea, and vomiting. Bleeding tendencies increase as a consequence of the reduced prothrombin synthesis by injured liver cells. Reduced bile in the intestines leads to reduced vitamin K absorption. Liver function tests (LFTs) are usually abnormal.

Prognosis

Life-threatening (fulminant) hepatitis resembles acute liver failure.

Most patients recover in 6 to18 weeks. However, liver function tests can stay abnormal for a longer period. The mortality rate is less than 1%. Possible complications of hepatitis include chronic hepatitis, chronic persistent hepatitis, chronic active hepatitis, chronic carrier state, and aplastic anemia.

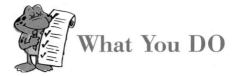

What You DO

Treatment

The treatment for hepatitis varies with the specific type, but generally centers on rest, medication therapy, dietary management, relief of pruritus, and postexposure prophylaxis. Dietary therapy with small, frequent meals that are high in calories and low in fats, as well as abstinence from alcohol, is recommended for all patients.

Few medications are available for treating hepatitis. Antibiotics are not used. Antiemetics may be given to control nausea and vomiting. Parenteral vitamin K is given to patients who have prolonged prothrombin times. Antihistamines are used to control pruritus. Certain antilipemic medications may be used to treat pruritus because they bind bile acids that are then excreted in the stool. Medications that are hepatotoxic, such as acetaminophen (Tylenol), phenobarbital (Luminal Sodium), phenytoin (Dilantin), chlorpromazine (Thorazine), morphine, paraldehyde, codeine, and alcohol, should be avoided.

Postexposure prophylaxis and vaccines are used for primary and secondary prevention of hepatitis. Immune globulin provides protection from hepatitis A. Hepatitis B vaccines promote immunity to hepatitis B and D. No vaccines for hepatitis C or E are available.

See Chapters 4B, 6B, 8A, 8B, 8C, and 12 in **RWNSG:** *Pharmacology*

Nursing Responsibilities

For the patient with hepatitis, the nurse should:
- Identify patients with risk factors to determine the possible type and cause of disease.
- Assess for jaundice (light-skinned patients), checking the sclera (dark-skinned patients), and checking the hard palate of the mouth and the inner canthus of the eye.
- Promote adequate nutritional intake and rest.
- Teach the patient to use tepid or emollient baths, avoid the use of alkaline soap, and apply lotion frequently to help with the pruritus. Encourage the patient to wear loose, soft clothing and to keep the room cool.
- Monitor complete blood count, liver function (alanine aminotransferase [ALT], aspartate aminotransferase [AST], bilirubin, alkaline phosphatase), gamma globulins, and prothrombin time.
- Provide patient and family teaching regarding the risk for transmitting infection.
- Reassure the patient and family that jaundice is usually a temporary condition and will resolve as the patient's condition improves. Encourage the patient to discuss feelings about self-image.

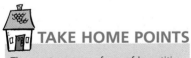

TAKE HOME POINTS

The most common form of hepatitis is the viral form. Health care workers must understand the importance of protecting themselves and others from this disease.

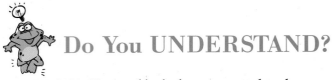

Do You UNDERSTAND?

DIRECTIONS: **Unscramble the letters to complete the sentence.**

1. One cause of hepatitis is _____ _____.
   (*citxo stbusacsen*)
2. The part of the liver that is responsible for protein and steroid synthesis is

   _____ _____.

   (*mpedlnaicos cirultume*)
3. One way to contract hepatitis is _____

   _____.

   (*icnfetde yodb udifsl*)

What IS Cirrhosis?

Pathogenesis

Cirrhosis is an irreversible, progressive liver disease characterized by inflammation, cell death, scarring, and fibrosis. Cirrhosis is the final stage of many types of liver problems. Extensive destruction of liver cells occurs, which are then replaced by nodular scar tissue. The scarring alters the biliary and vascular flow within the liver, resulting in bile stasis and portal hypertension (the portal vein receives blood from the intestines and spleen). As a result of the pressure increase in the portal vein, fluid accumulates in the peritoneum (ascites), varicose veins develop in the esophagus (esophageal varices), and protein metabolic wastes are not adequately cleared, resulting in an increase in ammonia levels and degenerative changes in the brain (encephalopathy).

Four major types of cirrhosis have been identified: alcoholic cirrhosis, postnecrotic cirrhosis, biliary cirrhosis, and cardiac cirrhosis. Alcoholic cirrhosis is related to excessive alcohol intake, which results in an accumulation of fat in the liver. The fatty deposits are eventually replaced by scar tissue. Postnecrotic cirrhosis is a complication of hepatitis, which results in scarring of liver tissue. Biliary cirrhosis is also chronic, characterized by obstruction and infection, which results in fibrosis scar formation. Cardiac cirrhosis is related to severe, right-sided heart failure, which ultimately causes liver scarring.

At-Risk Populations

Persons at primary risk for developing cirrhosis are those who abuse alcohol, particularly in the absence of proper nutrition. However, cirrhosis can also develop in patients with chronic obstructive biliary disease, long-standing heart failure, and chronic hepatitis.

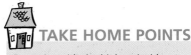

TAKE HOME POINTS

Countries with the highest incidence of cirrhosis also have the greatest per capita consumption of alcohol. However, do not be misled into believing that all patients who have cirrhosis are alcoholic. Many patients have the disease as a result of other GI problems.

Answers: 1. toxic substances; 2. endoplasmic reticulum; 3. infected body fluids.

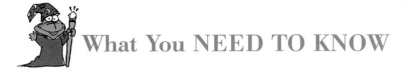

What You NEED TO KNOW

Clinical Manifestations

The signs and symptoms of cirrhosis include ascites, jaundice, dependent edema, bleeding tendencies, esophageal varices, hemorrhoids, anemia, and encephalopathy. An enlarged spleen (splenomegaly) indicates severe portal hypertension. Anemia, leukopenia, or thrombocytopenia can result from splenomegaly. Laboratory testing reveals impaired liver function—elevated liver serum enzymes (AST, ALT, lactate dehydrogenase [LDH]), low serum albumin, anemia, and elevated prothrombin time.

Prognosis

The outcome of cirrhosis depends on the severity of the disease and the extent to which it responds to treatment. Progression of the disease causes liver failure, gram-negative bacterial infections, infection of the peritoneum (peritonitis), liver tumors, and death in a significant number of patients.

Cirrhosis is the leading cause of liver-related death in the United States.

What You DO

Treatment

The treatment of cirrhosis includes abstaining from all alcohol, reducing dietary protein, restricting fluid, and preventing infection. Drug therapy with vitamins, particularly fat-soluble and B complex and Vitamin K, helps maintain nutritional status. Diuretics are used to decrease ascites and edema. Neomycin and lactulose help decrease serum ammonia levels. Corticosteroids decrease inflammation. Vasopressin may be needed to control bleeding from esophageal varices. Histamine 2 antagonists decrease gastric upset caused by ammonia build up. For some patients, a liver transplant may be needed to sustain life.

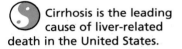

See Chapters 7, 8, 9, 12, and 13B in RWNSG: *Pharmacology*

Some patients may require a portacaval shunt inserted to reduce portal hypertension. A portacaval shunt involves the surgical anastomosis of the portal vein from the liver to the vena cava, which helps reduce the pressure in the portal circulation. Inserting a peritoneovenous shunt (LeVeen shunt) helps remove ascitic fluid from the peritoneal cavity. A peritoneovenous shunt consists of insertion of a peritoneal tube leading from the abdominal cavity to the superior vena cava or the jugular vein. For some patients, a liver transplant may be needed to sustain life.

Nursing Responsibilities

For the patient with cirrhosis, the nurse should:
• Help the patient maintain nutritional intake sufficient to meet metabolic needs—decreased protein and sodium and increased calories.

- Help the patient avoid drugs that are toxic to the liver while administering required medications (e.g., diuretics, vitamins).
- Maintain skin integrity.
- Monitor daily weights, intake, and output.
- Monitor for edema and ineffective breathing patterns related to pressure on the diaphragm from ascites (by measuring abdominal girth).
- Monitor for signs and symptoms of infection related to decreased white blood cell count.
- Monitor for potential complications, such as encephalopathy (orientation, speech patterns, ammonia levels, and blood pH); bleeding (hemoglobin, hematocrit, and prothrombin times); and nosebleeds (epistaxis), bruising, blood in the urine (hematuria), and blood in the stool (melena).

Do You UNDERSTAND?

DIRECTIONS: **For the following symptoms of cirrhosis, explain why they occur in the patient and provide two nursing interventions appropriate when the patient experiences these symptoms.**

1. Ascites
   a. Occurs because: _____
      _____
   b. Appropriate nursing interventions: _____

2. Portal hypertension
   a. Occurs because: _____
      _____
   b. Appropriate nursing interventions: _____

3. Jaundice
   a. Occurs because: _____
      _____
   b. Appropriate nursing interventions: _____

Answers: 1. a, decreased metabolism of proteins leads to decreased plasma proteins; b, semi-Fowler's to Fowler's position decreases pressure on diaphragm from ascites, daily abdominal girths; monitor daily intake and output and daily weights; administer diuretics as ordered to decrease edema; 2, a, destruction of hepatic tissue with resultant scarring leads to obstruction of blood and lymph; b, monitor vital signs frequently; maintain low-protein diet; monitor daily intake and output and daily weights; 3, a, of decreased bilirubin metabolism, which results in hyperbilirubinemia, leading to jaundice; b, assess for appearance and amount; assess urine and stool; provide skin care.

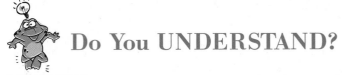

What IS Cholecystitis?

Pathogenesis

Cholecystitis is an inflammation of the gallbladder and is associated most frequently with gallstones (cholelithiasis). In the absence of stones, bacteria that reach the gallbladder via the vascular or lymphatic system may be the cause. Inflammation of the gallbladder is accompanied by an increase in peristalsis and contraction within the biliary system. When gallstones are present, distention of the gallbladder can occur, venous and lymphatic drainage becomes impaired, and proliferation of bacteria, localized irritation, and ischemia are present. This process can lead to pus (empyema) in the gallbladder. The inflamed gallbladder is edematous and thickened. Areas of gangrene or necrosis may also be present. Recurrent episodes of acute cholecystitis can cause fibrosis of the walls of the gallbladder.

At-Risk Populations

Obese, caucasian, multiparous women over the age of 40 are most at risk for cholecystitis.

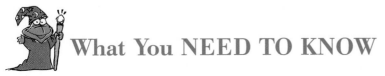

What You NEED TO KNOW

Clinical Manifestations

Assessment of the patient may reveal a history of flatulence, bloating, dyspepsia, eructation, intolerance to fatty foods, and vague upper abdominal sensations. Nausea, pain in the upper right quadrant of the abdomen (biliary colic), fever, and leukocytosis are frequent. If gallstones are present and causing an obstruction, the patient may develop obstructive jaundice, dark amber urine, and clay-colored stools.

Prognosis

Removal of the gallbladder and the obstructing gallstones is usually effective in reducing symptoms. After the patient is symptomatic, intervening to prevent progression to a more severe, occasionally fatal, complication of gallbladder disease is essential. Approximately one third of complications are a result of perforation of the gallbladder. A gangrenous area becomes necrotic, and bile leaks into the peritoneal cavity. Peritonitis with systemic distribution of pepsin has a mortality rate of approximately 20%. Pericholecystic abscess accounts for 50% of the complications, although it is the least severe of the complications, having a mortality rate of approximately 15%. In some cases, a fistula develops when the gallbladder becomes attached to a portion of the gastrointestinal tract and perforates it. The duodenum is the most common site for fistula formation, followed by the colon.

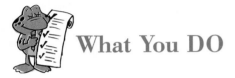

What You DO

Treatment

The treatment of cholecystitis includes promoting comfort. Meperidine is the drug of choice for pain control. Morphine and its derivatives are more likely to cause spasms in the biliary system and should be avoided. Cholesterol-dissolving agents are especially useful in dissolving cholesterol gallstones. Two medications are used for this purpose: chenodeoxycholic acid and ursodeoxycholic acid.

Obese, Caucasian, multi-parous women over the age of 40 are most at risk for cholecystitis.

Genetics appears to play a role in the development of gallstones for some patients, which is evident in Pima and Chippewa native American, Chinese, Jewish, and Italian populations, all of whom have an increased incidence of the disease.

TAKE HOME POINTS

A higher incidence of gallbladder disease is present in large women who have had multiple pregnancies. Symptoms related to intolerance of a fatty diet should alert the health care provider of the possibility.

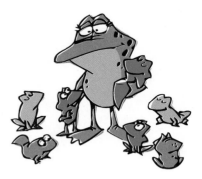

See Chapter 14 in **RWNSG:** *Pharmacology*

Surgical intervention may become necessary for patients with acute cholecystitis. Extracorporal shock wave lithotripsy may be used when a handful of small stones are producing symptoms. This procedure requires general anesthesia. The patient is placed in a large tub of water and shock waves are directed to the stones. These waves are administered repeatedly until the stones are crushed. The patient is then able to pass the stones through the feces.

Percutaneous cholecystolithotomy removes gallstones using endoscopy and stone baskets. General anesthesia is not required for this procedure.

A laparoscopic cholecystectomy involves making four small incisions into the abdomen: one near the umbilicus to visualize the gallbladder, one for grasping the gallbladder, one for suction and irrigation, and the last one for the dissection instruments and applying clips. This procedure is performed under general anesthesia, and patients are usually able to leave within 24 hours.

An open cholecystectomy removes the gallbladder through an upper right midline incision of the abdomen. This procedure usually involves insertion of a T tube into common duct to ensure adequate bile drainage after surgery. The procedure is performed under general anesthesia and usually requires up to a 6-week postoperative healing time.

Nursing Responsibilities

For the patient with cholecystitis, the nurse should:
- Assess for pain, usually upper right quadrant pain that frequently radiates to the back. The pain may appear in "waves" (biliary colic) or it may be steady, consistent pain that is related to inflammation.
- Institute measures appropriate to treat nausea and vomiting. Distention of the bile ducts and fat intolerance trigger the vomiting center in the brain. Antiemetics, NPO status, and possible NG decompression may be used.
- Modify diet, such as limiting the amount of fat in the diet, which decreases the amount of bile released from the inflamed gallbladder thus decreasing symptoms.
- Monitor for signs of infection; fever and leukocytosis are common in acute cholecystitis.
- Monitor for jaundice, as evidence of biliary obstruction.
- Provide patient and family teaching regarding the disease and possible treatment options.
- Provide postoperative care and monitoring for postoperative complications.

See Chapter 8B in **RWNSG:** *Pharmacology*

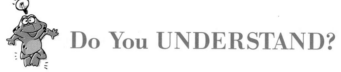

Do You UNDERSTAND?

DIRECTIONS: **Fill in the blanks.**

1. Postoperative symptoms to monitor that might indicate an infection are fever and _____.

2. _____ is the drug of choice for pain control in the patient with cholecystitis.

3. A surgical procedure that involves four small incisions into the abdomen for the treatment of cholecystitis is termed a _____ cholecystectomy.

4. The pain frequently experienced by patients with acute cholecystitis is termed _____ colic.

5. Stones in the gallbladder are termed _____.

6. _____ is inflammation of the gallbladder.

7. A complication of a perforated gallbladder is _____, which is inflammation of the peritoneal cavity.

8. The population most at risk for developing cholecystitis is obese _____ women over the age of 40.

9. Measures to treat nausea and vomiting during an acute attack of cholecystitis include antiemetics, _____, decompression, and NPO status.

10. The pain of cholecystitis is usually found in the upper right _____ of the abdomen.

Section F
MALIGNANCIES OF THE GI TRACT

Squamous (scaly or platelike) cell carcinomas involve the epidermis of the skin and linings of the mouth, pharynx, esophagus, anus, and vagina. Adenocarcinomas arise from glandular tissues or when the tumor cells form recognizable glandular structures.

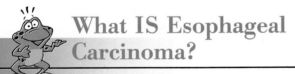

What IS Esophageal Carcinoma?

Pathogenesis

Although squamous cell carcinoma is the most common form of cancer of the esophagus, adenocarcinoma of the esophagus is also common. The cause of cancer of the esophagus is unknown. Esophageal carcinoma usually begins as benign tissue changes that are frequently associated with chronic esophagitis. Most squamous cell carcinomas are found in the upper third of the esophagus. Adenocarcinomas are usually found in the lower third of the esophagus. The glandular tissue in the esophagus and lymph node extension promote early and rapid metastasis.

At-Risk Populations

GERD and chronic ingestion of hot food and beverages are risk factors. Alcohol abuse and nutritional deficiencies have also been indicated. Smoking tobacco and opium are known causative factors.

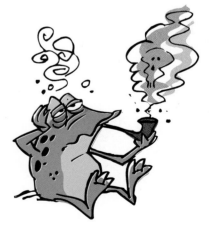

Answers: 3. laparoscopic; 4. biliary; 5. cholelithiasis; 6. cholecystitis; 7. peritonitis; 8. multiparous; 9. nasogastric; 10. quadrant.

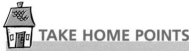 In northern China, the rate of esophageal carcinoma is extremely high. The rate in men is twice that found in women.

TAKE HOME POINTS

Esophageal cancer can be mistaken for GERD. Early identification and treatment is essential for a positive prognosis.

What You NEED TO KNOW

Clinical Manifestations

The first symptoms of esophageal carcinoma are usually difficulty swallowing (dysphagia) or the sensation of burning or squeezing pain when swallowing (odynophagia). A sore throat, a feeling of choking, and hoarseness may also occur. Weight loss is common.

Prognosis

Unfortunately, by the time significant symptoms are apparent, the cancer has usually invaded the deep layers of the esophagus and metastasized to adjacent tissues and lymph nodes. Because of this characteristic, the overall 5-year survival rate is 15%.

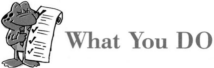

What You DO

Treatment

Treatment of esophageal carcinoma depends on the location of the tumor and the extent of growth and metastasis. Unfortunately, most tumors are discovered in the advanced stages, thus treatment is palliative and directed at allowing the patient to continue to eat. Radiation therapy is especially useful to treat tumors in the upper third of the esophagus. Radiation is used to shrink the tumor thus providing a larger lumen in the esophagus. Radiation may be used before surgical intervention as well. Esophageal dilation with various dilators or the placement of stents or prostheses enlarges the lumen of the esophagus thus relieving dysphagia and allowing for improved nutritional intake.

Surgical intervention may be needed for some patients. Laser therapy may be used to vaporize the tumor through endoscopy. An esophagectomy removes all or part of the esophagus followed by insertion of a graft to replace the resected esophagus. An esophagogastrostomy removes all or part of the esophagus with anastomosis to the stomach. An esophagoenterostomy removes all or part of the esophagus with anastomosis to the intestine.

Nursing Responsibilities

For the patient with esophageal carcinoma, the nurse should:
- Promote and monitor nutritional status, including small frequent feedings of soft foods. Placement of a feeding tube may be necessary. Keep the head of bed elevated at least 30 degrees.
- Monitor intake, output, and daily weights.
- Promote effective respiratory function while assessing for potential aspiration.
- Promote effective coping and use of stress-management techniques.
- Monitor for postoperative complications.

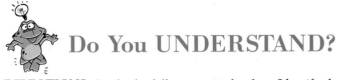

Do You UNDERSTAND?

DIRECTIONS: **Study the following set of orders. Identify the order from the health care provider in which you would question the patient diagnosed with esophageal cancer. Provide rationale for your answer.**

1. Nutritional status is a priority for clients with esophageal cancer. Your patient has lost 5 pounds this week.

   _____ a. Order 1: Elevate head of bed no more than 15 degrees.
   Insert NG tube.
   Initiate tube feeding at 300 cc per hour.

   _____ b. Order 2: Check swallowing reflex each shift.
   Provide soft, bland diet.
   Eat 6 small meals per day.

   Rationale: _____

   _____

   _____

   _____

DIRECTIONS: **Explain in lay terms what is removed during each of the following surgical procedures. How would these surgeries benefit the patient with esophageal cancer?**

2. Endoscopic laser therapy: _____

   _____

   _____

3. Esophagoenterostomy: _____

   _____

   _____

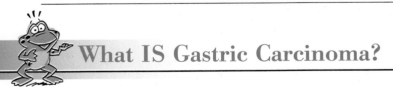

What IS Gastric Carcinoma?

Pathogenesis

Gastric carcinoma is characterized by malignant neoplasm in the stomach. No single causative agent has been identified for gastric carcinoma. Adenocarcinomas comprise the majority (90%) of gastric carcinomas. The pyloric and antral areas of the stomach are most frequently involved. Metastasis occurs early, frequently to the pancreas.

At-Risk Populations

Gastric carcinoma is found twice as often in men than it is in women. Chronic gastritis, presence of *H. pylori*, a diet with large amount of smoked fish and meat, and exposure to radiation and trace metals have been identified as predisposing factors. Genetic predisposition appears evident.

Answers: 1. a, head of the bed should be elevated at least 30 degrees; 300 cc per hour is too rapid a rate for beginning tube feeding; the patient would experience side effects from this rate; 2. from a tube inserted through the patient's mouth and into the throat, a laser would be directed at the tumor and liquefy or remove it; the patient would be sedated during the procedure; this will remove the visible tumor from the patient's esophagus; 3. all or part of the patient's esophagus (feeding tube) is removed, with the remainder attached to the patient's intestine, bypassing the stomach; this procedure will remove the tumor and surrounding tissue.

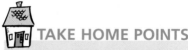

What You NEED TO KNOW

Clinical Manifestations

Early detection of gastric carcinoma is difficult because of its vague symptoms. The symptoms in many cases are identical to peptic ulcer disease (PUD) with indigestion, feeling of fullness, and mild discomfort are common. Anemia related to chronic blood loss is common, although bleeding into the stool is usually occult. Weight loss is also common. Frequently, the disease is not diagnosed until metastasis has occurred and symptoms become more pronounced.

Prognosis

The prognosis for gastric carcinoma depends on the stage of the disease at diagnosis. Most tumors are identified late in the course of the disease. The 5-year survival rate is approximately 15%.

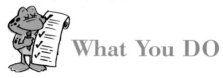

What You DO

Treatment

The only effective treatment for gastric carcinoma is surgery. The invasiveness of the tumor determines the extent of surgery. When significant metastasis is present, the surgery may be palliative. A Billroth I or II procedure removes lesions in the atrium and pylorus. A total gastrectomy with esophagojejunostomy is used to treat lesions in the cardia or high in the fundus. Radiation and chemotherapy are adjunctive therapies, along with blood transfusions, to treat anemia. Gastric decompression is required.

Nursing Responsibilities

For the patient with gastric carcinoma, the nurse should:
- Promote and monitor nutritional status, including daily weights, intake, and output.
- Maintain TPN or jejunostomy feedings while monitoring for complications.
- Maintain the patient's comfort level. Assess pain frequently and administer analgesics before they are needed. Use adjunctive measures when possible.
- Monitor the patient's activity level. Institute safety measures as needed while providing for rest and activity.
- Educate the patient and family regarding diagnosis, treatment, and home care.
- Provide support related to diagnosis and condition.

TAKE HOME POINTS

Gastric cancer is diagnosed late in the course of the disease because the symptoms frequently mimic PUD.

See Chapters 1D and 3A in RWNSG: *Pharmacology*

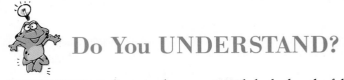

Do You UNDERSTAND?

DIRECTIONS: **Indicate in the space provided whether the following statements are *true* or *false*. If false, then correct the statement in the margin space to the right to make it true.**

_____ 1. No single causative agent has been identified for gastric carcinoma.

_____ 2. Squamous cell carcinomas comprise the majority of gastric cancers.

_____ 3. A risk factor for gastric cancer of which most people may be unaware is consumption of smoked fish.

_____ 4. The symptoms of gastric cancer are frequently confused with gallbladder disease.

_____ 5. Anemia is a frequent finding in patients who have gastric cancer.

_____ 6. A Billroth I surgical procedure involves a subtotal gastrectomy.

_____ 7. The prognosis for gastric cancer is excellent because few tumors metastasize.

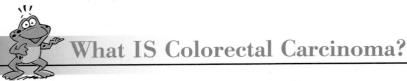

What IS Colorectal Carcinoma?

Pathogenesis

The term *colorectal carcinoma* refers to a malignant neoplasm found in the colon. The causes of colorectal cancer remain unclear, although several risk factors have been identified.

Adenocarcinomas are the most common type of colorectal cancers. These malignancies usually arise from colon polyps. The vast majority of tumors are found in the rectal and sigmoid areas of the colon. Metastasis is common related to the vascularity and the lymphatic system surrounding the intestines.

Colorectal cancer is the second leading cause of death from cancer in the United States.

At-Risk Populations

Risk factors for colorectal cancer include advancing age, familial polyposis, colorectal polyps, chronic inflammatory bowel disease, and family history of colorectal cancer. A low-residue, high-fat diet has also been indicated as a risk factor.

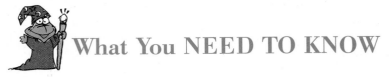

What You NEED TO KNOW

Clinical Manifestations

Symptoms are generally vague until the disease is advanced; they also differ depending on the location of the tumor. Rectal bleeding is the most common symptom of left-sided colorectal cancer. Additionally, alternating constipation, diarrhea, and a change in stool (ribbonlike and narrow) are common. Symptoms

Answers: 1. true; 2. false; adenocarcinomas make up the majority of gastric cancers; 3. true; 4. false; the symptoms of gastric cancer are frequently confused with peptic ulcer disease; 5. true; 6. true; 7. false; the prognosis for gastric cancer is 15% for 5-year survival as most tumors metastasize.

of obstruction occur as the tumor grows. Right-sided lesions are usually asymptomatic. Nonspecific abdominal pain, anemia, and occult bleeding may be present. Arterial bleeding (bright, bright red) from the rectum is most frequently a result of one of two causes: colorectal cancer or diverticular disease. In both cases, the sign is grim.

Prognosis

The prognosis of colorectal cancer depends on the degree of cancer involvement at the time of diagnosis. Unfortunately, most colorectal cancer remains unrecognized until it is in the advanced stages. The overall 5-year survival rate is 50%.

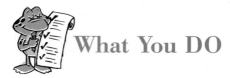

What You DO

Treatment

Surgery is the only curative treatment available for colorectal cancer. The type of surgery depends on the location and extent of cancer growth. The tumor and a section of colon on either side of the tumor are removed. This procedure is known as a colon resection. When the tumor is located within the intestine, a colostomy may be created during the surgical procedure. A colostomy is a connection between the bowel and an opening on the abdominal wall through which bowel contents can be excreted. A colostomy can be either temporary or permanent, depending on the surgical procedure required.

A temporary colostomy allows the bowel to rest and repair when attachment of the proximal bowel to the remaining segment of distal bowel (reanastomosis) is anticipated. A permanent colostomy provides fecal diversion for the rest of the patient's life. An abdominal perineal resection (APR) is performed when invasive rectal tumors require removal of surrounding tissue and the development of a permanent colostomy. Radiation and chemotherapy are used as adjuncts to decrease tumor size and prevent further metastasis.

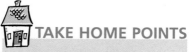

See Chapter 1D in RWNSG: *Pharmacology*

Nursing Responsibilities

For the patient with colorectal carcinoma, the nurse should:
* Promote nutritional status while monitoring intake, output, and daily weights.
* Monitor for postoperative complications, such as infection, deep vein thrombosis, hemorrhage, and wound healing.
* Provide education for the patient and family regarding the diagnosis and treatment regimen.
* Provide education for the patient and family regarding the care and maintenance of a colostomy.
* Support the patient and family during diagnosis and treatment of disease.
* Help the patient and family develop effective coping mechanisms.
* Provide support to the patient and family regarding changes in body image.

TAKE HOME POINTS

Patients with colorectal cancer require a great deal of support and education to deal with both the diagnosis and the treatment.

Do You UNDERSTAND?

DIRECTIONS: **Complete the following crossword puzzle.**

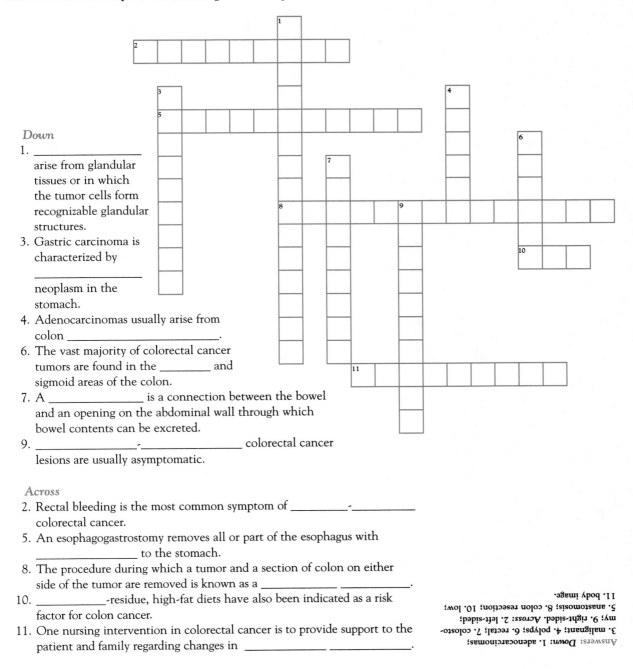

Down

1. _____ arise from glandular tissues or in which the tumor cells form recognizable glandular structures.
3. Gastric carcinoma is characterized by _____ neoplasm in the stomach.
4. Adenocarcinomas usually arise from colon _____.
6. The vast majority of colorectal cancer tumors are found in the _____ and sigmoid areas of the colon.
7. A _____ is a connection between the bowel and an opening on the abdominal wall through which bowel contents can be excreted.
9. _____-_____ colorectal cancer lesions are usually asymptomatic.

Across

2. Rectal bleeding is the most common symptom of _____-_____ colorectal cancer.
5. An esophagogastrostomy removes all or part of the esophagus with _____ to the stomach.
8. The procedure during which a tumor and a section of colon on either side of the tumor are removed is known as a _____ _____.
10. _____-residue, high-fat diets have also been indicated as a risk factor for colon cancer.
11. One nursing intervention in colorectal cancer is to provide support to the patient and family regarding changes in _____ _____.

Genitourinary and Renal Systems

SECTION A
INFECTIOUS DISEASES OF THE GENITOURINARY TRACT

Urinary tract infections (UTIs) are commonly occurring disorders that result from pathogenic microorganisms. UTIs are classified according to the site of the infection. The two UTIs that are important to understand are cystitis (bladder infection) and pyelonephritis (kidney infection).

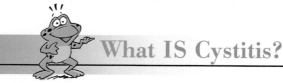

What IS Cystitis?

Pathogenesis

The bladder is the second most common infection site in the body, second only to the respiratory tract. Cystitis is an inflammation of the bladder wall, usually resulting from ascending bacteria. *Enterobacter, Klebsiella, Proteus, Serratia,* and *Pseudomonas* are present in some patients. Fungal infections of the bladder are on the rise because of the overuse of antibiotics that alter the normal flora and fauna of the urinary tract.

The bladder and urine are normally resistant to infection because the lining of the bladder is composed of mucin-producing cells. These cells maintain the integrity of the bladder lining, which prevents inflammation and damage. However, the presence of pathogenic organisms in the bladder acts as an irritant. The irritation triggers the inflammatory response with an inappropriate need to void (micturition).

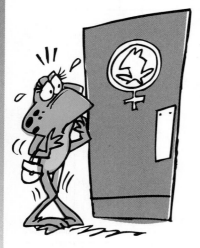

At-Risk Populations

Cystitis is more common in women; 25% of women develop cystitis sometime in their lives. The female urethra is short and close to the anus and vaginal opening, thus increasing the possibility of bacterial contamination. Cystitis is uncommon in adult men, except for those with a sexually transmitted disease, prostate enlargement, or those with structural deformity of the genitourinary (GU) tract that contributes to urinary stasis. The length of the urethra and perhaps the antibacterial properties of prostatic fluid reduce the risk of cystitis in men.

Individuals also at risk for cystitis include patients with urinary stasis and alkaline urine because these factors provide a favorable environment for microorganisms to grow. Anything that breaks down the integrity of the bladder lining leads to possible infection, such as an indwelling catheter, urinary tract instrumentation, and frequent or traumatic sexual intercourse. People with diabetes mellitus, a neurogenic bladder, poor hygiene, or a history of recurrent bladder infections are at risk.

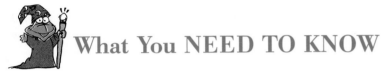 **What You NEED TO KNOW**

Clinical Manifestations

The cardinal signs and symptoms of infection are frequency, urgency, burning pain on urination (dysuria), voiding in small amounts, incomplete emptying of the bladder, and low back or suprapubic pain. The patient may also have malaise, chills, fever, and nausea; vomiting can occur when the ureters are also inflamed. Assessment may reveal cloudy urine, blood in the urine (hematuria), and abdominal or flank pain, which may indicate pyelonephritis.

Bacterial counts of 1000 to 10,000/ml (for voided specimens) may indicate cystitis, particularly when the patient has the cardinal signs and symptoms of infection. A colony count of 10,000/ml indicates an active infectious process in a catheterized specimen. In contrast, one third of patients with symptoms of cystitis have no bacteria in the urine. This finding is then known as interstitial cystitis and is not considered as an infectious disease of the urinary tract.

Asymptomatic cystitis occurs most commonly in older adults, with the only clinical manifestation being a change in their mental status. Of those with positive urine cultures, 10% are asymptomatic.

Prognosis

Generally, cystitis infections are uncomplicated and resolve spontaneously. The prognosis for cystitis depends on whether it is an uncomplicated or complicated case of cystitis, as well as on the patient's clinical manifestations, immune status, and presence of risk factors. The prognosis is good in a patient who exhibits mild symptoms. Complicated cystitis is characterized by the presence of more serious clinical manifestations. Prolonged, advanced cases of cystitis can lead to bladder ulceration or necrosis.

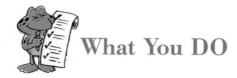

What You DO

Treatment

The treatment for cystitis depends on its severity. Ordinarily, no treatment is required for the patient who has asymptomatic bacteruria. Urinary tract antimicrobials (e.g., sulfamethoxazole-trimethoprim [Bactrim]) are provided to patients with asymptomatic bacteruria who are scheduled to undergo urologic surgery. Urinary tract antimicrobial or antiseptic medications (e.g., nitrofurantoin [Macrodantin]) are used for patients who have an acute but uncomplicated infection. Urinary tract analgesics (e.g., phenazopyridine [Pyridium]) may be used for symptom relief.

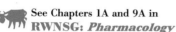

See Chapters 1A and 9A in RWNSG: *Pharmacology*

An additional intervention includes minimizing the use of indwelling catheters. Acidifying urine and optimizing hydration are also important measures in treating the underlying causes of the cystitis. Surgical intervention may be required for the patient who has a structural defect of the GU tract that predisposes the patient to cystitis.

Nursing Responsibilities

For patients with cystitis, the nurse should:

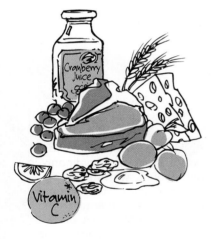

- Identify patients who are at risk for cystitis and assess for signs and symptoms of cystitis.
- Maintain optimal hydration (at least 3 L daily) while monitoring intake and output.
- Teach the patient about the importance of an acid-ash diet (e.g., cranberry juice, meats, eggs, cheese, prunes, cranberries, plums, whole grains, vitamin C) to help acidify the urine.
- Administer medications as ordered.
- Monitor the results of urinalysis, urine culture, and sensitivity tests.
- Provide patient and family teaching regarding primary prevention strategies, such as wiping front to back after bowel movements; showering rather than bathing in a tub; voiding and drinking a glass of water after intercourse; wearing cotton underwear and avoiding wearing pantyhose with slacks, tight jeans, or sitting around in a wet bathing suit; avoiding feminine hygiene sprays and other irritants, such as perfumed toilet paper or sanitary pads; voiding every 2 hours; using a water soluble lubricant for coitus, especially after menopause; inserting urinary catheters using strict aseptic techniques; and maintaining closed urinary drainage systems for patients with indwelling catheters.

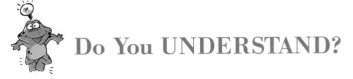

Do You UNDERSTAND?

DIRECTIONS: **Indicate in the space provided whether the statement is** *true* **or** *false*. **If false, then correct the statement in the margin space to the right to make it true.**

_____ 1. People with symptoms of interstitial cystitis rarely have bacteria in the urine.

_____ 2. No treatment is required for acute uncomplicated infection.

_____ 3. Generally, cystitis is uncomplicated and resolves spontaneously.

_____ 4. Cystitis is more common in men.

What IS Pyelonephritis?

Pathogenesis

Pyelonephritis is an inflammation of the kidney pelvis and parenchyma from a bacterial infection. Pyelonephritis can occur as an acute episode or progress into a chronic, persistent, or recurrent disorder. The two forms differ, primarily in their clinical manifestations and long-term effects. One or both kidneys can be affected.

The most common cause of pyelonephritis is *Escherichia coli*, although viruses or fungi can also cause the infection. *Proteus* or *Pseudomonas* may also be isolated in a urine culture. Causative organisms spread to the kidney through the bloodstream, or they ascend through the urinary tract. The presence of pathogenic organisms in the kidney acts as an irritant. The irritation triggers the inflammatory response with an increase in the number of white blood cells. The inflammation leads to edema and swelling of the involved tissues. The inflammatory response is usually focal and irregular, affecting the kidney pelvis, calyces, and medulla. As the infection is treated, fibrosis and scar tissue form. If the infection recurs, more and more scar tissue develops, which leads to fibrosis and altered tubular reabsorption and secretion.

At-Risk Populations

Pyelonephritis is most common in women, and the risk increases with age. Other individuals at risk for pyelonephritis include those who have alkaline urine. Alkaline urine, particularly when associated with a kidney stone or neurogenic bladder, provides a favorable environment for organisms to grow.

Risk factors for acute pyelonephritis include urinary tract instrumentation and female sexual trauma. People with a history of recurrent bladder infections or chronic urinary tract obstruction with reflux are at an increased risk.

Bacteruria is more common among pregnant women, as compared with nonpregnant women in the same age group. Pregnancy is also associated with increased risk for pyelonephritis because of urinary stasis from mechanical obstruction and ureteral relaxation.

Answers: 1. true; 2. false; treatment is needed for an acute uncomplicated infection; 3. true; 4. false; cystitis is more common in women.

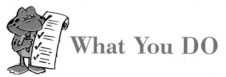

What You NEED TO KNOW

Clinical Manifestations

The signs and symptoms of acute pyelonephritis are related to the degree of infection and include frequency, dysuria, costovertebral angle (CVA) tenderness, flank or groin pain, headache, muscular pain, and general prostration. The pain is described as colicky, radiating down the ureter or toward the epigastric region in the abdomen. The patient typically appears to be in acute distress and may appear intoxicated. The patient frequently experiences symptoms of cystitis for several days. Urine may be cloudy or bloody, foul smelling, and contain a large number of white blood cell casts and white blood cells. Older adults with pyelonephritis may experience gastrointestinal (GI) and respiratory symptoms but no fever.

The signs and symptoms of chronic pyelonephritis are similar to those present in the acute phase of pyelonephritis, although early symptoms are frequently minimal or vague. Chronic pyelonephritis is frequently diagnosed incidentally when the patient is evaluated for hypertension or its complications. Hypertension is the most common sign of the disease. Chronic pyelonephritis gradually progresses to diffuse scarring, atrophy of functional units in the kidney, and renal failure.

Prognosis

Acute pyelonephritis rarely leads to renal failure but is associated with the development of perinephric abscesses, renal abscesses, emphysematous pyelonephritis, and chronic pyelonephritis. Chronic pyelonephritis can lead to renal failure.

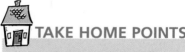

What You DO

Treatment

Treatment of pyelonephritis includes attention to the underlying cause. The use of urinary tract antimicrobial drugs is based on the results of urine culture and sensitivity. The usual routine involves parenteral antibiotics for 3 to 5 days until the patient has been without a fever (afebrile) for 24 to 48 hours. Oral antibiotics follow for a period of 2 to 4 weeks. Urinary tract analgesics are used as needed for symptom relief. Acidifying the urine and optimizing hydration aid recovery. Most importantly, hypertension must be controlled. Additional drug therapy may be required to correct any predisposing factors.

Surgical intervention may be needed for patients who have structural defects that predispose them to pyelonephritis. Intravenous (IV) pyelography and cystoscopy procedures are used to identify structural defects amenable to surgical correction.

TAKE HOME POINTS

A urine culture is needed to differentiate pyelonephritis from cystitis.

The kidneys of older adults are less able to recover from a severe infection, thus antibiotic therapy should be chosen and carefully administered. The normal changes of aging alter the distribution and concentration of drugs in the body.

 See Chapters 1A and 9A in RWNSG: *Pharmacology*

Nursing Responsibilities

For the patient with pyelonephritis, the nurse should:

- Identify patients who are at risk for the disorder and assess for signs and symptoms of pyelonephritis.
- Monitor the results of urinalysis and urine culture and sensitivity.
- Maintain optimal hydration, minimizing nausea and vomiting, and monitoring intake and output.
- Provide an acid-ash diet (e.g., cranberry juice, meats, eggs, cheese, prunes, cranberries, plums, whole grains, vitamin C) to acidify urine.
- Administer antibiotics and analgesic medications as ordered.
- Provide patient and family teaching about ways to prevent recurrent infections and the importance of follow-up care after the infection has been resolved.

Do You UNDERSTAND?

DIRECTIONS: **Indicate in the space provided whether the statement is *true* or *false*. If false, then correct the statement in the margin space to the right to make it true.**

_____ 1. Pyelonephritis is defined as an inflammation of the urethra.

_____ 2. Pyelonephritis can occur as an acute episode or progress into a chronic disorder that is persistent or recurrent.

_____ 3. The primary cause of pyelonephritis is fungal.

_____ 4. One or both kidneys can be affected in pyelonephritis.

SECTION B
OBSTRUCTIVE DISORDERS OF THE GENITOURINARY TRACT

What IS Renal Calculi?

Pathogenesis

Kidney stones (renal calculi) are hardened clusters of organic crystals. Although kidney stones can form anywhere in the urinary tract, the most frequent site of stone formation is in the kidneys.

Three factors must be present for a kidney stone to form: saturated urine, organic material to serve as the basis for stone formation, and deficiency of substances that hinder stone formation. Individuals born with abnormally high production of mucoproteins and a deficiency in substances that bind stone-forming material (inhibitors) are at an increased risk for forming kidney stones.

Answers: 1. false; pyelonephritis is an inflammation of the pelvis of the kidney; 2. true; 3. false; the primary cause of pyelonephritis is bacterial. 4. true.

Extremely high concentrations of stone-forming crystals also promote stone formation. Urine pH, temperature, ionic strength, and concentration of urine can increase the concentration of stone-forming substrates.

Calcium is the most common stone-forming substance, although stones can also form as a result of high concentrations of other substances, such as uric acid, cystine, and struvite. Struvite kidney stones are also called *infective stones*.

Urinary organic matter (mostly mucoproteins) provides a structure for the deposit of crystals. As crystals become trapped in the organic matter, a stone is formed. Stones that are sufficiently small to pass through the urinary tract have no medical consequences. However, larger stones may be unable to pass, causing the patient severe coliclike pain as these stones stretch the ureters. Kidney stones increase the risk of urinary obstruction and infection.

At-Risk Populations

Stone formation is more frequent in the patient with a family history of kidney stones or metabolic disorders (e.g., overactive parathyroid gland) that increases serum calcium levels. A previous kidney stone places the patient at an increased risk for forming another kidney stone. When no medical treatment is provided, 50% of patients will form another stone within 5 years. Anything that increases the concentration of the urine (e.g., dehydration) or that causes urinary stasis (e.g., immobility) places the patient at risk for stone formation. Certain medications can facilitate the formation of kidney stones. For example, patients with human immunodeficiency virus (HIV) who are taking indinavir (Crixivan), a protease inhibitor drug, are prone to forming kidney stones unless they can be properly hydrated.

The incidence of stone formation is greatest in the summer months and in areas of high humidity and high temperatures (southeastern United States). Massive doses of vitamin C and certain medications also contribute to high concentrations of stone-forming substances.

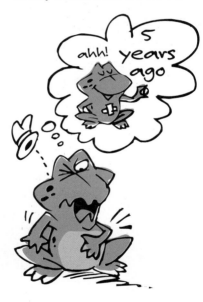

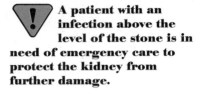

A patient with an infection above the level of the stone is in need of emergency care to protect the kidney from further damage.

Caucasian men between the ages of 20 and 40 are three times more likely to form kidney stones than are women.

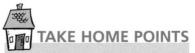

TAKE HOME POINTS

History of kidney stones, dehydration, and immobility increases the patient's risk of forming kidney stones.

What You NEED TO KNOW

Clinical Manifestations

The signs and symptoms of kidney stones are related to obstruction of the urinary tract. The manifestations include a sudden, severe pain in the back and side that may radiate to the abdomen and into the testis or labium. The pain may be described as colicky, cramping, dull, achy, or as having a heavy feeling. The patient may be restless and unable to find a position of comfort. Urgency and urinary frequency may be noted when the stone is lodged where the ureter joins the bladder. Blood is frequently present in the urine (hematuria). Nausea, vomiting, pallor, and sweating (diaphoresis) may be present with severe pain. Fever and chills indicate that an infection is present.

Prognosis

Most kidney stones pass spontaneously. Of those patients with kidney stones, 20% require medical intervention. The greatest dangers are obstruction and kidney infection; either could lead to the loss of a kidney.

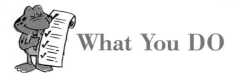

What You DO

Treatment

The goal of therapy is to prevent kidney damage from obstruction or infection and to prevent further stone formation. Treatment of acute episodes of kidney stones is based on the size of the stone. Stones that are less than 6 mm in diameter usually pass spontaneously. However, appropriate pain management is important. Because pain is thought to be related to prostaglandin E2, nonsteroidal anti-inflammatory drugs (NSAIDs) give as much or better pain relief as opioid analgesics. Antiemetic medications may be used if pain relief does not eliminate the nausea and vomiting. When required, IV medications may be given. The urine should be strained after each voiding for stones that have passed.

Stones greater than 6 mm in diameter are frequently removed using an instrument placed through the skin and into the kidney. The stones are broken down and the pieces removed. Kidney stones can also be removed through a procedure known as *extracorporeal shockwave lithotripsy* (ESWL), during which the stones are broken down using sound waves and then allowed to pass through the urinary system. Stone removal from the ureters may also be accomplished using a special instrument (ureteroscope). The ureteroscope is passed through the urethra and bladder and into the ureter for stone removal. Surgical removal of the stones may be needed if all other strategies for removal have failed.

When the kidney stones are infected, immediate drainage of the infected kidney is required. A special instrument is inserted through the skin and into the kidney. The kidney is then drained of the infectious materials. This procedure includes the use of IV antibiotics and the placement of a special drainage apparatus (ureteral stent) that allows infected material and urine to drain.

Modalities that are used to prevent further stone formation include developing a life-long habit of increased fluid intake (10 to 12 large glasses of water per 24 hours). Daily consumption of coffee, tea, beer, or wine may decrease the risk of stone formation; consumption of apple or grapefruit juice increases the risk of stone formation.

The patient may be given medications that control the acid or alkali nature of the urine. Allopurinol (Zyloprim) reduces the risk of forming kidney stones in patients with high urinary calcium or uric acid levels. Thiazide diuretics such as hydrochlorothiazide (HydroDIURIL) help increase the elimination of calcium. Sodium cellulose phosphate helps bind calcium in the intestines for elimination in the stool. A number of other drugs can be used to reduce the quantity of cystine or struvite in the body thus reducing the risk of stone formation.

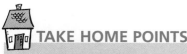
TAKE HOME POINTS
The severity of the signs and symptoms do not directly correlate with the size of the stone.

Kidney stones can be life threatening when associated with kidney infection; however, death related to kidney stones is rare.

See Chapters 8, 11, and 14 in RWNSG: *Pharmacology*

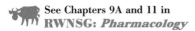
See Chapters 9A and 11 in RWNSG: *Pharmacology*

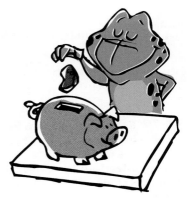

Nursing Responsibilities

For the patient with kidney stones, the nurse should:

- Obtain the patient's history, including dietary habits and risk factors such as medications, history of urinary tract infections or gout, and mobility status.
- Monitor the patient for signs and symptoms of obstruction or infections, such as fever and chills, pain, nausea, vomiting, and irritative voiding behaviors (e.g., frequency, urgency, incontinence).
- Monitor laboratory results of white blood cell counts and urinalysis for evidence of infection or the presence of blood.
- Provide adequate pain management through medication before pain is out of control.
- Encourage a high normal fluid intake (10 to 12 glasses of water per 24 hours).
- Strain all urine and save any stones that are captured for laboratory analysis.

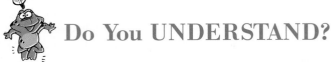

Do You UNDERSTAND?

DIRECTIONS: **Provide short answers to the following questions.**

1. Based on what you know about the formation of kidney stones, what do you think should be areas of research to prevent kidney stone formation?

2. What would you include in a teaching plan for a patient who has a kidney stone?

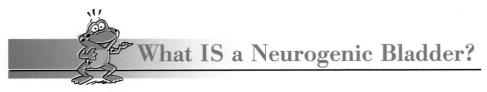

What IS a Neurogenic Bladder?

Pathogenesis

A neurogenic bladder is one that has lost its response to nervous system stimulation. When all nerve response is lost, the bladder does not receive the impulses that cause muscle relaxation or contraction. Additionally, the brain does not receive the message that the bladder is filling. The interruption causes the loss of voluntary bladder control or loss of bladder sensation, which results in urinary retention and, eventually, overflow incontinence. The patient is at risk for infection and backup of urine into the kidney.

Five classifications of a neurogenic bladder have been identified. The classifications are organized into those caused by upper motor neuron involvement and those caused by lower motor neuron involvement.

Answers: 1. Studies that examine how we predict or screen those at risk for getting stones; genetic studies to determine whether there are genes that increase the risk of stone formation; studies that examine the substances that inhibit stone formation and whether they should be given to patients who are at risk for stone formation. 2. Drinking at least 10 to 12 large glasses of water every day; monitoring for signs and symptoms of infection; teaching the importance of exercise, purpose of medications, and role of calcium and uric acid in stone formation.

Upper motor neuron–related neurogenic bladder disorders:

1. *Uninhibited.* Loss of cortical inhibition
2. *Reflex or automatic,* Reflex arc maintained below the level of the lesion with spontaneous voiding
3. *Autonomous.* Loss of cortical inhibition and interruption of spinal reflexes

Lower motor neuron–related neurogenic bladder disorders:

1. *Motor paralysis.* Intact sensory functions
2. *Sensory paralysis.* Intact motor functions

The causes, clinical manifestations, and treatments are displayed in the table that follows.

Treatments for Neurogenic Bladder

TYPE	CAUSES	CLINICAL MANIFESTATIONS	TREATMENT
Uninhibited	Lack of voluntary control in infancy Multiple sclerosis	Small urine volume Frequency, urgency, incontinence, enuresis	Anticholinergic medications
Reflex or automatic	Spinal cord transection Spinal cord tumors Multiple sclerosis above T12	Involuntary voiding Incomplete emptying of bladder Urinary retention and infection	Catheter or condom drainage Bladder training
Autonomous	Sacral cord trauma Herniated disk Surgeries with damage to pelvic parasympathetic nerves	Overflow incontinence	Catheter Urinary diversion surgery
Motor paralysis	Spinal cord lesions at S2-4 Poliomyelitis Trauma Tumors	Overflow incontinence	Manual compression of bladder (Crede's maneuver)
Sensory paralysis	Damage to lumbar nerve roots Diabetes mellitus Degeneration of dorsal column of spinal cord and sensory nerve trunks	Dribbling Overflow incontinence Loss of sensation of bladder fullness	Bladder training

At-Risk Populations

Individuals with trauma to the brain or spinal cord and those who have a neurologic condition, such as Parkinson's disease, multiple sclerosis, stroke, or damage to the nerves from tumors, are at risk for a neurogenic bladder. Patients who have poorly controlled diabetes and those with UTIs are also at risk.

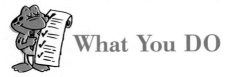

What You NEED TO KNOW

Clinical Manifestations

The signs and symptoms of a neurogenic bladder include incontinence or urinary retention, loss of sensation to void, and loss of the ability to void spontaneously.

Prognosis

The prognosis for a patient with neurogenic bladder depends on the cause of the nerve damage. Currently, no method is available to repair nerves that are damaged within the central nervous system.

What You DO

Madigan Army Medical Center: Neurogenic Bladder

http://www.mamc.amedd.army. mil/williams/GU/Bladder/ Neurogenic/Neurogenic.htm

See Chapter 2C in RWNSG: *Pharmacology*

Treatment

Treatment depends on the type of neurogenic bladder. The table on page 269 identifies possible treatment modalities.

For some patients, surgical intervention is indicated. An artificial sphincter can be created when the urinary sphincter is not working. Interrupting the nerve innervation to the bladder reflex may help the patient with an uninhibited bladder. Electrodes that interfere with reflex bladder contractions can be implanted. Drug therapy can also be used for some patients. The use of baclofen (Lioresal), a skeletal muscle-relaxing drug, may help some patients. The drug decreases the frequency and amplitude of bladder muscle spasms through an action in the spinal cord.

Nursing Responsibilities

For the patient with a neurogenic bladder, the nurse should:

- Teach the patient about ways to recognize a UTI and to perform self-catheterization; educate the patient about a bladder training program and ways to protect the skin from breakdown.
- Link the patient with effective support systems.
- Assess for signs and symptoms of urinary retention and infection.
- Assess for skin breakdown caused by urine leakage.
- Assess for signs of excessive autonomic response (e.g., hypertension, bradycardia, headache, blurred vision).

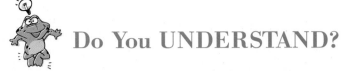

Do You UNDERSTAND?

DIRECTIONS: Provide short answers to the following questions.

1. A patient has had a stroke that results in the loss of the regulatory tracts for bladder control. What signs and symptoms will this patient have?

2. Why does a patient with paralyzed bladder muscles have incontinence?

3. What are the risks associated with a neurogenic bladder?

SECTION C

GLOMERULAR DISORDERS OF THE GENITOURINARY TRACT

What IS Glomerulonephritis?

Pathogenesis

Glomerulonephritis is usually an autoimmune response that results in inflammation of the glomeruli. Acute glomerulonephritis comes on rapidly and is self-limiting 95% of the time. For the remaining 5%, the disorder becomes chronic, and glomeruli damage is more gradual. However, one rare form of the disease progresses rapidly (rapidly progressive glomerulonephritis), resulting in end-stage renal disease (ESRD) within a few weeks. The most common cause of glomerulonephritis in the United States is IgA nephropathy (a deposit of IgA antibodies in the glomeruli). However, anything that causes inflammation of the glomeruli can cause glomerulonephritis, including drugs, toxins, vascular disorders, and systemic diseases (e.g., lupus erythematosus).

Two types of acute glomerulonephritis have been identified: infectious glomerulonephritis and postinfectious glomerulonephritis. Infectious glomerulonephritis develops within a few days of an infection. Bacterial, viral, or parasitic infections are the primary causes. Postinfectious glomerulonephritis occurs 14 to

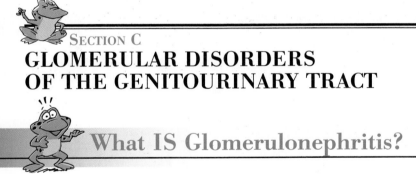

21 days after the infection that caused the damaging antigen-antibody complexes to be formed. It is frequently the result of a type A beta-hemolytic strep infection, although other organisms can also cause the immune response.

In glomerulonephritis, antigen-antibody complexes left over from an infection somewhere in the body are sent through the bloodstream to the kidneys for elimination. Most of the antigen-antibody complexes are filtered from the blood to become part of the urine. Occasionally, antigen-antibody complexes are simply the wrong size. Rather than passing into the urine, these complexes become lodged in the tiny openings of the glomerulus, the presence of which excites the immune system and an inflammatory response is initiated. White blood cells (macrophages) destroy antigen-antibody complexes.

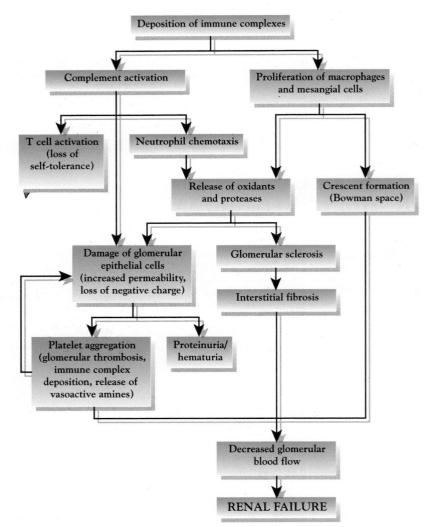

The cells and chemicals that are part of an inflammatory response injure the glomerulus. The damaged cells allow large molecules such as proteins and red blood cells to move from the circulation into the filtrate of the kidneys. The kidneys' tubule cells cannot move these large molecules back into the capillaries that surround the tubules and are thus lost to the urine.

At-Risk Populations

People with autoimmune diseases such as systemic lupus erythematosus are also at risk. The incidence of acute glomerulonephritis decreases with age, although adults between the ages of 40 and 60 are at the greatest risk for the rapidly progressing form of glomerulonephritis.

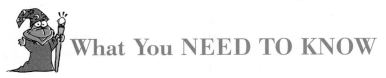

What You NEED TO KNOW

Clinical Manifestations

The patient with acute glomerulonephritis experiences a sudden onset of symptoms, including protein in the urine (proteinuria), blood in the urine (hematuria), and hypertension. The patient may have decreased or no urine output (oliguria or anuria) for several days. Signs of infection such as fever, chills, nausea, and vomiting may also be noted. Occasionally, generalized edema is observed.

Chronic glomerulonephritis develops slowly and may not be recognized for several years. Symptoms of chronic glomerulonephritis include the signs and symptoms of renal insufficiency or failure, such as fatigue, mental sluggishness, edema, and dizziness. Excessive urine output (polyuria) develops as a result of the kidney's inability to concentrate urine. High blood pressure, severe anemia, hematuria, proteinuria, and casts of white blood cells and kidney tubular cells in the urine may also be present.

Prognosis

In acute glomerulonephritis, symptoms start to subside in approximately 14 days, although full recovery may take from weeks to months. Generally, the damaged cells are repaired and normal kidney function returns. Of those patients with acute, self-limiting glomerulonephritis, 95% experience a full recovery.

With chronic glomerulonephritis, the damaged cells fail to heal and are gradually replaced with scar tissue. As more and more scar tissue forms, normal kidney function is lost. Although chronic glomerulonephritis progresses at variable rates, in some patients it can progress to ESRD.

Children have the highest risk for acute glomerulonephritis, although any individual with an untreated type A beta-hemolytic strep infection is susceptible. The incidence of acute glomerulonephritis decreases with age.

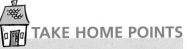

TAKE HOME POINTS

The longer oliguria lasts, the worse the chances are for a full recovery. Any damage remaining after 2 years is likely permanent.

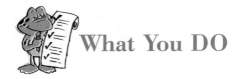

What You DO

Treatment

No specific treatment is available that will repair damaged kidneys. The goal is to prevent further damage and allow the kidneys to heal. Treatment includes antibiotics to treat infections, drug therapy to decrease immune system damage, and removal of antibodies from the circulation (plasmapheresis) to decrease immune response. Dialysis or kidney transplant may be required in some patients.

See Chapters 1A, 3, 7, and 9A in RWNSG: *Pharmacology*

Nursing Responsibilities

For the patient with acute glomerulonephritis, the nurse should:
- Obtain a complete history of recent infections or invasive procedures.
- Monitor and recognize complications.
- Assess the severity of the patient's edema.
- Monitor the patient's vital signs (particularly blood pressure), intake and output, and daily weights.
- Examine the urine for color, amount, and abnormal substances.
- Teach the patient and family about the disorder and the need to limit protein, sodium, and potassium intake, as appropriate.

For the patient with chronic glomerulonephritis, the nurse should:
- Monitor the patient for signs of renal failure (see Section D).
- Provide symptomatic relief.
- Assist the patient and family in developing support systems for coping with a chronic illness.
- Provide supportive therapy if the glomerulonephritis leads to kidney failure.

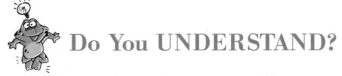

Do You UNDERSTAND?

DIRECTIONS: Provide short answers to the following questions.

1. Why is it important to treat strep infections early?

2. Why is protein found in the urine of patients with glomerulonephritis?

3. How would greater knowledge of the immune system help treat this disease?

Answers: 1. Antigen-antibody complexes that build up can cause an inflammatory response and damage the kidneys; 2. The inflammation and subsequent damage to the kidney by glomerulonephritis allows large molecules through the glomeruli that would ordinarily not be lost to the urine; 3. If ways to stop the inflammation from occurring could be found, the damage to the kidneys would not occur.

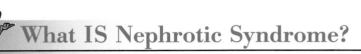

What IS Nephrotic Syndrome?

Pathogenesis

Nephrotic syndrome is not a disease; rather, it is the manifestation of protein wasting that occurs with glomerular damage. In a normal kidney, protein molecules are too large to enter the filtrate (what will become urine) and remain in the body. However, with glomerular damage from disease, "holes" in the glomeruli allow the large protein molecules to become part of the filtrate and eventually part of the urine. This protein loss is difficult to replace with dietary measures.

The cause of nephrotic syndrome is loss of plasma proteins, particularly albumin, to the urine. As much as 30 g of protein may be lost in a single day. The protein is lost because the glomeruli have been damaged from medications, toxins, or disease, which causes them to be abnormally permeable. The most common cause of nephrotic syndrome is glomerulonephritis. However, systemic disorders such as diabetes mellitus, systemic lupus erythematosus, hepatitis B, leukemia, infectious disease, or preeclampsia can also cause nephrotic syndrome.

When protein is lost from the plasma, the pressure that draws fluid from the spaces between cells (interstitial spaces) back into the circulation is greatly reduced. As the concentration of protein decreases intravenously, the *pressure* for water to move to the higher concentration of proteins increases. This causes loss of fluid in the circulation and leads to decreased fluid volume (hypovolemia) and low blood pressure. The excess fluid in the tissues results in edema.

A satisfactory blood pressure reading and adequate renal perfusion is required for the kidneys to filter blood. When blood pressure decreases, the kidneys release renin, which raises blood pressure and causes the release of aldosterone. Aldosterone increases the amount of sodium and water retained by the kidneys. This extra fluid also leaks out of the capillaries, which further contributes to the developing edema.

Complications of nephrotic syndrome include severe deficit of circulating fluids, blood clot formation in the renal vein, abnormal thyroid function, and softening of the bones (osteomalacia). The patient also has an increased susceptibility to infections.

At-Risk Populations

No specific age group is at higher risk than is any other group. Anyone with a disorder that permits the kidneys to filter plasma proteins into the urine is at risk for nephrotic syndrome. Predisposing risk factors to nephrotic syndrome include allergic drug reactions. Drugs that are associated with nephrotic syndrome include anticonvulsants, probenecid, captopril, gold salts, NSAIDs, penicillamine, and heroin.

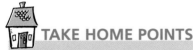

TAKE HOME POINTS

Nephrotic syndrome is the combination of signs and symptoms that occur with protein wasting from kidney disease. The major problems are hypovolemia and edema.

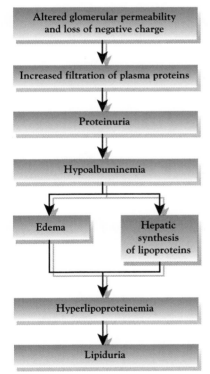

See Chapter 12 in **RWNSG:** *Pharmacology*

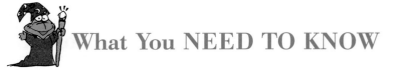

What You NEED TO KNOW

Clinical Manifestations

The signs and symptoms of nephrotic syndrome are the result of protein loss and accumulation of extracellular fluid. The classical signs include protein in the urine, a decrease in the amount of protein (particularly albumin) in the plasma, and edema. Edema is usually the patient's primary complaint.

High levels of fats in the blood are thought to result from the liver's increased synthesis of lipoproteins. Depending on the severity of kidney involvement, patients have some degree of anemia. Other manifestations of nephrotic syndrome include loss of appetite, fatigue and malaise, irritability, abnormal menses or stoppage of menstrual periods (amenorrhea), and depression.

Serum albumin concentrations may drop as low as 1.0 to 2.5 g/dl. Some hematuria may be present. Large amounts of protein are present in the urine. The amount of protein lost in the urine may reflect losses of 4 to 30 g/day.

Prognosis

The prognosis for the patient with nephrotic syndrome depends on the extent of kidney damage, degree of protein wasting, and extent of edema.

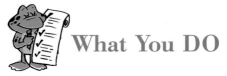

What You DO

Treatment

The goal of treatment is to heal the glomerulus and stop the loss of protein in the urine. Through attention to these two goals, the cycle of edema is broken. Treatment includes mild dietary restrictions of sodium and potassium with a daily intake of 1.0 to 1.5 g of high–biologic-value protein per kilogram of body weight. The protein requirement is designed to prevent further protein breakdown.

Drug therapy includes loop diuretics, such as furosemide (Lasix) and IV administration of protein-based plasma-volume expanders such as albumin (Dextran). Depending on the cause of the disorder, glucocorticosteroids such as prednisone may be used to reduce inflammation. Anticoagulants may be needed to prevent further clot formation if a renal vein thrombosis is present.

See Chapters 3, 7A, and 9A in RWNSG: *Pharmacology*

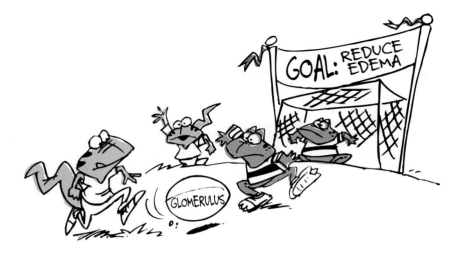

Nursing Responsibilities

For the patient with nephrotic syndrome, the nurse should:

- Teach the patient and family about the underlying cause or causes of the disorder, the importance of diet therapy, and the prevention of infection.
- Monitor vital signs for fluid volume deficit. Assess breath sounds for pulmonary edema as fluid moves into interstitial spaces in the lungs.
- Assess for signs and symptoms of electrolyte imbalance and infection.
- Monitor intake, output, and daily weights.
- Promote adequate dietary intake by monitoring the patient's degree of anorexia, depression, and malaise.
- Assist the patient and family in developing adequate coping skills for a chronic illness.

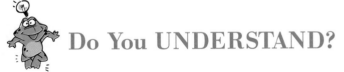

Do You UNDERSTAND?

DIRECTIONS: Select the correct option from the italicized words that makes each statement correct.

1. Nephrotic syndrome is the result of _____ damage and is manifested as the loss of _____ to the urine. (*glomerular/tubular*) (*albumin/red blood cells*)

2. The most common cause of nephrotic syndrome is _____. (*pyelonephritis/glomerulonephritis*)

3. The loss of albumin from the circulation leads to _____ and a subsequent drop in . _____ _____. (*hypervolemia/hypovolemia*) (*blood pressure/heart rate*)

Answers: 1. glomerular; albumin; 2. glomerulonephritis; 3. hypovolemia; blood pressure.

4. When blood pressure _____, the kidneys release _____, which in turn causes the release of (renin/aldosterone). There is a subsequent increase in the amount of _____ that is retained by the kidneys. The extra fluid leaks out of the capillaries into the _____ spaces contributing to the edema seen in nephrotic syndrome.
(increases/decreases) (renin/aldosterone) (sodium/potassium) (interstitial/intravascular)

5. The high levels of fats in the blood are thought to be the result of the liver's _____ synthesis of lipoproteins.
(increased/decreased)

DIRECTIONS: Complete the following sentences.

6. Serum albumin concentrations in the patient with nephrotic syndrome may drop as low as _____.

7. The prognosis for the patient with nephrotic syndrome depends on the extent of _____, degree of _____, and the extent of the _____.

8. Drug therapy for the patient with nephrotic syndrome may include the use of _____, _____, _____, and _____.

9. Assess the patient's _____ for evidence of pulmonary edema.

10. Monitor the patient's vital signs for evidence of _____ _____.

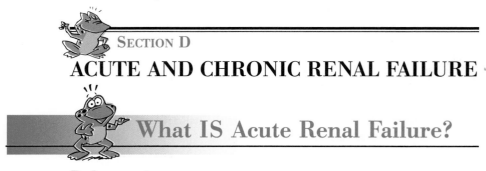

SECTION D

ACUTE AND CHRONIC RENAL FAILURE

What IS Acute Renal Failure?

Pathogenesis

Acute renal failure is the sudden inability of the kidneys to maintain normal function. This inability affects most of the body's systems because of the kidneys' important role in maintaining fluid balance, regulating electrolytes, providing constant protection against acid-base imbalances, and controlling blood pressure. The causes of acute renal failure are generally classified into three major areas: prerenal (associated with poor systemic perfusion and decreased renal blood flow), intrarenal (associated with renal ischemia or toxins), or postrenal (associated with the obstruction of urine flow out of the kidneys).

Answers: 4. decreases; renin; aldosterone; sodium; interstitial; **5.** increased; **6.** 1.0 to 2.5 g/dl; **7.** kidney damage; protein wasting; edema; **8.** furosemide; IV albumin; prednisone; anticoagulants; **9.** breath sounds; **10.** fluid volume deficit.

Prerenal disorders include factors that decrease the amount of blood going to the kidneys. Severe blood loss, burns, septic shock, or massive trauma are major causes of prerenal failure. Prerenal failure may also be related to the systemic inflammation that is present in burns, septic shock, or massive trauma. Decreased blood volume from dehydration, fluid shifting from the vascular tree to interstitial tissue, and congestive heart failure are also prerenal sources of acute kidney failure.

Intrarenal causes of acute renal failure include factors that damage the kidneys themselves. Intrarenal failure can occur as a result of ischemia, physical trauma, infection, inflammation, or exposure to toxic chemicals. Nephrotoxic drugs include the penicillins, sulfonamides, aminoglycosides, tetracyclines, radiographic iodine contrast materials, and heavy metals.

Death of the renal tubule cells (acute tubular necrosis) from decreased renal perfusion and ischemia or from nephrotoxins accounts for the majority of acute renal failure. Glomerulonephritis, pyelonephritis, diabetic sclerosis, thrombus, or narrowing of the renal arteries can also be responsible for acute renal failure.

A postrenal cause of acute renal failure is usually a result of an obstruction in the urinary tract below the level of the kidneys. The obstruction leads to a backup of urine and kidney damage. Obstructions can be from prostatic disease, tumors, narrowing of the ureters or urethra, kidney stones, or neurogenic bladder.

The exact pathogenesis of acute renal failure is unclear. Acute tubular necrosis (ATN) is a major contributing factor to acute renal failure. The renal tubular cells are injured and are no longer able to excrete waste products into the urine or reabsorb needed electrolytes and other molecules from the filtrate in an effective manner. The damaged tubular cells allow leakage of tubular fluid back

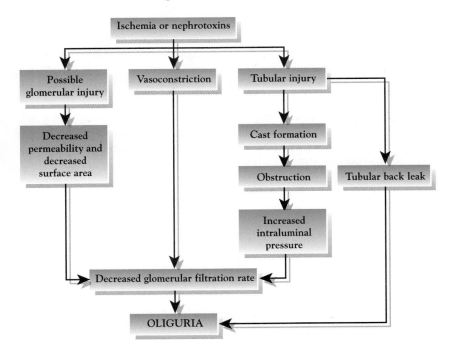

Any episode of severe hypovolemia increases the risk for acute renal failure.

into the interstitial area. Tubular cells may be obstructed by dead cells from tubular cell damage, or they may be damaged from a lack of sufficient blood flow (excessive vasoconstriction or extreme hypovolemia, usually secondary to severe blood or fluid loss). A buildup of waste products in the blood and a loss of important electrolytes to the urine are the result.

At-Risk Populations

The very young and very old are at highest risk for acute renal failure. Any patient who suffers decreased perfusion to the kidneys or who is exposed to kidney toxins is at risk. Patients experiencing trauma, sepsis, or acute blood loss are at the greatest risk for acute renal failure.

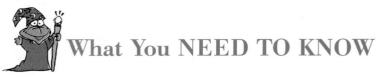 **What You NEED TO KNOW**

Clinical Manifestations

The signs and symptoms of acute renal failure include decreased urinary output (less than 400 to 600 ml/day for 8 to 15 days). Edema, weight gain, anemia, and hypertension develop. Protein in urine (proteinuria) develops, particularly when the cause is glomerulonephritis. The urine is mud-colored when the cause of renal failure is acute tubular necrosis. Elevated blood urea nitrogen (BUN) and creatinine levels and changes in electrolytes are present.

A *diuretic stage* develops at a later point in this disorder; the urinary output increases and the BUN and creatinine levels begin to fall. This stage lasts from 7 to 10 days. The inability to concentrate urine can lead to excessive fluid and electrolyte loss, which, in turn, leads to hypovolemia and hypoperfusion of the kidneys. A *convalescent stage* of renal failure starts the day the BUN is stable and may extend for several months.

Prognosis

The prognosis for the patient with acute renal failure depends on the cause and extent of renal damage. Patients who have decreased urinary output for longer than 15 days may never regain normal kidney function. When renal function has deteriorated to a point that it is no longer adequate to sustain life and the process is considered irreversible, the patient has ESRD.

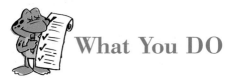 **What You DO**

Treatment

The treatment goal for acute renal failure is to prevent further renal damage and support the kidneys as they heal. Treating reversible problems, such as urinary obstruction, replacing fluid volume, and correcting anemia with the use of packed red blood cells (when anemia is great) provide the means to accomplish this goal. A high-caloric, low-protein diet helps decrease waste products, although protein replacement is used when protein wasting is also present. Electrolyte imbalances are corrected with restrictions in sodium and potassium. Hemodialysis may be necessary to correct fluid volume, electrolyte level, and acid-base imbalances.

Nursing Responsibilities

Prevention is the primary goal. Nurses can have a significant effect on preventing acute renal failure by closely monitoring patients at risk and by understanding the potential toxicity of medications. The nurse should:

- Assess fluid balance by accurately monitoring intake, output, daily weights, and edema.
- Check vital signs, particularly blood pressure.
- Evaluate mucous membranes and skin turgor for signs of dehydration.
- Teach the patient and family about protein intake and dietary restrictions of sodium and potassium.
- Provide or offer frequent oral hygiene techniques to reduce the effects of renal waste products on taste, smell, and integrity of mucous membranes.
- Treat any associated nausea, vomiting, and anorexia.
- Assess for complications of acute renal failure (e.g., pleural effusion, pericarditis, acidosis, uremia); monitor the patient's level of consciousness; assess breathing and heart sounds.
- Prevent secondary infection through good hand-washing practices, providing meticulous skin, respiratory, and central line care; assess for signs and symptoms of infection.
- Teach the patient basic hygiene skills, when necessary.
- Avoid the use of nephrotoxic drugs; use protocols to provide appropriate, adequate dosages.
- Provide psychologic support to help the patient cope with the disorder and required therapy.

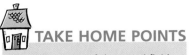

TAKE HOME POINTS

Always be aware of decreased fluid volume, and take precautions to prevent prolonged fluid volume deficit. Assess for urinary obstruction and kidney disease. Early assessment and early intervention can save lives.

Do You UNDERSTAND?

DIRECTIONS: **Match the causes in Column A with each type of renal failure in Column B.**

Column A

_____ 1. Prerenal
_____ 2. Intrarenal
_____ 3. Postrenal

Column B

a. Obstruction of urine flow out of the kidneys
b. Renal ischemia or toxins
c. Poor systemic perfusion and decreased renal blood flow

DIRECTIONS: Indicate in the space provided whether the statement is *true* or *false*. If false, then correct the statement in the margin space to the left to make it true.

_____ 4. Urine is red when the cause of renal failure is acute tubular necrosis.

_____ 5. The very young and the very old are at highest risk for acute renal failure.

_____ 6. Clinical manifestations of acute renal failure include a urine output of less than 400 to 600 ml/day for 8 to 15 days.

What IS Chronic Renal Failure?

Healthy People 2010: Chronic Renal Failure
www.ep.niddk.nih.gov/Divisions/ Kuh/KidneyHP2010.htm

Pathogenesis

Chronic renal failure is a slow, progressive, and irreversible loss of kidney function. Chronic renal failure may follow an episode of acute renal failure, depending on the extent of nephron loss. The causes of chronic renal failure are many but can generally be divided into three groups: (1) those that directly affect the kidney by infection, inflammation, and upper urinary tract obstruction; (2) those in which an obstruction of the lower urinary tract is present; and (3) those associated with systemic diseases and toxicities, such as elevated serum calcium levels, hypertension, disseminated lupus erythematosus, atheroma, and diabetes mellitus.

Whatever the cause, the result of renal failure is destruction of the functional units of the kidneys. The patient has no clinical manifestation of renal failure until 50% or more nephrons no longer function. When the nephrons are lost, body wastes accumulate and fluids and electrolytes become out of balance.

The clinical course of chronic renal failure is described in four stages. A glomerular filtration rate (GFR) between 30 and 75 ml/min suggests chronic renal insufficiency. (A normal GFR is between 100 and 150 ml/min.) In early chronic renal failure, the GFR declines to between 10 and 30 ml/min. The GFR in late renal failure is between 5 and 10 ml/min. In the terminal stages of renal failure, the GFR is less than 5 ml/min. Because all of the creatinine (a by-product of muscle energy metabolism) that is filtered by the kidneys in a given period appears in the urine, the creatinine is equivalent to the GFR.

A decreased production of erythropoietin—a hormone produced by the kidneys to increase red blood cell formation—is present, thus anemia develops. Additionally, a decrease in the activation of vitamin D is present, which leads to decreased absorption of calcium.

The BUN and serum creatinine levels rise. Sodium, calcium, phosphate, and potassium imbalances lead to hypertension, pulmonary edema, altered metabolism, loss of calcium from the bones (osteoporosis), changes in mental status, and peripheral nerve conduction delays. Decreased platelet factor III, decreased fat metabolism, and decreased white blood cell activity contribute to dermatologic problems.

At-Risk Populations

Patients who have diabetes mellitus are at a significant risk for chronic renal failure, particularly when blood sugar levels are not controlled. Patients with long-standing, untreated hypertension are also at risk.

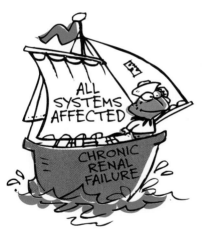

African Americans and Native Americans with diabetes mellitus or long-standing, untreated hypertension are especially at increased risk for developing chronic renal failure and ESRD.

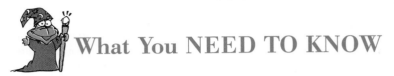

What You NEED TO KNOW

Clinical Manifestations

All body systems are affected by chronic renal failure. The signs and symptoms include the following:

Cardiovascular: Hypertension, arrhythmias, heart failure, pericarditis, atherosclerosis, anemia-clotting factor disorders

Genitourinary: Decreased creatinine clearance, oliguria, anuria

Musculoskeletal: Soft tissue calcifications; osteodystrophy related to phosphate and calcium imbalance; decreased absorption of calcium, which leads to increased stimulation of parathyroid glands; increased loss of calcium from bones; joint swelling and pain

Perceptual: Retinal changes related to hypertension, conjunctival calcification, blurred vision

Reproductive: Decreased libido, infertility, impotence, enlarged mammary glands (gynecomastia)

Dermatologic: Pallor, bruising, pruritus, edema, dry skin, dry hair, altered pigmentation

Gastrointestinal: Decreased appetite, nausea, vomiting, changes in taste and smell (uremic factor), stomatitis, an offensive breath odor (uremic fetor), bloody emesis, blood in the stools, diarrhea, constipation

Respiratory: Pleural effusions, pulmonary edema, deep rapid respirations (Kussmaul's respirations), lack of respirations (apnea).

Neurologic: Numbness, burning, tingling feet, jumpy feeling (peripheral neuropathy) insomnia, irritability, altered level of consciousness, changes in motor function, changes in cognition or behavior

Prognosis

The clinical manifestations of nephron loss are prominent in late renal failure and life threatening in ESRD.

> **Chronic renal failure affects every system in the body and, without treatment, will end in death within a short time.**

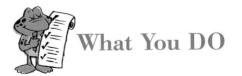

What You DO

Treatment

The care of the patient with chronic renal failure must emphasize interventions to conserve residual renal function, such as controlling blood pressure and blood sugar and avoiding nephrotoxins. Relieving symptoms and maintaining ideal body weight and fluid and electrolyte balance are important as the kidneys fail.

Dietary restrictions are aimed at minimizing urea toxicity, controlling various metabolic upsets, and providing optimal nutrition. Modifications involve adjustments to protein, carbohydrate, fat, sodium, potassium, and phosphate intake.

Drug therapies includes cation exchange resins, such as the following: Kayexalate to lower serum potassium levels, anticonvulsants to control seizures caused by elevated blood urea levels (when necessary), antihypertensive drugs to control blood pressure, diuretics to manage excessive circulating fluid volume (hypervolemia), antimicrobial drugs to treat infection, phosphate-binding drugs to prevent absorption of phosphorus from the intestinal tract, H2-receptor antagonists and antiemetics to control gastrointestinal upset, erythropoietin to manage anemia, cardiac drugs to manage heart failure, antipruritics to relieve pruritus caused by build up of urea on the skin, laxatives or stool softeners to manage diarrhea and constipation, and vitamins and minerals to promote nutritional status.

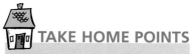

See Chapters 1A, 3, 6B, 9A, and 9B in RWNSG: *Pharmacology*

TAKE HOME POINTS

The only treatment for ESRD is dialysis or kidney transplantation.

Nursing Responsibilities

The nursing responsibilities of caring for the patient in chronic renal failure include recognizing changes in renal function, electrolyte balances, cardiovascular, skin, electrolytes, gastrointestinal, metabolic, neurologic, perceptual, reproductive, respiratory, and musculoskeletal systems, and to provide supportive care.

Medical and nursing interventions are aimed at providing the highest quality of life. To do so, the nurse should:

- Collaborate with the patient and health care team to provide optimal quality of life within the limitations of the disease.
- Accurately record intake and output with consideration to fluid and dietary restrictions.
- Obtain weights at the same time daily, on the same scale, and in the same type of clothing.
- Provide age-appropriate and culturally appropriate patient and family teaching regarding the disorder and the treatment regimen.
- Assess the extent of the patient's anorexia, nausea, vomiting, diarrhea, and constipation, taking measures to relieve symptoms.
- Assist in obtaining laboratory specimens.
- Administer medications as ordered and monitor for adverse effects.
- Monitor for clinical manifestations of infection, dehydration, overhydration, pruritus, petechiae, purpura, edema, and changing neurologic status.
- Maintain safety precautions, reorienting the patient to reality, when necessary.
- Assess the patient's fatigue and activity tolerance and adjust care to permit rest periods.
- Assess sexual dysfunction and effect on patient-spouse relationship.
- Offer emotional support, arrange for family counseling, teach coping strategies, and provide information about available support groups.

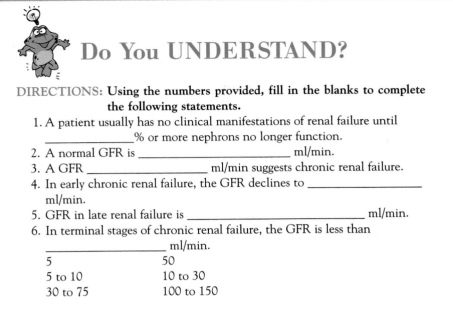

Do You UNDERSTAND?

DIRECTIONS: Using the numbers provided, fill in the blanks to complete the following statements.

1. A patient usually has no clinical manifestations of renal failure until _____% or more nephrons no longer function.

2. A normal GFR is _____ ml/min.

3. A GFR _____ ml/min suggests chronic renal failure.

4. In early chronic renal failure, the GFR declines to _____ ml/min.

5. GFR in late renal failure is _____ ml/min.

6. In terminal stages of chronic renal failure, the GFR is less than _____ ml/min.

5	50
5 to 10	10 to 30
30 to 75	100 to 150

SECTION E
HEREDITARY DISEASES OF THE GENITOURINARY TRACT

What IS Goodpasture's Syndrome?

Pathogenesis

Goodpasture's syndrome is a type of autoimmune disease in which antibodies destroy the basement membrane of glomeruli and pulmonary capillary membranes.

The causative factors for the development of the antibodies is unknown, although influenza A infections and genetic predisposition may be, at least in part, to blame. The disorder is associated with a number of glomerular diseases such as poststreptococcal glomerulonephritis.

By the time this rapidly progressing disease is diagnosed, renal insufficiency is apparent. The destruction leads to a rapidly progressing glomerulonephritis, pulmonary hemorrhage, and iron deficiency anemia.

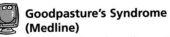
Goodpasture's Syndrome (Medline)
http://medlineplus.nlm.nih.gov/medlineplus/kidneydiseases general.html

At-Risk Populations

Although rare, Goodpasture's syndrome is most common in men between the ages of 20 and 30.

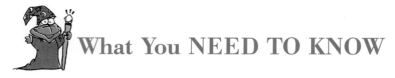

What You NEED TO KNOW

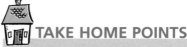

TAKE HOME POINTS

Goodpasture's syndrome causes a rapidly progressive form of glomerulo-nephritis and pulmonary hemorrhage. Currently, no successful way is available that will stop the damage being done to the kidneys and the respiratory tract by the immune system.

Clinical Manifestations

The clinical manifestations of Goodpasture's syndrome include blood in the urine, proteinuria, edema, hypertension, and signs and symptoms of renal failure.

Prognosis

The prognosis for the patient with Goodpasture's syndrome is poor. The glomerular injury is typically accompanied by a rapid decline in GFR, progressing to renal failure in a few weeks or months.

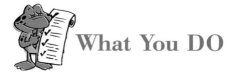

What You DO

Treatment

Few treatments have proven effective against Goodpasture's syndrome. Neither antiinflammatory drugs such as glucocorticosteroids (e.g., prednisone) nor immunosuppressant drugs such as cyclophosphamide or azathioprine have been effective. Anticoagulation therapy with heparin or warfarin has shown some promise in decreasing the buildup of fibrin within Bowman's capsule. Dialysis or transplantation may be required for patients who develop complete renal failure.

See Chapters 1C, 3, and 7B in RWNSG: *Pharmacology*

Nursing Responsibilities

The nursing responsibilities for the patient with Goodpasture's syndrome are primarily supportive. The nurse should:

- Assess vital signs, particularly changes in blood pressure and respiration, which are indicative of a worsening condition.
- Accurately record intake and output.
- Obtain weights at the same time daily, on the same scale, and in the same type of clothing.
- Provide age-appropriate and culturally appropriate patient and family teaching regarding the disorder.
- Examine urine for color, amount, and abnormal substances.
- Assist the patient and family in developing support systems and coping with chronic illness.

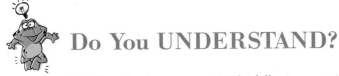

Do You UNDERSTAND?

DIRECTIONS: Provide short answers to the following questions.

1. How is Goodpasture's syndrome different from acute glomerulonephritis?

2. What community resources are identified in your textbook for patients with Goodpasture's syndrome? List the resources. Report your findings to your classmates.

What IS IgA Nephropathy?

Pathogenesis

IgA nephropathy (IgA glomerulonephritis) is a form of acute glomerulonephritis. IgA nephropathy is rare, affecting 2% to 4% of the population. Deposits of IgA, IgG, and complement in the glomeruli characterize IgA nephropathy, microscopically. A renal biopsy may be required for a diagnosis.

Evidence suggests that the disorder is a result of either increased production or reduced clearance of IgA and associated complexes that are ultimately deposited in the kidneys. IgA nephropathy is frequently associated with an upper respiratory infection or influenza-like illness with high serum IgA levels, although normal IgA may be present.

The glomeruli normally filter wastes and excess water from the blood, sending them to the bladder as urine. IgA causes "holes" in the glomeruli, which leads to blood and protein in the urine. Patients with IgA nephropathy have a marked deposit of IgA (and, occasionally, IgG with complement) in the glomeruli.

At-Risk Populations

Men are more susceptible than are women to this disease.

National Institute of Diabetes and Diseases of the Kidneys (IgA Nephropathy)
www.niddk.nih.gov/health/kidney/summary/iganeph/iganeph.htm
IgAN Foundation (IgA nephropathy)
www.igan.org

Adults with IgA nephropathy progress to loss of renal function more frequently than do children.

What You NEED TO KNOW

Clinical Manifestations

The symptoms of IgA nephropathy occur almost immediately. The urine is foamy and tea-colored for 2 to 6 days. Puffiness develops around the eyes, hands, or feet. Patients may complain of a pain in the small of the back immediately below the ribs that is not aggravated by motion. The urge to urinate becomes frequent, particularly at night, and a reduced amount of urine is produced. Hypertension is a complication of the disease.

Prognosis

This problem is a self-limiting, single-occurrence disorder for over 50% of patients. The remaining patients have a gradual progression of glomerular disease over a period of 10 to 20 years with recurrent episodes of hematuria and mild proteinuria. Patients with early hypertension and proteinuria that exceeds 3 g/day tend to progress to renal failure.

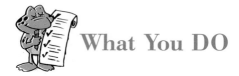

What You DO

Treatment

No widely accepted medical treatment for IgA nephropathy is available. The treatment is primarily supportive. Angiotensin-converting enzyme (ACE) inhibitor drugs can help control blood pressure and delay the deterioration of kidney function. Some evidence suggests that daily consumption of fish oil slows the progression of the disease. Reducing cholesterol through diet, medications, or both appears to help slow the progression of the disease.

See Chapter 4 in RWNSG:
Pharmacology

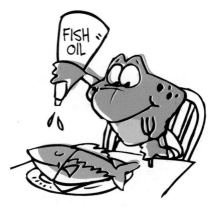

Nursing Responsibilities

The nursing responsibilities for patients with IgA nephropathy are similar to the care of the patient with glomerulonephritis. The nurse should:
- Obtain a complete history of recent infections or invasive procedures.
- Monitor for and recognize complications.
- Assess the severity of the patient's edema, vital signs (particularly blood pressure), and intake and output.
- Examine urine for color, amount, and abnormal substances.
- Obtain weight at the same time daily, on the same scale, and in the same type of clothing.
- Provide age-appropriate and culturally appropriate patient and family teaching regarding the disorder.
- Provide relief of symptoms.
- Assist the patient and family in developing support systems and coping skills when the disease becomes progressive.

Do You UNDERSTAND?

DIRECTIONS: **Indicate in the space provided whether the statement is**
true or _false._

_____ 1. IgA nephropathy in children results in loss of renal function more frequently than it does in adults.

_____ 2. Hypertension is a complication of IgA nephropathy.

_____ 3. ACE inhibitors can delay renal function deterioration in IgA nephropathy.

_____ 4. Urine is nonfoamy and greenish in the patient with IgA nephropathy.

What IS Polycystic Kidney Disease?

Pathogenesis

Polycystic kidney disease (PKD) is a genetic disorder characterized by the growth of numerous cysts in the kidneys. The grapelike cysts replace normal kidney tissue. People with PKD live decades without developing symptoms. The reasons for which the cysts form in the kidney are unknown.

Normal kidney cells are crowded out by groups of cysts filled with fluid, blood, or even urine. The kidneys enlarge along with the cysts, which can number in the thousands, while roughly retaining their kidney shape. In fully developed PKD, a cyst-filled kidney can weigh as much as 22 pounds.

High blood pressure occurs early in the disease, frequently before the cysts appear. Kidney stones usually develop and kidney infection is common because of the compression and obstruction of the urinary tract. Cysts may also form in other areas, such as the lung, liver, and pancreas.

At-Risk Populations

Patients at risk for PKD are those who carry the defective gene. Approximately 90% of all polycystic kidney disease is a genetic, autosomal dominant disorder. When one parent has the disease, the chances are 50% that the disease will pass to a child. In some rare cases, the cause of the autosomal dominant disease occurs spontaneously in the child soon after conception. In these cases, the parents are not the source of the disease. A genetic flaw different from that causing autosomal dominant PKD causes autosomal recessive PKD. Parents who do not have the disease can have a child with the disease when both parents carry the abnormal gene and both pass the gene to their baby. The chance of this happening, when both parents carry the abnormal gene, is one in four. When only one parent carries the abnormal gene, the baby cannot get the disease.

PKD is thought to occur more frequently in Caucasians than it does in African Americans and more frequently in females than it does in males.

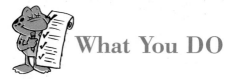

What You NEED TO KNOW

Clinical Manifestations

The symptoms of the autosomal dominant form of the disease usually develop between the ages of 30 to 40, but they can begin earlier, even in childhood. The most common clinical manifestations of PKD are pain in the back and sides, as well as headaches. The dull pain can be temporary or persistent, mild or severe. Additionally, patients with autosomal dominant PKD can experience the following: urinary tract infections, blood in the urine, liver and pancreatic cysts, abnormal heart valves, high blood pressure, kidney stones, bulges in the walls of blood vessels (aneurysms) in the brain, and small outpocketing of the wall of the colon (diverticulosis).

Symptoms of the autosomal recessive form of the disease begin in the earliest months of life, even *in utero*. Children with PKD experience high blood pressure, urinary tract infections, and frequent urination. The disease usually affects the liver, spleen, and pancreas, which results in low blood cell counts, varicose veins, and hemorrhoids.

Because kidney function is crucial for early physical development, children with autosomal recessive PKD are usually smaller when compared with the average child.

PKD is the fourth leading cause of kidney failure in the United States.

Prognosis

Many people with autosomal dominant form of PKD live for decades without developing symptoms. Adults show signs of hypertension and kidney failure 5 to 15 years after the onset of symptoms.

Children with autosomal recessive PKD usually develop kidney failure within a few years. The severity of the disease varies. Babies with the worst cases die hours or days after birth. Children with an infantile version may have sufficient renal function for normal activities for a few years. People with the juvenile version may live into their teens and twenties but usually have liver problems as well.

What You DO

Treatment

Currently, the course of PKD cannot be genetically altered. Treatment is aimed at preserving kidney function for as long as possible. Interventions include prompt treatment of UTIs, prompt recognition and treatment of urinary tract obstruction, and maintenance of fluid and electrolyte balance. Genetic counseling is vital to reduce the likelihood of transmission of the disease.

Nursing Responsibilities

For the patient with PKD, the nurse should:
- Accurately record intake and output and monitor laboratory tests that assess kidney function.

- Assess for and teach the patient to recognize the signs and symptoms of UTIs (urgency, frequency, dysuria).
- Assess vital signs, particularly blood pressure for hypertension.
- Avoid invasive procedures of the urinary tract.
- Evaluate the patient's level of pain from compression of internal structures.
- Administer analgesic medications as ordered, and monitor the patient's response to the drugs.
- Assist the patient and family in obtaining genetic counseling.
- Help the patient and family understand and cope with effects of the disease.
- Provide information about renal dialysis and transplantation when appropriate.

Do You UNDERSTAND?

DIRECTIONS: Fill in the blanks.

1. PKD leads to renal failure because the nonfunctioning _____ gradually replace the _____.
2. Patients at risk for PKD are those who carry the defective _____.
3. _____ counseling is important in reducing the transmission of PKD.

SECTION F
MALIGNANCIES OF THE GENITOURINARY TRACT

What IS Bladder Carcinoma?

Pathogenesis

Bladder carcinoma is a cancer of the cells that line the bladder. Of all bladder cancers, 90% are transitional cell carcinomas, 1% to 2% are adenocarcinomas, and approximately 8% arise from squamous cells. Transitional cell carcinomas develop from the epithelial lining of the urinary tract, thus they may occur in the ureters, renal pelvis, and urethra. The carcinomas frequently grow as stalks. Growths that are not papillary are more aggressive. All bladder cancer is capable of invading the bladder wall.

Damage to a cell irreversibly changes the structure of the cell, thus it no longer sends or receives normal cell messages; it does not know when to stop dividing. The abnormal cell undergoes uninhibited growth, which crowds out normal cells. Without treatment, the cancer cells invade nearby organs and spread to lymph nodes, bones, liver, and lungs.

Answers: 1. cysts, nephrons; 2. gene; 3. genetic.

Cigarette smoking may be a possible cause of bladder cancer. Industrial exposure to certain chemicals (e.g., textile chemicals, petroleum products, leather finishes, benzidine) has also been linked to bladder cancer. Genetic changes (i.e., mutations in gene p53—a tumor-suppressor gene—may also be a precursor for the development of bladder cancer.

At-Risk Populations

Men are twice as likely to develop bladder cancer as women, and the risk increases with age. Individuals over age 55 are at an increased risk, as well as people who smoke, those who have a long history of chronic bladder stones, or those with chronic bladder irritation.

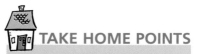

Caucasian men are at greater risk for bladder carcinoma than are African-American men.

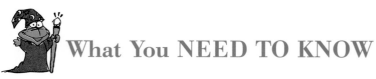

What You NEED TO KNOW

Clinical Manifestations

The signs and symptoms of bladder cancer are subtle in onset and include painless hematuria, with frequency and urgency appearing late in the disease. Pelvic pain develops in patients with advanced bladder cancer.

Prognosis

The prognosis for patients with bladder cancer depends on the extent to which the cancer has advanced at the time of diagnosis. Patients with localized bladder cancer have a 95% survival rate. Patients with tumors that extend beyond the bladder wall have a poorer prognosis (46% to 49%, 5-year survival rate).

TAKE HOME POINTS

Bladder cancer is a "silent cancer," meaning that it is usually asymptomatic until it invades nearby tissues. Blood in the urine, particularly painless blood in the urine, always warrants further evaluation.

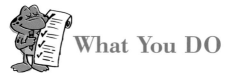

What You DO

Treatment

Choices of treatment for bladder cancer are limited. Surgical removal of the cancer cells can be performed using a procedure called transurethral resection of the bladder tumor. In some cases, the entire bladder may need to be removed (cystectomy). Radiation is not extremely effective but may be used in combination with antineoplastic therapy.

See Chapter 1D in RWNSG: *Pharmacology*

Nursing Responsibilities

The nursing responsibilities for the patient with bladder cancer are aimed at helping the patient cope with the diagnosis and treatment plan. Postoperative nursing care will be needed if the patient has had a surgical procedure; however, generally, the nurse should:

- Elicit a history of exposure to known cancer-causing chemicals (carcinogens).
- Assess the urine for quantity, color, and characteristics.

- Be aware of diagnostic tests, procedures, and side effects for diagnosing bladder cancer, including the fact that the kidneys are highly vascular and may bleed profusely after renal biopsy.
- Encourage the patient to increase fluid intake after a cystoscopy and to report any signs of infection (e.g., blood in the urine, burning, pain, increased frequency with urination).
- Observe for reactions to contrast medium used for the intravenous pyelogram (IVP). Contrast medium is renal toxic.
- Teach about the importance of follow-up care.
- Teach the patient and family about care of the skin after radiation therapy.
- Provide age- and culture-supportive, symptomatic care for the patient who is receiving chemotherapy.
- Provide perioperative care based on the surgical procedure performed.
- Evaluate the patient's and family's support systems, and assist with learning effective coping strategies.

Do You UNDERSTAND?

DIRECTIONS: **Fill in the blanks.**

1. The patient with bladder cancer may experience _____ _____.

2. _____ _____ is difficult to treat after the cancer metastasizes beyond the bladder.

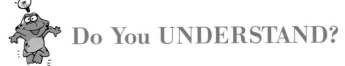

What IS Renal Cell Carcinoma?

Pathogenesis

Renal cell carcinoma is a cancer of cells that line the tubules of the kidneys and is the most common renal cancer. The right and left kidneys are at equal risk for development of cancerous tumors. At least 85% of all renal tumors are malignant.

Cancerous cells usually begin in the outer layer of the left or right kidney. Tumor growth is slow, usually developing in one kidney and spreading through lymph nodes and blood vessels to lymph nodes, liver, bones, lungs, thyroid gland, and central nervous system. Tumor growth places pressure on blood vessels and surrounding tissue, which contributes to tissue death and interruption of kidney function. Metastasis can occur even after the diseased kidney is removed.

At-Risk Populations

A genetic predisposition to renal cell carcinoma may exist. Tobacco use doubles the risk of renal cancer, although the exact mechanism of cell damage is unclear. Obesity and long-term use of dialysis also places the patient at greater risk.

Answers: 1. painless hematuria; 2. bladder cancer.

The population at risk for renal cell carcinoma is adult men between the ages of 50 and 70. Renal cell carcinoma occurs two times more frequently in men than it does in women.

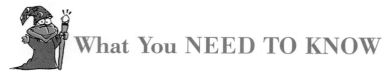

What You NEED TO KNOW

Clinical Manifestations

Because one kidney is able to maintain fluid and electrolyte balance, the signs and symptoms of renal cell carcinoma are usually not apparent until tumor growth is extensive. Hematuria is the most common symptom. Flank pain is described as dull and aching. Other findings may include a palpable mass, although tumor palpation is difficult in all but the thinnest people. The patient may note weight loss and develop an intermittent fever. Hypertension develops as a result of increased renin production. Liver function tests are altered with an elevated serum alkaline phosphatase, prothrombin, and bilirubin.

Prognosis

The prognosis for the patient with renal cell carcinoma depends highly on the tumor grade, tumor cell type, and extent of metastasis at the time of diagnosis (staging). At best, 5-year survival rates are approximately 65% for carcinoma in the early stages (stage I). Tumor contained within the kidney's capsule is known as stage I carcinoma. Stage II carcinoma is evidenced by spread of the cancer through the renal capsule but within the surrounding fascia. Stage III carcinoma involves regional lymph nodes, the renal vein, or vena cava. Stage IV carcinoma involves the spread of the cancer to distant sites. Survival beyond 5 years is rare for patients with stages III and IV.

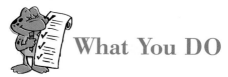

What You DO

Treatment

Treatment of renal cell carcinoma is usually surgical removal of the affected kidney (radical nephrectomy). The combination of antineoplastic drugs and biologic response–modifying drugs is frequently used. Interleukins and interferons (IL-2, INF-α) show promise in treating this cancer. Radiation therapy may be used preoperatively to shrink the tumors or postoperatively to destroy remaining tumor cells.

See Chapters 1C and 1D in RWNSG: *Pharmacology*

Nursing Responsibilities

For the patient with renal cell carcinoma, the nurse should:

- Increase fluid intake, when indicated, to ensure adequate excretion of waste products before surgery.
- Assure the patient that the remaining kidney will function sufficiently to meet the body's needs.
- Advise the patient of the importance of postoperative deep breathing and coughing. Coughing is difficult because the incision is near the diaphragm.
- Evaluate and manage the patient's pain with patient-controlled analgesia (PCA).
- Accurately record intake and output.
- Provide meticulous catheter care, which is necessary to prevent postoperative UTI.
- Postoperatively monitor the GI tract for evidence of failure of appropriate forward movement of intestinal contents (paralytic ileus).
- Provide age-appropriate and culturally appropriate patient and family teaching regarding the disorder, surgery, chemotherapy, and radiation therapy.
- Assist the patient and family with the grieving process and the development of coping skills.

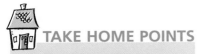

TAKE HOME POINTS

Kidney tumors are nearly always malignant and difficult to find in the early stages, which makes treatment particularly challenging.

Do You UNDERSTAND?

DIRECTIONS: Fill in the blanks.

1. The most common urinary tract tumor is _____ carcinoma.
2. The most common initial sign of bladder cancer is _____ _____.
3. The most common cancer that arises in the kidney is renal _____ _____.
4. The survival rate for renal carcinoma is lower than for many other cancers because _____ _____.

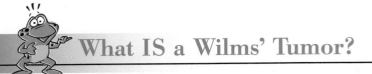

What IS a Wilms' Tumor?

Pathogenesis

A Wilms' tumor is a rapidly developing mixed tumor of the kidney that occurs in children. Because it is made up of embryonal elements, Wilms' tumor is also known as a *nephroblastoma*. The condition has been linked to the deletion or inactivation of suppressor genes on the short arm of chromosome 11. One of the three genes associated with the disorder has been associated with the familial form of Wilms' tumor.

Answers: 1. bladder; 2. gross hematuria; 3. cell carcinoma; 4. it has frequently reached the advanced stages before diagnosis.

The pathogenesis of both the sporadic and inherited forms of the tumor is similar to that of retinoblastoma. Inherited cases, which are relatively rare, are transmitted in an autosomal dominant fashion. The child inherits the loss of one copy of the Wilms' tumor-suppressor gene in all of the fetal renal cells that normally differentiate into the renal tubules and glomeruli. Loss of the other copy of the gene is all that is needed for the tumor to develop. Tumors can develop in both kidneys in the inherited form because the fetal kidney cells are vulnerable to the loss of the second copy of the gene. Because normal kidney development occurs during the eighth to the thirty-fourth week of gestation, gene loss likely occurs during this time.

At-Risk Populations

Wilms' tumor usually develops in children before age 5. The peak incidence is between 2 and 3 years of age. One in every 10,000 children will develop a Wilms' tumor. Of the children who have a Wilms tumor, 18% also demonstrate a number of congenital abnormalities, including lack of an iris in the eye, asymmetry of the body, and GU malformations. Children with a combination of congenital anomalies and Wilms' tumor are more likely to have the inherited bilateral form of the disease.

 What You NEED TO KNOW

Clinical Manifestations

The clinical manifestation of Wilms' tumor is an enlarging, asymptomatic upper abdominal mass at the time of diagnosis. Many tumors are found by the parent who notices an abdominal swelling during bathing or dressing the otherwise healthy, thriving child. The firm, nontender, smooth mass is generally confined to one side of the abdomen. Other signs and symptoms include vague abdominal pain, hematuria, and fever. Either encroachment by the tumor on the blood supply or secretion of renin by the tumor elevates the blood pressure. An abdominal ultrasound, computerized tomographic (CT) scan, or magnetic resonance imaging (MRI) may be used for initial examination. Diagnosis is based on surgical biopsy.

Prognosis

Metastasis of Wilms' tumor is to regional lymph nodes, lungs, liver, brain, and bone. In the past, the mortality from this type of cancer was extremely high; however, aggressive treatment approaches have been extremely effective in controlling the tumor. With modern treatment modalities, the overall cure rate is as high as 80% to 95%, as long as no metastasis has occurred. The prognosis is generally poor for children with metastases.

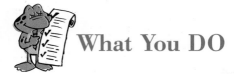

What You DO

Treatment

Surgical exploration and resection begin the treatment of Wilms' tumor. Intervention may include removal of a portion of the less involved kidney and total removal of the other. Radiation therapy is most effective when administered 1 to 3 days after surgery. Radiation is unnecessary for the early stages of the disease but may be used in the later stages. Radiation therapy is also used for areas of metastases, should they be present.

Antineoplastic therapy with both vincristine and actinomycin D appears to be more effective than is either drug alone. Doxorubicin (Adriamycin) may also be added to the regimen for some children. Cyclophosphamide has been used to treat highly aggressive tumors. High-dose antineoplastic therapy followed by autologous bone marrow transplant has been used for patients with advanced disease.

See Chapter 1D in **RWNSG:**
Pharmacology

Nursing Responsibilities

The nursing responsibilities for the patient with Wilms' tumor includes much of the same care as for any patient with cancer. In addition, the nurse should:
- Use age-appropriate methods for evaluating and managing the patient's pain.
- Accurately record intake and output.
- Provide age-appropriate and culturally appropriate patient and family teaching regarding the disorder, surgery, chemotherapy, and radiation therapy.
- Use play therapy in helping the child cope with the disease and its treatment.
- Assist the patient and family with the grieving process and the development of coping skills.

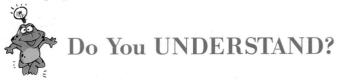

Do You UNDERSTAND?

DIRECTIONS: **Provide short answers to the following questions.**
1. What is the peak age for a Wilms' tumor to surface?

2. What are the signs and symptoms of Wilms' tumor?

3. What is the primary treatment for Wilms' tumor?

Answers: 1. 2 to 3 years of age; 2. firm, smooth, nontender abdominal mass, vague abdominal pain, hematuria, and fever; 3. surgical removal of the primary affected kidney and partial removal of the less-affected kidney, followed by radiation 3 days later.

Male and Female Reproductive Systems

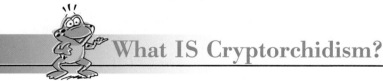

SECTION A
MALE REPRODUCTIVE DISEASES

The male reproductive system produces, sustains, and transports sperm; introduces sperm into the female vagina; and produces hormones. The male gonads (testes) develop within the abdominal cavity and descend into the scrotum before birth. Their position within the scrotum is necessary for the production of viable sperm. Sperm production begins at puberty and continues throughout life.

The male urethra, which is composed of the prostatic urethra, membranous urethra, and penile urethra, is the passageway for sperm, fluids from the reproductive tract, and urine. The seminal vesicles, prostate, and bulbourethral glands secrete fluids that nourish sperm and enhance the motility and viability of the sperm. These structures also help neutralize the acidity of the urethra and vagina, providing lubrication during intercourse.

Three hormones are the primary regulators of male reproductive functioning. Follicle stimulating hormone (FSH) stimulates the development of sperm (spermatogenesis). Luteinizing hormone (LH) stimulates the production of testosterone. Testosterone, in turn, stimulates the development of male secondary sexual characteristics and sperm production.

 Two percent of male newborns have a congenital anomaly of the reproductive system.

What IS Cryptorchidism?

Pathogenesis

Failure of one or both of the testes to descend into the scrotum is known as cryptorchidism. As the male fetus grows, the testes develop in the abdomen. At approximately 7 months gestation, the testes descend to the upper part of the groin from which they move into the inguinal canal and then normally into the scrotum. However, the descent of the testes may be halted in the abdomen or within the canal. In most cases, only one testis is involved. Testes that remain in the abdomen may not produce the hormones that induce secondary sexual characteristics. A testis lodged in the inguinal canal can induce secondary sex characters but cannot produce spermatozoa. Most testes that have not descended spontaneously at birth do so during the first 6 to 9 months of life. After the first year, spontaneous descent is unlikely to occur.

Most undescended testes are a result of a short spermatic cord, fibrous bands, adhesions in the normal pathway of the testes, or a narrowed inguinal canal. Failure of the testes to descend can also be the result of a congenital gonadal defect that makes the testis insensitive to gonadotropins (the likely explanation for unilateral nondescent) or a lack of maternal gonadotropins (the likely explanation for bilateral nondescent of prematurity). Chromosomal studies do not support a genetic cause.

At-Risk Populations

Cryptorchidism is found in 3% of full-term and 30% of premature male infants. The incidence of cryptorchidism in adults is less than 1%.

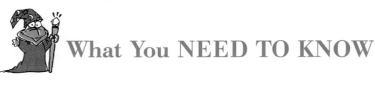

What You NEED TO KNOW

Clinical Manifestations

Cryptorchidism may be unilateral or bilateral. Examination of the male genitalia reveals an absence of one or both of the testes in the scrotal sac. The male adult with cryptorchidism may complain of infertility.

Prognosis

The prognosis for the child with cryptorchidism is good. Early repair decreases the risk of infertility, malignancy, and testicular torsion.

TAKE HOME POINTS

Patients with cryptorchidism or a history of undescended testes have a 35 to 50 times greater risk for testicular cancer in later life compared with the general male population.

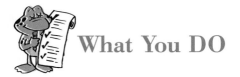

What You DO

Treatment

Because cell changes occur in the cryptorchid testis by 1 year of age, the most favorable age of treatment is 9 to 10 months. Treatment usually begins with the administration of human chorionic gonadotropin (HCG), a hormone that may initiate descent, making surgery unnecessary. If hormone therapy is unsuccessful, then the testis is located and surgically moved in young children (orchiopexy). The surgery is best performed before the patient is 5 to 7 years of age, because operating at a later age can involve more risk to the cells that produce spermatozoa.

The testes may be removed entirely (orchiectomy) in children over age 10 and in adults who fail hormone therapy. Testes that are properly placed in the scrotal sac provide adequate hormone function and give the scrotum a normal appearance. A testicular prosthesis is provided in the scrotal sac for patients who have an orchiectomy.

Nursing Responsibilities

Although care responsibilities for the child with an orchiopexy is limited, the nurse should:

- Teach the caregivers of young patients how to care for the surgical incision and to watch for the clinical manifestations of infection.
- Advise adult patients on ways to care for the scrotal incision and to notify the health care provider should signs and symptoms of infection appear.
- Elevate the scrotum with a scrotal support to reduce edema and discomfort caused by the surgical incision. Keep the wound clean and dry.

Do You UNDERSTAND?

DIRECTIONS: **Indicate in the space provided whether the statement is** *true* **or** *false*. **If false, then rewrite the statement in the margin space to the left to make it true.**

_____ 1. Cryptorchidism is caused by a genetic abnormality.

_____ 2. The treatment for cryptorchidism in a child under age 10 is referred to as an orchiectomy.

_____ 3. Surgical repair of cryptorchidism must be performed after puberty to preserve testicular function.

_____ 4. The risk of testicular cancer in the patient with a history of cryptorchidism is low compared with that of the general male population.

_____ 5. The most favorable age for treatment of cryptorchidism is 9 to 10 months.

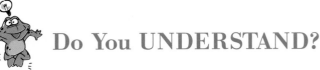

What IS Orchitis?

Pathogenesis

Orchitis is a rare, acute inflammation of one or both testes and may be associated with trauma or infection elsewhere in the body. Mumps is the most common cause of orchitis. Infectious organisms can reach the testis through the blood or lymphatics but most commonly by ascent through the urethra, vas deferens, and epididymis. Occasionally, in middle-age men, a nonspecific, apparently noninfectious inflammatory process can occur. The inflammation may contribute to the development of a painless collection of fluid along the spermatic cord (hydrocele).

Answers: 1. false; cryptorchidism is the result of a short spermatic cord, fibrous bands, or adhesions in the pathway of the testes or a narrowed inguinal canal; 2. false; treatment of cryptorchidism in a child under age 10 is known as an orchiopexy; 3. false; surgical repair is performed at age 9 to 10 months; 4. false; the risk of testicular cancer is 35 to 50 times greater than that of the general population; 5. true.

At-Risk Populations

Orchitis is uncommon except as a complication of systemic infection or as an extension of an associated epididymitis.

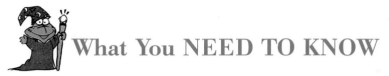

What You NEED TO KNOW

Clinical Manifestations

Orchitis is unilateral in 75% of cases. Orchitis presents with sudden onset of severe pain and a red, warm, and tender testis, usually occurring 3 to 4 days after the onset of the infection. Other signs and symptoms include high fever, marked prostration, bilateral or unilateral erythema, edema, and tenderness of the scrotum and leukocytosis. The acute phase lasts approximately 1 week. An acute hydrocele may develop. Orchitis is frequently difficult to diagnose because the inflammatory edema and pain of palpation prevent accurate distinction.

Prognosis

In patients with orchitis secondary to mumps, atrophy with irreversible damage to spermatogenesis may result. Bilateral orchitis does not affect androgenic function but may cause permanent sterility.

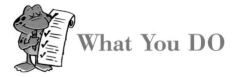

What You DO

Treatment

Treatment of orchitis is supportive and includes suspending the scrotum in a suspensory or toweling and using hot or cold compresses. Opioids and antiinflammatory medications are administered to reduce pain and inflammation. When an acute hydrocele develops, it is aspirated. Testicular abscess usually requires surgical removal of the testis. Antibiotics are used for bacterial orchitis. Corticosteroids may be necessary in cases of nonspecific, noninfectious inflammatory orchitis.

Nursing Interventions

Because patients may be reluctant to ask for help, skillful communication techniques are essential to help them express concerns. Be sensitive and give the patient permission to talk about the problem.

🍎 Teach the patient about using hot and cold compresses to control swelling.

• Be aware of the patient's discomfort, administering analgesic and other medications as ordered.

Orchitis occurs in approximately 25% to 38% of postpubertal men, but sterility is rare.

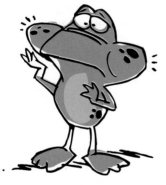

See Chapters 1A, 7A, 11, and 14 in RWNSG: *Pharmacology*

Do You UNDERSTAND?

DIRECTIONS: **Indicate in the space provided whether the statement is *true* or *false*. If false, then rewrite the statement in the margin space to the left to make it true.**

_____ 1. Orchitis is a common disorder of men.

_____ 2. The most common disorder associated with orchitis is mumps.

_____ 3. In all cases, orchitis occurs in both testes.

_____ 4. Bilateral orchitis does not affect androgenic function.

_____ 5. A hydrocele associated with the development of orchitis is treated by aspiration.

What IS Epididymitis?

Pathogenesis

Epididymitis is an inflammation of the epididymis. Infection causes most cases of epididymitis. Pathogens reach the epididymis through the vas deferens from infected urine, the posterior urethra, or seminal vesicles. In rare cases, heavy lifting or straining can result in reflux of urine from the bladder into the vas deferens and epididymis with the subsequent development of epididymitis. Urine is also irritating to the epididymis and may initiate an inflammatory response.

At-Risk Populations

Epididymitis generally occurs in sexually active young men under the age of 35 but is rare before puberty.

In young men, the cause of epididymitis is usually a sexually transmitted organism such as *Neisseria gonorrhoeae* or *Chlamydia trachomatis* (see Chapter 10C). Nonsexually transmitted forms typically occur in older men and are associated with intestinal bacteria and *Pseudomonas aeruginosa* from urinary tract infections and prostatitis. Although uncommon, tuberculosis epididymitis can occur in regions in which the incidence of pulmonary tuberculosis is high.

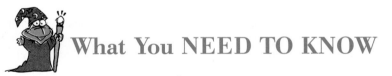

What You NEED TO KNOW

Clinical Manifestations

The main symptom of epididymitis is pain. Acute, severe pain develops in the scrotum and can radiate to the spermatic cord. The spermatic cord may be swollen and tender to palpation. Flank pain can occur as the urethra passes over the spermatic cord. Pain relief when the inflamed testis and epididymis are elevated is a diagnostic sign of epididymitis (Phren sign).

Swelling of the spermatic cord obstructs the urethra. The patient may have pyuria and bacteruria and a history of urinary symptoms, including urethral discharge. The scrotum on the involved side is red and edematous as a result of the inflammatory changes and is tender during palpation. The tail of the epididymis near the lower pole of the testis usually swells first, followed by the head of the epididymis. Fever occurs in approximately 50% of patients, with accompanying nausea and vomiting. A hydrocele may accompany epididymitis.

Prognosis

Complete resolution of swelling and the pain of epididymitis can take from several weeks to months. Complications of epididymitis include abscess formation, testicular necrosis, recurrent infection, and infertility.

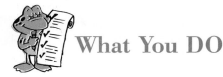

What You DO

Treatment

Treatment of epididymitis is directed toward the identified pathogen. Appropriate antibiotic therapy, bedrest, and scrotal elevation are integral parts of treatment. Scrotal elevation facilitates maximal lymphatic and venous drainage. The patient's sexual partner should be treated with antibiotics if the causative organism is a sexually transmitted pathogen. Although rare, when an abscess develops, it is drained surgically. An orchiectomy may be necessary in some cases.

See Chapter 1A in **RWNSG:**
Pharmacology

Nursing Responsibilities

For the patient with epididymitis, the nurse should:
* Advise the patient to avoid straining while voiding.
* Encourage the patient to elevate the scrotum to minimize discomfort.
* Counsel patients with epididymitis from sexually transmitted organisms to contact their partner thus treatment may be initiated.

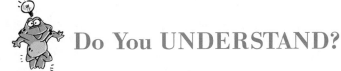

Do You UNDERSTAND?

DIRECTIONS: Fill in the blanks.

1. Sexually transmitted organisms such as _____ and _____ cause epididymitis.
2. Epididymitis usually occurs in sexually active men under the age of _____.
3. The main symptom of epididymitis is _____.
4. Epididymitis unresponsive to antibiotic therapy may require a surgical procedure known as _____.

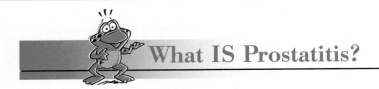

What IS Prostatitis?

Pathogenesis

Prostatitis is an inflammation or infection of the prostate gland and occurs in four common forms: acute bacterial, chronic bacterial, nonbacterial, and prostatodynia (pain in the prostate). Prostatitis can result from an ascending urethral infection, reflux of infected urine, extension of a rectal infection, or from hematogenous spread. Pathogens associated with acute and chronic bacterial prostatitis include gram-negative bacilli, *Enterobacter, Klebsiella, Pseudomonas,* and *Proteus.* Gardnerella, chlamydia, and mycoplasma are organisms associated with nonbacterial prostatitis. In nonbacterial prostatitis, the cause may be unknown, or it may be associated with an autoimmune process, an allergic reaction, neuromuscular dysfunction, or a psychologic factor. Prostadynia is not be caused by a pathologic condition but by spasms in the genitourinary tract, disorder of the bladder outlet, or tension in the muscles of the pelvic floor.

At-Risk Populations

> Approximately 50% of older adult men have prostatic inflammation.

Some degree of prostatic inflammation is present in 4% to 36% of the male population.

What You NEED TO KNOW

Clinical Manifestations

The signs and symptoms of acute bacterial prostatitis are those of urinary tract infection. Symptoms include painful or difficult urination (dysuria) and excessive urinary frequency. The patient may also have a slow, small urinary stream, an inability to empty the bladder, and the need to void frequently during the night (nocturia). An acute inflammation can cause a urinary obstruction that compresses the urethra. Systemic signs of infection include high fever, fatigue, and joint and muscle pain. Prostatic pain may be present when the patient is in an upright position. Some patients experience low back pain, painful ejaculation, and rectal or perineal pain. Physical examination reveals an extremely tender, swollen, firm, indurated, warm prostate.

Chronic bacterial prostatitis is characterized by recurrent urinary tract infections and persistence of pathogenic bacteria. This form is the most common recurrent urinary tract infection in men. The clinical manifestations are variable and similar to that of acute bladder infection: frequency, urgency, dysuria, perineal discomfort, low back pain, and muscle and joint pain. Physical examination reveals the prostate to be only slightly enlarged or boggy, but fibrosis can cause it to be firm and irregular in shape.

Men with nonbacterial prostatitis may complain of a continuous or sporadic dull ache in the suprapubic, infrapubic, scrotal, penile, or inguinal areas. Other clinical manifestations include pain during ejaculation and urinary symptoms. The prostate gland feels normal during palpation.

Prognosis

The complications associated with acute bacterial prostatitis include urinary retention, prostatic abscess, epididymitis, bacteremia, and septic shock.

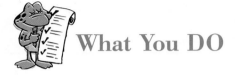

What You DO

Treatment

The treatment for prostatitis is based on the cause; thus management of the disease begins with making an accurate diagnosis.

In severe cases, the patient is hospitalized and treated with aminoglycoside antibiotics and ampicillin. Analgesics, antipyretics, bed rest, and adequate hydration are also therapeutic. An indwelling, urethral catheter is contraindicated in patients with acute bacterial prostatitis and urinary retention, thus a suprapubic catheter may be required. No generally accepted treatment for nonbacterial prostatitis is available. Alpha-blocking agents or anticholinergic drugs may be helpful in some patients. Other treatments include muscle relaxants, nonsteroidal antiinflammatory drugs, low-dose anxiolytic drugs, biofeedback, diathermy, exercise, and sitz baths. Evidence of obstruction, an elevated creatinine level, and recurrent infection are clear indications for referral to a urologist.

Nursing Responsibilities

Generally, patients with prostatitis are treated on an outpatient basis. For those patients hospitalized with the condition, the nurse should:
- Monitor creatinine levels. An increase in creatinine levels should be reported to the urologist.
- Encourage the patient to drink plenty of fluids.
- Administer medications as ordered.

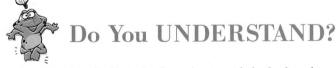

Do You UNDERSTAND?

DIRECTIONS: **Indicate in the space provided whether the statement is
true or *false*. If false, then rewrite the statement in the
margin space to the right to make it true.**

_____ 1. Pathogens associated with acute and chronic bacterial prostatitis include gram-negative bacilli, *Enterobacter*, *Klebsiella*, *Pseudomonas*, and *Proteus*.

TAKE HOME POINTS

Fluoroquinolone medications or trimethoprim-sulfamethoxazole are used for at least 30 to 42 days to treat patients with acute prostatitis. Men with chronic prostatitis may require continuous, low-dose suppressive therapy, or they may benefit from a radical transurethral prostatectomy.

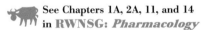
**See Chapters 1A, 2A, 11, and 14
in RWNSG: *Pharmacology***

Answer: 1. true.

_____ 2. Gardnerella, chlamydia, and mycoplasma are organisms associated with nonbacterial prostatitis.

_____ 3. The clinical manifestations of acute bacterial prostatitis are those of urinary tract infection.

_____ 4. The pain of prostatitis may be present when the patient is supine.

_____ 5. An indwelling, urethral catheter is contraindicated in patients with acute bacterial prostatitis and urinary retention.

What IS Benign Prostatic Hyperplasia?

Pathogenesis

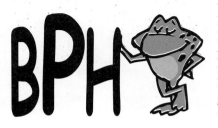

Benign prostatic hyperplasia (BPH) is an enlargement of the prostate gland. BPH begins in the periurethral glands, the inner portion of the prostate. The prostate enlarges as nodules form and grow, and glandular cells enlarge. The resulting hyperplasia leads to hypertrophy of the gland. Because hyperplasia, not hypertrophy, causes the major prostatic changes, the term *benign prostatic hyperplasia* is preferred. The hyperplastic process results in mechanical obstruction of the urethra as it passes through the prostate.

During the early stages of BPH, the detrusor muscle hypertrophies to help the bladder force urine out against increasing resistance. As obstruction progresses, the detrusor muscle decompensates, and the bladder is unable to empty all of the urine. Increasing volumes of urine are retained until urinary retention becomes a chronic problem. The amount of urine that is retained can be large to the extent that it produces uncontrollable overflow incontinence with any increase in abdominal pressure.

Progressive bladder distension causes outpouchings in the bladder wall, and some neural degeneration of smooth muscle cells occurs. The ureters may become obstructed with subsequent development of hydroureters, hydronephrosis, bladder calculi, and bladder or kidney infections.

The etiologic factors of BPH are uncertain, but several agents appear to play a role. Increased testosterone, increased estrogen, stimulation of alpha adrenergic nerve endings that interfere with opening of the bladder sphincter, and smoking may all have effects on the gland. Although dihydrotestosterone (DHT) is necessary for normal prostate development, its role in BPH remains unclear.

At-Risk Populations

BPH is the most common benign tumor in men, and its incidence is age-related. The main risk factors are age and the presence of androgens.

Answers: 2. true; 3. true; 4. false; the pain of prostatitis is present when the patient is in an upright position; 5. true.

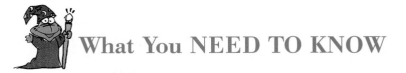

What You NEED TO KNOW

Clinical Manifestations

The symptoms of BPH include reduced or interrupted urinary flow, an inability to empty the bladder, and increased frequency of urination. Most patients have a gradual worsening of obstructive symptoms, including a weak urinary stream, abdominal straining to void, hesitancy, intermittency, incomplete bladder emptying, terminal dribbling, frequency, nocturia, and urgency. Urinary obstruction can occur in patients who have a small prostate; and conversely, large prostates do not necessarily cause obstruction, which makes diagnosis and treatment difficult. The palpated prostate does not always reflect the degree of BPH because a substantial portion of the enlargement is within the gland itself.

Symptoms of BPH usually begin after age 55, with approximately 25% of men reporting obstructive voiding. At age 75 years, 50% of men report a decrease in the force of the urinary stream.

Prognosis

The development of BPH occurs over a prolonged period. Changes within the urinary tract are slow. Reversing progressive BPH is impossible.

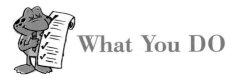

What You DO

Treatment

Because BPH is not always progressive, the timing of intervention is variable and depends on the severity of symptoms and the presence of complications. The treatment of BPH ranges from watchful waiting to medication therapy or surgery. BPH is treated with alpha-adrenergic blocking drugs (prazosin and terazosin) to relax the smooth muscle of the bladder and prostate. Antiandrogen drugs such as finasteride selectively block androgens at the prostate cellular level and cause the prostate gland to shrink. Hormonal therapy may also be used for less severe symptoms.

See Chapters 2A and 10 in RWNSG: *Pharmacology*

Patients with prostate glands weighing over 60 grams are treated with transurethral resections of the prostate (TURP) or laser therapy. Even larger glands are surgically removed (prostatectomy). A urinary catheter may be used. The length of time the catheter remains in use depends on the type of surgery, patient's recovery, and health care provider's preference. A permanent, indwelling urinary catheter may be inserted for the patient who cannot undergo surgery.

Nursing Responsibilities

For the patient with benign prostatic hypertrophy, the nurse should:
- Assess the patient's ability to empty the bladder.
- Preoperatively assess both physical and psychosocial aspects.

- Assess the patient's knowledge base regarding treatment options. The patient may not understand the implications of the many treatment options.
- Encourage the patient and significant other to discuss concerns about sexuality while providing empathetic listening, accurate information, and ongoing support. Referral for sexual counseling may be helpful.
- Encourage patients to manage rather than treat postoperative pain.
- Instruct the patient on the proper way to manage urinary irrigation devices and collection bags.
- Teach the patient the proper way to care for the urinary or suprapubic catheter postoperatively. Increase fluid intake while the catheter is in place to promote free flow of urine and minimize clot formation.
- Advise the patient to avoid straining for defecation for 6 weeks after surgery, which this can lead to bleeding from the operative site. Administer stool softeners or laxatives as ordered.
- Advise the patient to avoid strenuous activity for 4 to 6 weeks after discharge.

Do You UNDERSTAND?

DIRECTIONS: **Fill in the blanks.**

1. Benign prostatic hypertrophy is defined as _____.
2. Benign prostatic hypertrophy is the most common _____ tumor in men.
3. Treatment of BPH includes conservative treatment with _____ _____, _____ therapy, or _____.
4. TURP is used for patients whose prostate gland weighs over _____ grams.

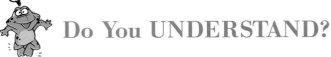

What IS Testicular Carcinoma?

Pathogenesis

Germ cells are responsible for sperm production and are the site of most testicular tumors. Metastasis occurs primarily through lymphatic spread. Drainage from the right testis is to the interaortic lymphatic system, whereas the left testis drains to the preaortic lymph nodes. Retroperitoneal lymph nodes are commonly affected. Distance metastasis is commonly to the lung. The cause of testicular carcinoma is unknown, but congenital and acquired factors have been associated with tumor development.

At-Risk Populations

Lack of descent of the testicles and damage to the testicles appear to be common risk factors. The incidence of testicular carcinoma is approximately 2 to 3 cases per 100,000 men in the United States each year.

Factors that appear to increase the risk of testicular carcinoma are Caucasian heritage, high socioeconomic status, family history, gonadal dysgenesis, fetal exposure to DES, a synthetic estrogen or oral contraceptives, and a history of orchitis.

Answers: 1. enlargement of the prostate gland; 2. benign; 3. watchful waiting, medication, surgery; 4. 60.

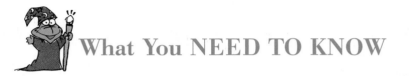

What You NEED TO KNOW

Clinical Manifestations

Men with testicular tumors experience a painless enlargement in the testis. Some men describe the sensation as a dragging sensation. Pain is rare unless the tumor is found during an examination after injury. A hydrocele or hematocele may develop. Back pain, vague abdominal pain, nausea and vomiting, changes in bowel or bladder patterns, anorexia, and weight loss are common and suggest metastasis to the retroperitoneal lymph nodes. When the lungs are involved, manifestations may include cough, dyspnea, and hemoptysis. Testicular cancer is slightly more common on the right side than it is on the left side.

Prognosis

Tumors of the sexually undifferentiated embryonic gonads (seminomas) generally have a favorable prognosis with a 90%, 5-year survival rate because they are usually localized and metastasize late.

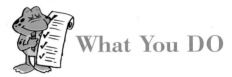

What You DO

Treatment

A removal of the entire testis is the major intervention for testicular carcinoma. Surgery is used because a needle or open biopsy would lead to rapid spread and because after a tumor has been shown to be a solid mass (through ultrasound imaging), the chance of it being malignant is nearly 100%. A decision must be made as to whether to do a lymph node dissection in addition to testicular removal. Antineoplastic or radiation therapy may also be indicated.

Nursing Responsibilities

The nursing responsibilities for the patient at risk for testicular carcinoma are to teach testicular self-examination (TSE). In addition, the nurse should:

- Carefully assess the patient's understanding of and readiness for surgery, because the time between diagnosis and surgery may be a few days at most.
- Discuss sperm banking with the patient, because fertility may be impaired postoperatively or as a consequence of antineoplastic or radiation therapy.
- Teach the postoperative patient to monitor for complications (e.g., hematoma, infection) and self-care strategies.
- Recommend the use of ice bags to control scrotal edema. Analgesics are ordered for pain management, usually through the use of a patient-controlled analgesic (PCA) pump or epidural infusion.
- Encourage ambulation as soon as possible to help prevent postoperative phlebitis.

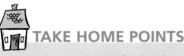
Primary testicular carcinoma is the most common solid tumor in men ages 15 to 35. Testicular carcinoma seldom occurs in men younger than age 15 or older than age 40.

TAKE HOME POINTS

A testicular mass is considered malignant until proven otherwise; however, malignant tumors of the testis are rare.

The overall survival rate from all types of testicular cancer is approximately 89% in Caucasians and 78% in African Americans.

See Chapter 1D in **RWNSG:** *Pharmacology*

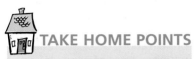
TAKE HOME POINTS

TSE is the most effective strategy for early detection of testicular carcinoma.

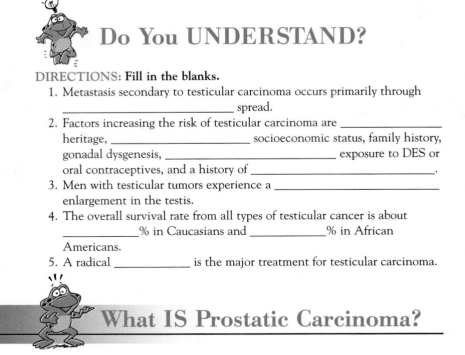

Do You UNDERSTAND?

DIRECTIONS: Fill in the blanks.

1. Metastasis secondary to testicular carcinoma occurs primarily through _____ spread.
2. Factors increasing the risk of testicular carcinoma are _____ heritage, _____ socioeconomic status, family history, gonadal dysgenesis, _____ exposure to DES or oral contraceptives, and a history of _____.
3. Men with testicular tumors experience a _____ enlargement in the testis.
4. The overall survival rate from all types of testicular cancer is about _____% in Caucasians and _____% in African Americans.
5. A radical _____ is the major treatment for testicular carcinoma.

What IS Prostatic Carcinoma?

Pathogenesis

The majority of prostatic cancers are adenocarcinomas. The prostatic tumor begins in the periphery of the posterior lobe of the gland in contrast to BPH in which the disorder occurs centrally. The lesions are confined to the prostatic capsule and grow slowly. Occasionally, the tumor grows rapidly, with metastasis occurring through direct extension to the bladder neck and seminal vesicles. Other spread occurs through lymphatic and circulatory routes. With advanced disease, metastasis to the bone, lungs, and liver is common.

At-Risk Populations

Prostatic cancer is the most common male cancer and the third leading cause of death among men in the United States.

African Americans, men with a family history of prostate cancer, a history of high dietary fat intake, and perhaps men who have undergone vasectomy are at an increased risk for developing prostatic cancer. Japanese men have low rates of prostate cancer until they migrate to the United States, which suggests dietary habits as a possible risk factor to the disease. A higher incidence is found in urban areas, which suggests an environmental consideration. Occupations linked to higher rates of prostate cancer include employment in fertilizer, textile, and rubber industries, as well as working with cadmium-containing batteries. Gonorrhea is also associated with an increased incidence of prostate cancer.

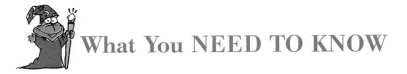

What You NEED TO KNOW

Clinical Manifestations

Unless BPH is present at the same time, manifestations of prostate cancer are absent at the time of digital examination. The presenting findings are those of prostatitis. Urinary obstruction is rare unless BPH is present. Rectal pressure or obstruction from local tumor growth can produce stool changes and painful bowel movements. Painful ejaculation may also be noted. Many men present at a late stage in their disease, complaining of hip or back pain and possible sensory or motor changes from spinal cord pressure. Lymphatic metastases are usually identified in the obturator lymph node chain. Late in the disease, thrombophlebitis and lower extremity lymphedema may develop.

Prostate-specific antigen (PSA) is a glycoprotein that is produced in the cytoplasm of benign and malignant prostate cells. The PSA can be useful in detecting and staging prostate cancer, monitoring response to treatment, and detecting recurrence before it becomes clinically evident. Approximately 24% of men with moderate elevations of PSA are found to have prostate cancer. Patients with urinary retention or ureteral obstruction from local or regionally advanced prostatic cancers may present with elevations in blood urea nitrogen (BUN) or creatinine levels. Patients with bony metastases may have elevations in alkaline phosphatase or hypercalcemia. Prostatic biopsy and imaging are also used to evaluate and detect prostatic cancer.

Prognosis

Prostate cancer tends to be diagnosed in men over the age of 50, many of whom will die of other causes before they become symptomatic from prostate cancer.

TAKE HOME POINTS

Few forms of prostate cancer become metastatic.

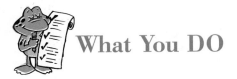

What You DO

Treatment

Treatment of prostatic cancer remains controversial. The side effects of treatment combined with the relatively long life expectancy of many patients with prostate carcinoma make aggressive treatment an option for only certain patients. Some patients may have a life expectancy equal to or better than that of patients who are treated.

Treatment decisions are based on staging and grading of the tumor and the patient's age. Most patients with an anticipated survival in excess of 10 years should be considered for treatment with irradiation or surgery. Radiation therapy and radical prostatectomy allow for acceptable levels of local control.

Patients who are candidates for radical prostatectomy are those who have no other serious medical problems, those who have a discrete tumor involving less than one lobe of the prostate, and those who have an expected survival of at least 10 to 15 years.

Antineoplastic drugs given singly or in combination have been used to treat or occasionally stabilize the disease. Examples of drugs used include cyclophosphamide, fluorouracil, doxorubicin, and mitomycin, to name a few.

Palliative therapy with oral androgen blockers (e.g., flutamide) and gonadotropin-releasing hormone analogs (e.g., leuprolide) are used in symptomatic patients with advanced disease. Antineoplastic therapy and radiation can also provide additional symptomatic disease relief to patients with advanced disease.

Nursing Responsibilities

Nursing responsibilities for the patient with prostate carcinoma is essentially the same as that for the patient with BPH. However, the psychosocial and emotional care of these patients is different because the issues of cancer must be addressed. Some patients may refuse treatment because of the fear of impotence. These patients need a great deal of emotional support to understand the options available to them. In addition, the nurse should:

- Advise the patient who is undergoing radiation therapy about the possibility of radiation cystitis or proctitis. The patient must learn about the need to control diarrhea and ways to protect the perianal skin surfaces that can become excoriated. Antidiarrheal drugs may help control diarrhea.
- Teach the patient who is undergoing antineoplastic therapy about the adverse effects of the drugs. Make suggestions about ways to cope with and manage the adverse effects.
- Encourage patients who are receiving antineoplastic therapy to have their blood counts assessed as recommended.
- Provide preoperative and postoperative care as needed. The specifics of care will depend on the procedure used. Generally, care involves close monitoring of surgical wounds, fluid intake, urinary output, and vital signs.
- Teach patients who are going home with a urinary catheter ways to care for the device. Urinary incontinence usually occurs after removal of the catheter, but leakage subsides within approximately 6 months in the majority of patients.
- Provide bladder retraining, which may be required for the patient who undergoes laser or cryosurgery of the prostate.
- Instruct patients to prevent strain on the perineal incision. Recommend the use of a scrotal support, T-binder, or mesh pants to prevent wound trauma and to hold the dressing in place.

See Chapter 1D in RWNSG: *Pharmacology*

See Chapter 8C in RWNSG: *Pharmacology*

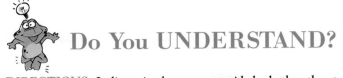

Do You UNDERSTAND?

DIRECTIONS: **Indicate in the space provided whether the statement is true or false. If false, then rewrite the statement in the margin space to the right to make it true.**

_____ 1. The majority of prostatic cancers are seminomas.

_____ 2. With advanced prostate carcinoma, metastasis to the bone, lungs, and liver is common.

_____ 3. The PSA can be useful in detecting and staging prostate cancer, monitoring response to treatment, and detecting recurrence before it becomes clinically evident.

_____ 4. The adverse effects of treatment combined with the relatively long life expectancy of many patients with prostate carcinoma make aggressive treatment an option for only certain patients.

_____ 5. Nursing responsibilities for the patient with prostate carcinoma is essentially the same as that for the patient with BPH.

SECTION B
FEMALE REPRODUCTIVE DISEASES

The uterus is a pear-shaped organ that consists of two parts: the body and the cervix. The uterus secures and protects the fertilized ovum, provides an optimal environment while the ovum develops, and pushes the fetus out during delivery.

The inner lining of the uterus (endometrium) thickens and becomes rich with blood vessels to prepare for the implantation of the fertilized egg. When fertilization does not occur, the endometrium sloughs off as part of the menstrual flow.

The cervix is located at the lower one third of the uterus. The cervix acts as a barrier to microorganisms that may be present in the vagina. The cervical os opens into the vagina to allow menstrual blood to flow out of the uterus during menstruation. The cervical os dilates during labor and through which the child will be born.

The fallopian tubes serve as a pathway for the ova from the ovaries to the uterus. Near the end of each fallopian tube is an ovary. The ovaries contain the necessary materials needed to produce ripened eggs (ova). Because hormones regulate ovarian function, any disorder that disrupts hormone secretion or reception by target cells can result in ovarian dysfunction and infertility.

For the menstrual cycle to remain normal, consistent, synchronized interaction between the brain and reproductive organs must be present. The interaction of six hormones produced by the hypothalamus, anterior pituitary gland, and the ovaries controls menstruation. The way in which hormones control endometrial and ovarian reactions to implement appropriate diagnostic testing and identify the correct treatment for certain disorders is important to understand.

Answers: 1. false; the majority of cancers are adenomas; 2. true; 3. true; 4. true; 5. true.

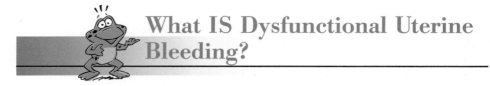

What IS Dysfunctional Uterine Bleeding?

Pathogenesis

Dysfunctional uterine bleeding (DUB) is excessive, prolonged, irregular bleeding that is unrelated to structural or systemic disease.

DUB can originate as a primary disorder of the ovaries or as a secondary defect in ovarian function that is related to hypothalamic-pituitary stimulation. The latter can be initiated by emotional stress, marked variation in weight, or nonspecific endocrine or metabolic disturbances. Organic causes of DUB include reproductive tumors, infection, pregnancy complications, endometrial polyps, polycystic ovary syndrome, and pregnancy. Blood dyscrasias (e.g., thrombocytopenia, aplastic anemia, von Willebrand's syndrome) and systemic diseases such as hyperthyroidism, hepatic, adrenal, or pituitary disorders, diabetes, and colorectal cancers can also alter menstrual patterns. Iatrogenic causes of DUB include contraceptives, androgens, anabolic agents, and hypothalamic depressants.

DUB can occur normally in women at the beginning or end of their reproductive years.

At-Risk Populations

Dysfunctional bleeding patterns occur in any woman of childbearing age.

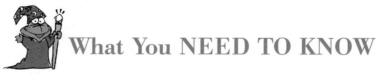

What You NEED TO KNOW

Clinical Manifestations

DUB can occur in the following patterns:
- Absence of menses for 6 months or longer than three of the patient's normal menstrual cycles (amenorrhea)
- Bleeding in which the interval varies from 36 days to 6 months (oligomenorrhea)
- Profuse or prolonged bleeding occurring at regular intervals, lasting more than 7 days and resulting in a blood loss of more than 80 ml in volume (menorrhagia)
- Excessive uterine bleeding that occurs at irregular intervals (menometrorrhagia)
- Bleeding that occurs at regular intervals of less than 21 days (polymenorrhea)

Prognosis

The prognosis for DUB is generally good but is relative to the severity of the disorder. Most patients respond well to medication therapy.

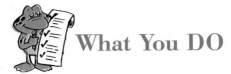

What You DO

Treatment

When no organic pathologic factor is found for the abnormal bleeding pattern, medical therapy is preferred over surgery. The treatment of choice for DUB is drug therapy. Treatment is based on the need to interrupt the growth of the endometrium and create a hormonal environment that is not conducive to endometrial thickening. The medication regimens may include progestins, estrogens, and nonsteroidal antiinflammatory drugs. Progestins (e.g., medroxyprogesterone) not only stop endometrial growth, but also support and organize the endometrium thus sloughing occurs in an organized fashion. When contraception is required, an oral contraceptive accomplishes the same purpose.

When tissue for progestational action is insufficient, or when prolonged intractable bleeding has occurred, estrogen therapy is warranted. Estrogen causes rapid growth of the endometrium and also stimulates clotting at the capillary level. Medroxyprogesterone should be given following the estrogen therapy or concomitantly.

Nonsteroidal antiinflammatory drugs alter the balance between the platelet aggregating substance thromboxane A2 and the antiplatelet substance prostacyclin. Blood loss has been shown to be reduced by as much as 50%.

Other methods used to treat DUB include antifibrinolytic drugs, androgenic steroids, ergot derivatives, desmopressin, and GnRH analogues.

The choice of drug therapy is based on factors such as the patient's desire for fertility, extent of bleeding, accompanying symptoms, other medical conditions, side effects, cost, and patient preference.

See Chapters 3A, 7A, 10A, 11, and 14 in RWNSG: *Pharmacology*

Nursing Responsibilities

For the patient with DUB, the nurse should:
- Obtain a thorough history that includes the woman's age; age at menarche; a thorough history of menses, including flow, pattern, frequency, duration, sexual history, pregnancies, contraception, and medications (including over-the-counter medications); any type of violence; surgical history; family history; and all lifestyle patterns. The number of pads or tampons used during each period should be estimated. The patient should also be questioned about other symptoms experienced during menses or any abnormal bleeding, premenstrual syndrome, premenstrual breast tenderness, bloating, or cramping.
- Assess the meaning of menses to the patient and the way in which it affects her view of body image.
- Encourage the patient to achieve a balance between diet and exercise and to keep a chart of each menstrual cycle.
- Instruct the patient on the relationship of emotional stress to the menstrual cycle.

Do You UNDERSTAND?

DIRECTIONS: **Indicate in the space provided whether the statement is *true* or *false*. If false, then rewrite the statement in the margin space to the left to make it true.**

_____ 1. The most common treatment for DUB is surgical removal of the ovaries and uterus.

_____ 2. DUB occurs only in postmenopausal women.

What IS Amenorrhea?

Pathogenesis

Amenorrhea is the absence of menses. Primary amenorrhea is the failure to menstruate by age 16 or by age 14 when accompanied by the absence of secondary sex characteristics. Faulty gonadal development, congenital agenesis, testicular feminization, or a hypothalamic-pituitary-ovarian axis disorder is usually the cause of primary amenorrhea.

Secondary amenorrhea is the cessation of menses for at least 6 months in a woman who has established normal menstrual cycles. The leading cause of secondary amenorrhea is pregnancy. Other causes of secondary amenorrhea include ovarian, pituitary, or hypothalamic dysfunction, intrauterine adhesions, infections, pituitary tumor, anorexia, nervosa, or strenuous physical exercise. When abnormalities in the hormonal function or the structure of the reproductive organs are present, amenorrhea can occur.

At-Risk Populations

The majority of women experience amenorrhea at some time in life.

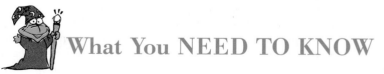

What You NEED TO KNOW

Clinical Manifestations

The major manifestation of primary and secondary amenorrhea is the absence of menses for 6 months or longer than three of the patient's normal menstrual cycles.

Prognosis

Successful treatment of amenorrhea depends on the underlying pathologic factors. Amenorrhea may require long-term therapy. Without treatment, infertility can result.

Answers: 1. false; the most common treatment is medication therapy; 2. false; DUB can occur in any woman of childbearing age.

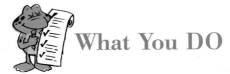

What You DO

Treatment

Treatment for primary amenorrhea involves the correction of any underlying disorder and hormonal replacement to induce the development of secondary sexual characteristics. Depending on the cause of the amenorrhea, treatment may involve hormonal replacement or surgical removal of any adenoma. Surgical alteration of the genitalia may be required to correct abnormalities. Before treatment for secondary amenorrhea can be implemented, pregnancy must be ruled out.

See Chapter 10A in **RWNSG:**
Pharmacology

Nursing Responsibilities

For the patient with amenorrhea, the nurse should:
- Educate the patient on the importance of following all treatment plans.
- Teach the patient about the causes and treatment for amenorrhea and the importance of an adequate diet and exercise.
- Instruct the patient to take hormonal replacement therapy as prescribed.

Do You UNDERSTAND?

DIRECTIONS: **Indicate in the space provided whether the statement is**
true **or** *false*. **If false, then rewrite the statement in the margin space to the right to make it true.**

_____ 1. Amenorrhea is the occurrence of irregular periods.
_____ 2. The leading cause of amenorrhea is menopause.

What IS Dysmenorrhea?

Pathogenesis

Dysmenorrhea is painful menses or severe menstrual cramps. Prostaglandin synthesis at the time of menses produces strong uterine contractions. The contractions constrict blood vessels that supply the uterus, causing ischemia and pain. Excess prostaglandins in smooth muscle also contribute to the gastrointestinal manifestations of dysmenorrhea, such as nausea, vomiting, or diarrhea. Headache is also common.

Primary dysmenorrhea is pain associated with ovulation but not a result of any disease process. Regardless of the cause, the outcome is the same: dysmenor-

Answers: 1. false; amenorrhea is the lack of periods; 2. false; the leading cause of amenorrhea is pregnancy.

rhea. Secondary dysmenorrhea is pain resulting from an abnormal medical condition. The most common cause of secondary dysmenorrhea is endometriosis. Other causes include pelvic inflammatory disease, uterine prolapse, fibroids, polyps, invasion of the uterine tissue by endometrial tissue, or the use of an intrauterine device (IUD).

At-Risk Populations

The true incidence and prevalence of dysmenorrhea are unknown, although most women are affected to some degree at one time or another during their lifetime.

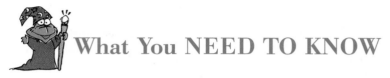

What You NEED TO KNOW

Clinical Manifestations

Primary dysmenorrhea begins with the onset of ovulatory cycles, increases in severity until the woman is in her mid-20s, and then begins to decline. The symptoms appear within a few hours of the onset of menses and can last from 1 to 2 days. Most discomfort is ordinarily experienced during the first 24 hours of flow. The pain is usually located in the lower abdomen and may radiate to the lower back, labia majora, or inner thighs. Headache, fatigue, nausea, vomiting, or diarrhea may accompany the discomfort. The pain of secondary dysmenorrhea may begin after many years of relatively pain-free menstruation.

Prognosis

Dysmenorrhea may ultimately affect women's productivity and increase absenteeism.

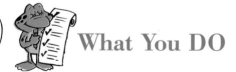

What You DO

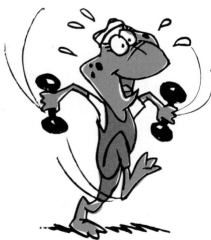

Treatment

The treatment of primary dysmenorrhea emphasizes prevention and education. Women who wish to avoid medications use nondrug therapies, such as biofeedback, therapeutic touch, or acupuncture. Exercise has been used as a remedy for dysmenorrhea because it increases blood flow of beta-endorphins thus making them available for pain relief. Nonsteroidal antiinflammatory drugs such as ibuprofen, indomethacin, and naproxen are commonly used to provide relief because they decrease prostaglandin activity.

Treatment of secondary dysmenorrhea is directed toward the underlying cause. When pelvic inflammatory disease causes dysmenorrhea, identifying the causative organism and selecting the appropriate antimicrobial drug is important. When dysmenorrhea results from the use of an IUD, removal may be warranted. Nonsteroidal antiinflammatory drugs may provide relief for some women.

See Chapters 1A and 11 in
RWNSG: *Pharmacology*

Nursing Responsibilities

Assessment, education, and the use of supportive measures are important nursing responsibilities in the care for women with primary dysmenorrhea. The nurse should:

- Determine the relationship between pain and bleeding, including the frequency, amount, and duration of menses, and the effect on the patient's activities of daily living.
- Encourage regular exercise, a diet low in fat, and appropriate rest and sleep.
- Advise the patient that local application of heat, massage, relaxation techniques, and orgasm are common comfort measures.
- Teach the patient mechanisms involved in dysmenorrhea and the actions and side effects of drugs used for therapy.
- Explain the importance of taking all medication as prescribed and to report any increase in physical discomfort.
- Assess the patient's need for sex education, including the mode of disease transmission, pathologic factors, and consequences of acquiring a sexually transmitted disease.

Do You UNDERSTAND?

DIRECTIONS: Fill in the blanks.

1. Prostaglandin synthesis at the time of menstruation produces strong

    _____ _____ .

2. The most discomfort associated with dysmenorrhea is ordinarily experienced during the first _____ of flow.

3. The primary treatment for dysmenorrhea emphasizes

    _____ and _____ .

4. Advise the patient that local application of _____ ,

    _____ , _____ _____ ,

    and _____ are common comfort measures.

What IS Endometriosis?

Pathogenesis

Endometriosis is a condition in which the tissue that normally lines the uterus (endometrium) escapes the uterus and migrates to other area of the body where it grows. The abnormal tissue growth can develop outside the uterus in the pelvic area, on the ovaries, fallopian tubes, bowel, rectum, and bladder. Endometriosis frequently occurs in other areas of the body as well.

Endometrial cells implant outside of the uterus where they respond to menses in a manner similar to that of uterine endometrium. At the end of every cycle,

Answers: 1. uterine contractions; 2. 24 hours; 3. prevention, education; 4. heat, massage, relaxation techniques, orgasm.

when hormones cause the uterus to shed the endometrial lining, endometrial tissue outside the uterus breaks apart, migrates to other areas, and bleeds. The blood has no place to go thus the surrounding tissues become inflamed or swollen. The continuous cycle of bleeding and healing causes scar tissue to form. Endometrial cells can also penetrate the ovary and multiply, causing ovarian cysts. Repeated episodes of bleeding cause adhesions during which, in time, one peritoneal surface becomes fixed to another.

At-Risk Populations

Endometriosis is a major cause of dysmenorrhea and infertility, affecting 7% of women, regardless of socioeconomic class, age, or race during the reproductive years.

Endometriosis appears to be hereditary, occurring more commonly in women whose mothers had the disorder.

Factors that increase the risk for endometriosis are hereditary factors, higher estrogen levels, prolonged heavy menses, low weight, and smoking. Oral contraceptive use and pregnancy may reduce the risk of developing endometriosis.

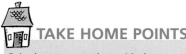 Endometriosis is found most frequently in pre-menopausal women ages 30 to 40 and rarely occurs in women under the age of 20.

The highest incidence of endometriosis is in nulli-parous Caucasian women.

TAKE HOME POINTS

Pain does not correlate with the severity of the endometriosis.

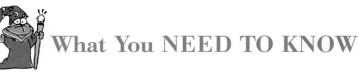 # What You NEED TO KNOW

Clinical Manifestations

Many women are unaware that they have endometriosis, although many experience significant symptoms. Over the years, symptoms tend to gradually increase as endometriosis increases in size. Pain is the most common symptom in 50% of patients. The pain occurs as cramping before and during menses, pain after sexual activity, and heavy or irregular bleeding.

Other symptoms include fatigue, painful bowel movements, low back pain with menses, diarrhea or constipation with menses, and intestinal upset. When the bladder is affected, pain during urination and blood in the urine may be present.

Prognosis

Endometriosis is a progressive disease, but the rate of progression and the nature of the lesions vary from patient to patient. The disease can be life long when symptoms are untreated. Infertility occurs in approximately 25% of patients.

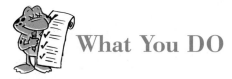 # What You DO

Treatment

The objectives of treatment are to remove or destroy the lesions, relieve symptoms, maintain or restore fertility, and avoid or delay recurrence of the disease.

The treatment chosen depends on the manifestations, age, parity, and extent of the disease. In determining the treatment option for endometriosis, the woman's reproductive goals should also be evaluated.

When endometriosis is mild, the woman is provided support, information about the disease, and suggestions for coping with the disorder. Analgesics and nonsteroidal antiinflammatory drugs can be helpful for women with mild discomfort that is associated with endometriosis. Drug treatment can last from 2 to 6 months. When a woman is infertile or wishes not to become pregnant, a progesterone containing oral contraceptive may be used. Progesterone causes the ectopic endometrium to slough off. This medication controls the endometriosis and works as long as the hormone is taken. In some instances, endometriosis can be forced into remission for months or years after this hormone medication is discontinued.

When progesterone therapy is ineffective, danazol may be used. Danazol is a synthetic androgen that suppresses the ovarian-pituitary axis by inhibiting the release of gonadotropins from the pituitary gland.

When severe symptoms are present, removal of the uterus and ovaries may be recommended, which stops menses and therefore stops the symptoms. Although this procedure is considered by some to be an absolute cure, nonetheless, some women experience a recurrence of the disease.

See Chapters 10A, 11, and 14 in
RWNSG: *Pharmacology*

See Chapter 7B in RWNSG:
Pharmacology

Nursing Responsibilities

Nursing responsibilities in the care for the woman with endometriosis are individualized, based on the severity of the patient's manifestations, the severity of the disease, the patient's age, and her childbearing status. The nurse should:

🍎 Discuss the nature of endometriosis, its treatment, and ways to cope with the manifestations.

🍎 Provide information and support in decision making when infertility is present.

Do You UNDERSTAND?

DIRECTIONS: Indicate in the space provided whether the statement is
true or false. If false, then rewrite the statement in the
margin space to the right to make it true.

_____ 1. Mild endometriosis is treated with support and mild analgesics.

_____ 2. Danazol, a synthetic androgen used to treat endometriosis, suppresses the ovarian-pituitary axis by inhibiting the release of gonadotropins from the pituitary gland.

_____ 3. The prognosis for endometriosis has no relationship to the rate of progression and the extent of the lesions.

_____ 4. Pain is the most common symptoms of endometriosis.

Answers: 1. true; 2. true; 3. false; the prognosis is related to the rate of progression and the nature of the lesions; 4. true.

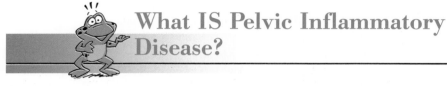

What IS Pelvic Inflammatory Disease?

Pathogenesis

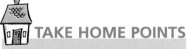

TAKE HOME POINTS

Many different organisms can cause PID, including *Chlamydia trachomatis*, gonococci, staphylococci, streptococci, and other pus-producing organisms.

Pelvic inflammatory disease (PID) is a nonspecific term used to identify a variety of problems found in the upper female genital tract that are characterized by inflammation and infection. PID can affect the ovaries, uterus, fallopian tubes, and other related structures. PID occurs when bacteria or other disease-causing organisms migrate upward from the urethra and cervix into the upper genital tract.

Chlamydia trachomatis, gonococcal, and staphylococcal organisms spread along the uterine endometrium to the fallopian tubes. An acute inflammation of the fallopian tubes (salpingitis) develops with the tubes becoming partially blocked (occluded). The tubes may drain pus, leukocytes, and other debris into the pelvic cavity, causing peritonitis. The material may also form a pocket around the ovaries, causing an abscess.

Streptococcal infections spread in a similar manner, except they tend to travel via the uterine or cervical lymphatic system to the fallopian tubes or ovaries. A pelvic cellulitis and, occasionally, thrombophlebitis of the pelvic veins can occur as a result of the organism's spread.

At-Risk Populations

Patients who are at risk for PID include women who have sex with more than one partner, those who were young at first intercourse, those who have intercourse frequently, those who had a new partner within 30 days of diagnosis of the disease, and women who have been previously diagnosed with the disease. Other risk factors for the development of PID are use of an IUD and douching.

What You NEED TO KNOW

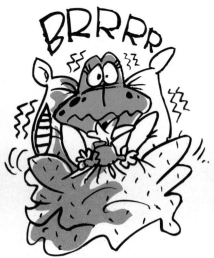

Clinical Manifestations

Women with PID frequently complain of fever and abnormal vaginal or cervical discharge. Other signs and symptoms include generalized infection, such as malaise, fever, chills, anorexia, nausea, vomiting, aching, and tachycardia. Additionally, acute, sharp, severe aching of the abdomen or pelvis may be present. Pain is aggravated with bowel movements and is accompanied by a heavy, purulent, foul-smelling discharge. Vaginal bleeding occasionally occurs. Cervical motion tenderness and adnexal tenderness are noted during pelvic examination. However, not all episodes of PID produce symptoms. Many women with PID have had sex with asymptomatic partners even though the partner is infected with the offending organism.

Prognosis

When PID is diagnosed and treated promptly, the patient experiences complete recovery. Without treatment, PID can cause scarring, pelvic pain, tubal pregnancy, infertility, and other serious complications. Although septic shock can occur, the most common complication is a pelvic abscess.

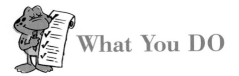

What You DO

Treatment

Many women with PID are asymptomatic. Because many organisms exist that can cause the infection, treatment requires a broad-spectrum antibiotic. Hospitalization may be required for the woman who is extremely ill. Pain management is important. Sitz baths or heat applied periodically to the lower abdomen or back can help relieve pain. All sex partners should be treated, even when no symptoms are reported. Surgical intervention may be required when a pelvic abscess develops. The type of surgical intervention varies with the presenting problem but may include laparotomy or total hysterectomy.

See Chapter 1A in RWNSG: *Pharmacology*

Nursing Responsibilities

The care of women with PID is directed toward providing health teaching and psychosocial support. The nurse should:

- Provide supportive care because guilt feelings and problems with significant others that center on the woman contacting the infection may be present.
- Plan for and allow time for expression of feelings because some women may be infertile after contracting PID.
- Advise female patients to avoid sexual activity, douches, and other activities that can worsen the infectious process.
- Tell the patient to return for reevaluation if her condition worsens or her manifestations continue.
- Place the hospitalized patient in a semi-Fowler's position to promote downward drainage of the pelvic cavity. Document the amount, color, odor, and appearance of any vaginal discharge.

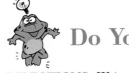

Do You UNDERSTAND?

DIRECTIONS: **Write the letter in the space provided that corresponds to the phrase that accurately complete each of the following statements.**

_____ 1. Patients with PID _____.
   a. do not experience symptoms.
   b. always experience symptoms.

Answer: 1. a.

_____ 2. The treatment of choice for PID is a _____.
   a. vaginal suppository
   b. vaginal douche
_____ 3. The most common organism that causes PID is _____.
   a. *Chlamydia trachomatis*
   b. *Staphylococcus aureus*
_____ 4. PID _____ cause scaring, pelvic pain, tubal pregnancy, infertility, and other serious complications without treatment.
   a. can
   b. does not
_____ 5. Sex partners of a woman with PID _____ treated even when no symptoms are reported.
   a. should be
   b. should not be

What IS Vulvovaginitis?

Pathogenesis

Vulvovaginitis is the inflammation of the vulva and vaginal area. Normal vaginal function depends on a balance between hormones and bacteria. Disturbance of the balance can precipitate infection. The most common causes of vulvovaginitis are bacterial vaginosis, candidiasis, and trichomoniasis. Sexually transmitted diseases (e.g., genital herpes) and bacterial infections with single organisms (e.g., *Escherichia coli, Staphylococcus aureus,* group A or B streptococcus) can also cause vulvovaginitis. Infections of Bartholin's gland, Skene's glands, the endometrium, and the fallopian tubes, although infrequent, can also cause increased vaginal discharge and inflammation. Additionally, various chemicals that are found in bubble bath, soaps, perfumes, and allergens, as well as poor hygiene, can cause inflammation and irritation.

At-Risk Populations

Sexual abuse should be considered in children with unusual, recurrent episodes of unexplained vulvovaginitis.

Most women will experience vulvovaginitis. Predisposing factors to vulvovaginitis include diabetes mellitus, pregnancy, antibiotic therapy, high-dose oral contraceptives, immune suppression, and, possibly, constricting clothing. Women with symptomatic human immunodeficiency virus (HIV) infection can present with oral, esophageal, or vaginal yeast infections.

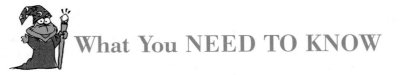

What You NEED TO KNOW

Clinical Manifestations

Vulvovaginitis is characterized by a change in vaginal discharge, irritation, itching, odor, swelling, and soreness or pain, particularly after intercourse. Some patients may not complain of symptoms despite the presence of discharge and other findings.

Prognosis

Maintenance of healthy lactobacilli and low vaginal pH are mutually reinforcing factors that reduce infections from various organisms. Consequences of bacterial vaginosis (BV) are increasingly recognized as common and serious. The bacteria and the virulence factors they produce are associated with the ascent and establishment of BV-associated organisms in the endometrium and fallopian tubes. Unless treated effectively, BV is associated with ascending reproductive tract infection during pregnancy, PID, and infection following pelvic surgery.

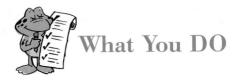

What You DO

Treatment

Treatment is dependent on the specific disorder. BV and trichomoniasis are commonly treated with oral or vaginal metronidazole or clindamycin. Topical clotrimazole suppositories may be used if the woman is pregnant. Recent sexual partners (previous 2 months) should also be treated despite the absence of symptoms. Gentian violet solution may be applied to the vagina in the form of swabs or tampons for some patients. Boric acid soaks to the vulva and potassium sorbate douches have also been found to be effective treatments.

See Chapters 1A and 1B in
RWNSG: *Pharmacology*

Vulvovaginitis caused by strains of Candida is usually treated with a 3- to 7-day course of topical antifungal drugs, such as miconazole or ketoconazole. Avoidance of tight-fitting clothing and improved perineal hygiene are traditional recommendations.

Nursing Responsibilities

The care of the patient with vulvovaginitis is primarily supportive. The nurse should:

- Advise the patient to get adequate rest, eat nutritious foods, and exercise at least three times per week.
- Teach the patient to wipe from front to back to avoid spreading bacteria, changing tampons or sanitary pads at least four times daily during menses, and washing the hands before and after each change.

- Instruct the patient that periodic douching is unnecessary and, in fact, may be detrimental because it washes away normal protective mucus and bacterial flora of the vagina. Douching may also introduce other bacteria.
- Encourage the patient to avoid feminine hygiene sprays because they can be irritating. Soap and water are appropriate for cleansing the perineal region.
- Advise the patient to avoid wearing tight-fitting pants, pantyhose, and nylon, satin, or thong underwear.
- Encourage the patient to seek early treatment for changes in vaginal drainage, particularly when the drainage is profuse or has a foul odor.
- Encourage women who are familiar with vulvovaginitis caused by candida to self-treat with over-the-counter medications.
- Advise the patient to avoid tampon use to avoid the risk of toxic shock syndrome. Patients who are experiencing vulvovaginitis for the first time should be advised to seek assistance from the health care provider.

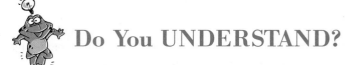

Do You UNDERSTAND?

DIRECTIONS: Write the letter in the space provided that corresponds to the phrase that accurately completes each of the following statements.

_____ 1. Vulvovaginitis _____ preventable.
    a. is
    b. is not

_____ 2. Repeated vulvovaginitis in young girls is _____ in this age group.
    a. common
    b. uncommon

_____ 3. BV and trichomoniasis _____ treated with metronidazole or clindamycin.
    a. are
    b. are not

_____ 4. Vaginal candidiasis is most commonly treated with antifungal drugs administered _____.
    a. orally
    b. vaginally

_____ 5. Vulvovaginitis is characterized by a change in vaginal discharge, irritation, itching, odor, swelling, and soreness or pain, especially after _____.
    a. intercourse
    b. menstrual cycle

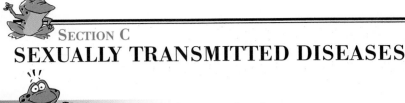

SECTION C
SEXUALLY TRANSMITTED DISEASES

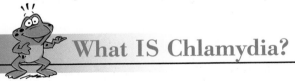

What IS Syphilis?

Pathogenesis

Syphilis is a systemic disease caused by the spirochete *Treponema palladium*, which penetrates intact skin or mucous membranes during sexual contact, multiplies, and rapidly spreads to regional lymph nodes. The spirochete then enters the blood stream within hours and is transported to other tissues and is capable of infecting almost any organ or tissue in the body. The incubation period for primary syphilis is approximately 3 weeks but ranges from 10 to 90 days after exposure. Syphilis can be transferred via the placenta from mother to fetus after the tenth week of pregnancy (congenital syphilis).

At-Risk Populations

Factors such as limited access to health care, decreases in health department clinical services, increased use of illicit drugs, and contact with multiple sexual partners increase the risk of contracting syphilis. Women of childbearing age, sexually active teens, drug users, inmates of penal institutions, and persons with multiple sex partners are most at risk.

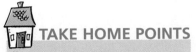

TAKE HOME POINTS

Sexually transmitted diseases (STDs) present a major public health problem. STDs include over 25 infectious organisms that are transmitted through sexual activity (vaginal, oral, and anal intercourse).

What IS Chlamydia?

Pathogenesis

Chlamydia trachomatis infection is the most common STD in the United States. A bacterium with at least 15 variations, Chlamydia spreads to lymph channels and lymph nodes. Typically, the site of infection in women is the genital tract in the transition zone of the endocervix. In men, the urethra is the most common site of infection. Incubation is variable but is usually at least 1 week.

Co-infection with gonococci and chlamydiae is common, and postgonococcal urethritis may persist following successful treatment of the gonococcal component. For this reason, the Centers for Disease Control and Prevention (CDC) recommends treating for both chlamydia and gonorrhea when either STD is present.

At Risk Populations

Chlamydia is common in the United States, particularly among adolescents and young adults.

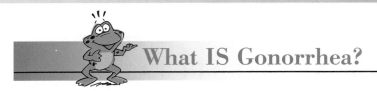

What IS Gonorrhea?

Pathogenesis

Gonorrhea is transmitted almost exclusively sexually, because the organism, *Neisseria gonorrhoeae*, cannot survive outside the body. The incubation period is 2 to 7 days. Gonorrhea is the major cause of PID, tubal infertility, ectopic pregnancy, and chronic pelvic pain.

At-Risk Populations

The infection rate is highest in sexually active young adults. The transmission risk from an infected man to a woman is 70% after one exposure.

Newborns are at risk for gonococcal ophthalmia from contact with infected vaginal discharge during vaginal birth.

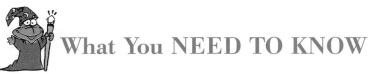

What You NEED TO KNOW

Clinical Manifestations of Syphilis

Primary syphilis produces a painless chancre at the site of inoculation. The chancre is a solitary macule with a well-defined, indurated border and a clear, red base that becomes encrusted. The chancre is frequently unnoticed and heals spontaneously. Chancres outside the genitals, such as the breasts and lips, are usually painful.

Secondary syphilis develops 6 to 8 weeks after exposure and is characterized by enlarged lymph nodes, generalized rash, and influenza-like symptoms. The rash may be macular, maculopapular, or papular, extending to palmar and plantar surfaces. Fever, headache, malaise, fatigue, muscle, or joint pain usually accompanies the rash.

The latent phase begins with healing of the lesions from the secondary stage and may last a few years or a lifetime. After a variable period, approximately 33% of untreated cases develop into tertiary syphilis. Neurologic and cardiovascular disease, soft tumors, auditory or ophthalmic involvement, and cutaneous lesions are characteristics of tertiary syphilis.

Prognosis for Syphilis

Although syphilis is treatable, reinfection is possible with continued exposure. An infection does not provide lasting immunity to the disease. Blindness is possible in late congenital syphilis, and approximately 28% of patients will die.

Clinical Manifestations of Chlamydia

Most persons who are infected with chlamydia are asymptomatic. Symptoms of chlamydial infection in women are mucopurulent cervicitis, urethritis, salpingitis, and proctitis. Women may present with complaints of vaginal discharge, dysuria, abnormal vaginal bleeding, and pelvic pain.

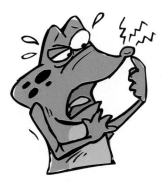

Congenital syphilis involves multiple organ systems with the stage of syphilis in the mother, which determines the effects on the fetus. Early congenital syphilis occurs from birth to age 2 and is characterized by mucocutaneous lesions, runny nose, and other symptoms. Congenital syphilis can be asymptomatic, particularly in the first weeks of life. Late congenital syphilis is characterized by bone and joint disorders, cardiovascular disease, cranial neuropathies, soft tumors of the liver and respiratory system, and interstitial iritis, which can cause blindness if untreated.

In men, chlamydial infection can cause nongonococcal urethritis (NGU) and acute epididymitis. Men may complain of discharge of mucopurulent or purulent material from the urethra and burning during urination. Reiter's syndrome (reactive arthritis, conjunctivitis, and urethritis) is a complication of untreated chlamydial infection that occurs primarily in men.

Prognosis for Chlamydia

Chlamydia is the leading cause of PID in women. Without adequate treatment, 20% to 40% of infected women will develop PID, which can result in infertility, potentially fatal ectopic pregnancy, and chronic pelvic pain.

Clinical Manifestations of Gonorrhea

In women, the common sites of infection are the pharynx, urethra, endocervix, upper genital tract, and rectum. Presenting symptoms include increased vaginal discharge, abnormal uterine bleeding, and dysuria. Vaginitis and cervicitis with inflammation of the Bartholin's glands are common. Symptoms of widespread disease include inflammation of the tendon sheath (tenosynovitis), skin lesions, fever, and multiple joint pains. Widespread disease usually occurs when acquired during menses or pregnancy. Less common manifestations include endocarditis and perihepatic involvement.

In men, the common sites of infection are the pharynx, urethra, epididymis, prostate, and rectum. Typically, men note urethritis and a purulent penile discharge. Without treatment, the infection can spread to the urethra, prostate, seminal vesicles, and epididymis. The result is urethral stricture and obstruction. Proctitis can occur after anal intercourse. Conjunctivitis and progressive corneal ulceration can occur as a result of inoculation into the conjunctiva.

Prognosis for Gonorrhea

The prognosis for gonorrhea is good with adequate treatment and reduced exposure. Without treatment, the disease may progress to PID.

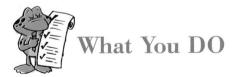 ## What You DO

Treatment for Syphilis

The most commonly used tests for syphilis are provided by the Venereal Disease Research Laboratory (VDRL) and rapid plasma reagin (RPR). The fluorescent treponemal antibody absorption (FTA-ABS) test is most widely used. All patients with syphilis should have an HIV test at the time of diagnosis.

Treatment of syphilis is parenteral penicillin G. Sexual contacts of patients who are being treated should be evaluated and treated presumptively if their exposure to the patient was within the previous 90 days. Patients with syphilis must abstain from sexual activity until they are found to be uninfected.

Overall, the prevalence of gonorrhea has declined but continues to be one of the most prevalent STDs in the United States.

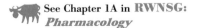 **See Chapter 1A in RWNSG:** *Pharmacology*

Treatment for Chlamydia

Chlamydia culture is most definitive, but other tests, such as direct immunofluorescence assay, enzyme-linked immunoassay, and a DNA probe, may also be used to diagnose this disorder. A ligase chain-reaction (LCR) test for chlamydia has superior sensitivity compared with all other methods and can be performed on urine. Concurrent testing for gonorrhea is also recommended for patients with a suspected chlamydia infection.

Treatment for uncomplicated urethral, endocervical, or rectal chlamydia infections includes doxycycline or azithromycin. Erythromycin is the treatment of choice in pregnant patients.

Treatment for Gonorrhea

Diagnostic tests for gonorrhea include cell cultures from the site of exposure, urethra, endocervix, throat, and rectum. Gram-stained specimens can be diagnostic in clinical settings. Nonculture tests such as DNA probes are reliable.

Treatment of adults with uncomplicated gonococcal infections of the cervix, urethra, and rectum include regimens of ceftriaxone, cefixime, ciprofloxacin, or ofloxacin. Retesting following treatment is usually unnecessary.

All symptomatic sexual contacts made within 30 days of the onset of symptoms should be evaluated and treated. With asymptomatic patients, all sexual contacts made within 60 days should be evaluated and treated. The CDC recommends screening for and treating chlamydia for all persons diagnosed with gonorrhea because the two infections are commonly found together.

Nursing Responsibilities

For the patient with a syphilis, chlamydia, or gonorrhea infection, the nurse should:

- Provide the patient with accurate information about transmission, early detection, treatment, follow-up, reinfection, sequelae, proper hygiene, and safe sexual practices.
- Individualize teaching to meet the patient's needs and psychosocial situation.
- Encourage the patient to complete the entire course of medication therapy and to return for follow-up evaluation.
- Advise the patient to abstain from all sexual contact (intercourse, oral-genital contact, oral-anal contact, or anal penetration) until after the treatment period is completed. All sexual contacts identified within the previous 60 days of exposure should be examined, cultured, and treated.

See Chapter 1A in RWNSG: *Pharmacology*

The CDC recommends that all pregnant women be screened for gonorrhea.

See Chapter 1A in RWNSG: *Pharmacology*

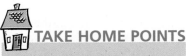

TAKE HOME POINTS

Advise the patient with gonorrhea to refrain from oral sexual activity when a pharyngeal infection is present. A primary measure for controlling gonorrhea is the screening of high-risk women for both chlamydia and gonorrhea.

Do You UNDERSTAND?

DIRECTIONS: **Fill in the blanks.**

1. Syphilis is caused by the spirochete known as _____.
2. Persons at high risk for syphilis include the following groups:

   _____
   _____
   _____
   _____
   _____

3. Primary syphilis is characterized by a painless _____ at the site of inoculation.
4. Secondary syphilis occurs approximately 6 to 8 weeks after sexual exposure and is characterized by _____,
   _____, and _____.

DIRECTIONS: **Write the letter in the space provided that corresponds to the phrase that accurately complete each of the following statements.**

_____ 5. Most persons infected with chlamydia are _____.
   a. symptomatic
   b. asymptomatic
_____ 6. The site of infection in women typically is the genital tract in the transition zone of the _____.
   a. endocervix
   b. ovaries
_____ 7. Anyone with whom the patient has had ongoing sexual exposure within _____ days of a positive test result should be treated.
   a. 60
   b. 120

DIRECTIONS: **Fill in the blanks.**

8. Treatment for uncomplicated urethral, endocervical, or rectal chlamydia infections is _____
   or _____.
9. The causative organism of gonorrhea is _____
   _____.
10. Common sites of infection with the gonococcal organism are the following:

    _____
    _____
    _____
    _____
    _____

Answers: 1. Treponema pallidum; 2. women of childbearing age, sexually active teenagers, drug users, inmates of penal institutions, persons with multiple sex partners; 3. chancre; 4. lymphadenopathy, generalized rash, influenza-like symptoms; 5. b; 6. a; 7. a; 8. doxycycline, azithromycin; 9. Neisseria gonorrhoeae; 10. pharynx, urethra, endocervix, upper genital tract, rectum.

11. Treatment of adults with uncomplicated gonococcal infections of the cervix, urethra, and rectum include regimens of the following:

_____

_____

_____

12. All sexual contacts identified within the previous _____ days of exposure should be examined, cultured, and treated presumptively.

What IS Genital Herpes?

Pathogenesis

An infant can become infected with genital herpes as the newborn passes through the birth canal. Genital herpes have also been implicated as a cause of cervical cancer.

Genital herpes is the result of the type II herpes simplex virus (HSV). Two types of herpes simplex viruses exist, both of which cause painful blisterlike lesions. Type I HSV ordinarily affects the oral cavity but can affect other body areas; type II HSV most often affects the genitalia. After gaining access to the body, HSV enters the nervous system, invading nerve cells located in the sacral ganglia where it remains indefinitely. The presence of the virus predisposes the patient to recurrent outbreaks.

At-Risk Populations

The incidence of active genital herpes is difficult to determine. The difficulty arises because many patients have mild symptoms that are self-limiting and thus not called to the attention of the health care provider. However, genital herpes affects both genders, is highly contagious, and is transmitted by direct person-to-person contact. Transmission is not limited to sexual contact. Transmission from one person to another via the hands is possible; for example, from a lip ulcer to the genital area or from the lip or genitals to the eye.

Factors that contribute to recurrent herpes outbreaks are not well understood, but exposure to sunlight, local trauma, fever, or emotional stress may precipitate an outbreak. Hormonal changes that precede menses have been associated with recurrences in women.

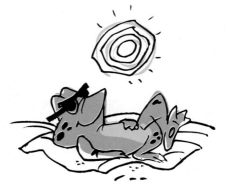

What You NEED TO KNOW

Clinical Manifestations

A genital rash and mild itching are usually the earliest signs of genital HSV infection. Eventually, blisters form on the skin surface, enlarge, break open, and ulcerate. The lesions are painful, particularly during intercourse, and can cause intense itching. When the urethra is involved, painful urination can result. In men, the blisters are found on the glans, shaft of the penis, prepuce, scrotum, and inner thighs. In women, the blisters usually involve the vulva, vagina, cervix, perineum, inner thighs, and buttocks. The blisters may or may not be present with first exposure to the virus. The blisters usually last from 1 to 3 weeks, with recurrent episodes becoming milder and less frequent. Possibly, however, some patients have weekly or monthly outbreaks that are quite painful and severe. Other symptoms include anorexia, malaise, and fever.

Because the virus lives in the blisters and nerve cells and not in the blood, antibody titers and cultures taken from the lesions are helpful in identifying the stage of the disease. A culture of the blisters is sensitive and specific for HSV. The presence of HSV antibodies at the time of an initial episode indicates a previous HSV infection. High antibody titers are usually found in patients with recurrent HSV.

Prognosis

Primary genital herpes is usually self-limiting, and immediate complications are rare, barring secondary infection and neurologic damage. Women with genital herpes are eight times more likely to develop carcinoma in situ than are those who lack HSV-II antibodies in their serum.

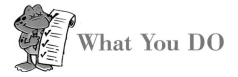 # What You DO

Treatment

Medication currently used for genital herpes includes topical, oral, or IV acyclovir (Zovirax), famciclovir (Famvir), or valacyclovir (Valtrex). These drugs help shorten the outbreak but do not provide a cure. Treatment goals include keeping the blisters clean and dry, controlling pain with analgesics, promoting healing with frequent sitz baths, and preventing secondary bacterial infections.

See Chapters 1A and 14 in RWNSG: *Pharmacology*

Nursing Responsibilities

For the patient with genital herpes, the nurse should:
- Provide accurate information, support, and counseling to help the patient cope with the disease and its effects, including the usual frequency of recurrence, asymptomatic shedding, and mode of transmission. Inform the patient that the attacks are less frequent and severe as time passes. Recommend abstension from sexual activity while symptoms or lesions are present. Advise patient to inform all sexual partners from time of suspected exposure. Encourage the use of condoms during sexual activity with any new or uninfected partners. Note, however, that condom use does not always prevent viral transmission. Recommend that all sexual partners be evaluated for mild or atypical signs of infection and treated appropriately.
- Instruct the patient to wear loose, cotton clothing to avoid trapping moisture in the genital area. Help the patient find effective coping mechanisms to help control outbreaks.

Mothers with HSV who have had two negative cervical smears for the virus within 1 week of delivery and those who have no active lesions at the time they go into labor can safely deliver their child vaginally.

- Advise the patient to avoid the use of perfumed soaps, feminine deodorant sprays, and douches.
- Assist patients in finding support groups that allows them to express anger and talk about their guilt. The American Social Health Association sponsors self-help groups and provides educational materials.
- Encourage female patients to have a Papanicolaou's smear every 6 months.
- Instruct the pregnant patient to abstain from intercourse during the last trimester when there is a history of genital herpes in either partner.

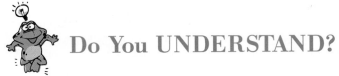

Do You UNDERSTAND?

DIRECTIONS: **Circle the correct answer.**

1. Which of the following are symptoms of herpes?

blisters	painless chancre	enlarged lymph nodes
fever	vaginal discharge	pelvic pain
genital rash	dysuria	abnormal vaginal bleeding

Answers: blisters, genital rash.

11 Musculoskeletal System

The musculoskeletal system is composed of muscles and bones together with associated structures, such as joints, ligaments, cartilage, and tendons. The purpose of the musculoskeletal system is to protect internal organs, provide structure and motion, store minerals, and form blood cells. Bone is composed of 90% to 95% collagen fibers, which provide strength. Bone is the hardest tissue in the body; 65% to 75% of bone is composed of mineral salt, such as calcium and phosphorus. Cells in bone tissue include fibroblasts, fibrocytes, osteocytes, osteoblasts, and osteoclast cells. Fibroblasts and fibrocytes are used for collagen formation. Osteocytes maintain bone matrix. Osteoblasts form new bone tissue, while osteoclasts break down bone tissue.

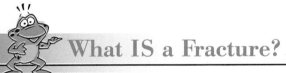

What IS a Fracture?

Pathogenesis

A fracture is a break or alteration in the normal contour of a bone. Fractures typically occur as a result of trauma but may also occur from muscle spasm or bone disease. Direct force is the most common cause of fractures.

Bone healing is a five-stage process. The first stage (hematoma stage) begins immediately after the injury and lasts approximately 1 day. Bleeding into tissues that surround the fracture site occurs from ruptured vessels in the bone, torn connective tissue that covers the bone (periosteum), and soft tissue. Blood from the area clots, forming a hematoma around the injured site. The body's normal inflammatory response to injury results in vasodilation and edema.

The second stage (cellular proliferation stage) occurs 2 to 6 days after the fracture when the hematoma changes. Fibroblasts from periosteum and nearby connective tissue enter the injured site and change into fibrous connective tissues or granulation tissue. A fibrin mesh is formed that protects the damaged bone

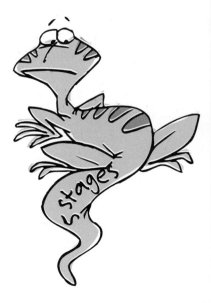

and provides structure for capillaries, fibroblast activity, and new bone growth. White blood cells migrate into the injured area to contain the inflammation caused by phagocytosis of the red blood cells and tissue debris.

The third stage (callus formation stage) lasts from 6 to 10 days. Osteoblasts, which arise from fibroblasts, invade the clot and granulation tissue to form a soft tissue around the injured site. The granulation tissue changes into newly formed cartilage (callus) and bone matrix. The newly formed callus is sufficiently strong to hold bones together but not for weight bearing.

The fourth stage (callus ossification stage) lasts 2 to 10 weeks after the injury. Calcium salts and cartilage are deposited in the soft-tissue callus, leading to rigid calcification and permanent callus formation.

The fifth stage (consolidation and remodeling stage) lasts 2 months to 1 year. Through osteoclastic (i.e., a cell associated with resorption of bone) activity, bone tissue overgrowth and excess calcium are remolded to the normal bone contour.

Older adult women (over age 65) are the group most at risk for osteoporosis, which weakens bone and leaves this group more prone to fractures.

At-Risk Populations

Fractures occur in all age groups. The highest incidence of fractures occurs in men age 15 to 24 and in elderly persons, particularly women over age 65.

What You NEED TO KNOW

Clinical Manifestations

Many possible manifestations of a fracture occur. The major symptom of a fracture is pain or tenderness on palpation. Tenderness at the site of the fracture is related to the rubbing, stretching, and swelling of the periosteum. Fracture pain is usually immediate, continuous, and severe during movement. The severity generally increases until the fracture site is splinted and protected. Other symptoms of a fracture include abnormal sensations as a result of nerve injury from a pinched or severed nerve (paresthesia). A grating sound or sensation (crepitus) may be noted from jagged bone ends rubbing together. Muscle spasms are common and related to sudden involuntary muscle contractions resulting from nerve irritation. Edema is usually present because of the leakage of blood into the tissues (extravasation) and an accumulation of serous fluid at the injury site, both of which contribute to a bruised appearance. When the break involves an arm or leg, the extremity may have an internal or external rotation. The extremity may appear shorter because of an overlapping of bone fragments.

An avulsion fracture occurs when a sudden pull on the tendon occurs. The bone to which the tendon is attached will break (tendons are stronger than bones). Common places for avulsion fractures include the lateral and medial malleolus (from twisted ankles) and phalanges of the hand (from sports objects being thrown and hitting the ends of the fingers).

Prognosis

The prognosis for the patient with a fracture is usually good. Factors that affect healing are many and include the amount of trauma to surrounding soft tissue, the type of fracture, size of the broken bone, and adequacy of immobilization. Infection, underlying pathologic conditions, bone death (avascular necrosis), age, fracture location, stress, accurate fracture reduction, early remobilization, the amount of circulation and nutrition to injured site, and the general condition of the patient all affect healing. When any of these factors are absent, the prognosis may be diminished.

An adequate amount of exercise stimulates healing. Healthy patients who have adequate nutrition and an exercise regimen heal more quickly than do malnourished patients.

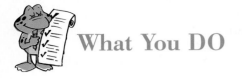

What You DO

Treatment

Treatment of a fracture includes realignment (reduction) of the fractured bone and pain management. A fracture should be reduced as soon as possible because soft-tissue swelling tends to increase for 6 to 12 hours after injury and becomes inelastic with time, making reduction more difficult.

Realignment of bone can be achieved with open or closed reduction or with traction. Closed reduction is accomplished through manual manipulation or reduction traction, which allows for realignment of the broken bones without direct visualization. Closed reduction is indicated when patients are unable to tolerate open reduction. Open reduction involves surgery with direct visualization of the injury. Surgery is usually performed within 24 to 48 hours in medically stable patients. Some patients may be unable to undergo open reduction because of the dangers associated with surgical anesthesia.

Traction may also be used to realign a broken bone. After the fracture is in a normal anatomic position, alignment is maintained by immobilizing the

Reduction traction

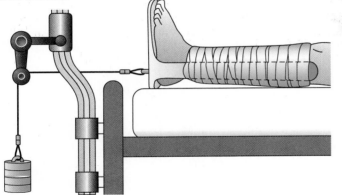

A fracture in an older adult takes longer to heal. Corticosteroids and the lack of estrogen after menopause tend to decrease the body's ability to form new bone tissue and to heal injured bone.

See Chapters 11 and 14 in RWNSG: *Pharmacology*

In an older adult with a fractured femur, fragile bones, and who is a poor surgical candidate, realignment may be achieved by Buck's traction.

extremity with a cast or splint. Initially, a splint is applied after reduction to allow the injured soft tissue to swell and expand. After the danger period for swelling has passed, a rigid cast that completely encircles the injured part is applied.

Nursing Responsibilities

The nursing responsibilities for a patient with a fracture begin with the initial assessment at the scene of injury or emergency department. In addition, the nurse should:

- Evaluate the ABCs (airway, bleeding, and circulation) and potentially life-threatening injuries.
- Assess the fracture site for deformity, shortening of extremity, limited or abnormal movement, pain, swelling, diminished neurovascular status, discoloration, soft-tissue damage, or crepitus.
- Immediately immobilize the fracture site and preventing movement of the injured part before moving the patient.
- Carefully handle the fractured part because movement and palpation can aggravate pain and cause further damage.
- Avoid improper handling of a newly applied plaster cast to avoid leaving indentations in the cast and pressure areas under the cast.
- Instruct the patient to keep the plaster cast dry. When a plaster cast becomes wet, strength and integrity are lost thus the function of support and immobilization is lost.
- Closely monitor and preserve neurovascular status, which prevents complications and restores independent function.
- Control the patient's pain to ensure that exercise and the activities of daily living can be accomplished with ease. Mobilize the patient with an adequate exercise regimen designed to increase circulation, promote healing, and assist in restoring function.

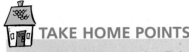

TAKE HOME POINTS

A wet plaster cast should be handled with the palms rather than with the fingertips and placed on a soft surface.

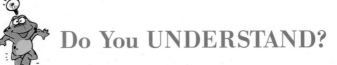

Do You UNDERSTAND?

DIRECTIONS: **Number the five stages of bone healing in order.**

_____ a. Callus ossification
_____ b. Consolidation with remodeling
_____ c. Cellular proliferation
_____ d. Hematoma formation
_____ e. Callus formation

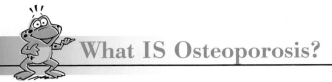

What IS Osteoporosis?

Pathogenesis

Osteoporosis is the most common bone disease and is defined as a reduction in bone density. Estrogen stimulates bone growth activity and limits bone breakdown. The bone density is below the level required for mechanical support and can lead to fragile bones and fractures. Osteoporosis results from bone breakdown that exceeds the rate of bone formation. The bones are left porous and weaker than is normal. The natural drop of estrogen in postmenopausal women is primarily responsible for osteoporosis.

At-Risk Populations

Women who have small, thin-framed bodies and who smoke are especially prone to osteoporosis. Men who work underground in large cities and who lead a sedentary life style are also at risk for osteoporosis. These people have limited exposure to sunlight and frequently have significant osteoporosis.

Additional factors predisposing a person to osteoporosis include the natural aging process, a deficiency of vitamin D and calcium, high intake of caffeine or alcohol, genetics, and hyperthyroidism. More than two cups of caffeine in the form of coffee or soft drinks per day and daily alcoholic beverages cause calcium loss. Excessive corticosteroid therapy also contributes to bone demineralization and breakdown.

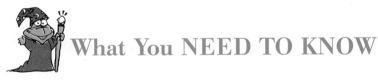

What You NEED TO KNOW

Clinical Manifestations

The reduction in bone mass that is associated with osteoporosis is asymptomatic. Frequently, the first manifestation of osteoporosis is a fracture of the wrist, forearm, hip, or vertebrae. Pain is a common complaint.

Prognosis

The prognosis of an individual with osteoporosis is poor because the associated fractures lead to significant morbidity and mortality. Approximately 25% of patients over age 65 die within 1 year of a hip fracture. Of those who survive, 20% require institutional care with an average length of stay of 7 years.

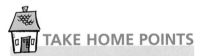

TAKE HOME POINTS

Patients with osteoporosis have a bone density that is inadequate for mechanical support and are at risk for fractures.

The population at highest risk for osteoporosis is postmenopausal Caucasian women over age 65.

European and Asian women are at high risk for osteoporosis.

TAKE HOME POINTS

As osteoporosis progresses, the vertebrae become weak and collapse, resulting in a decrease in height and hump back (kyphosis).

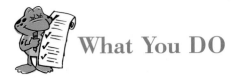

What You DO

Treatment

The treatment for osteoporosis includes biphosphonates, such as alendronate (Fosamax), calcitonin, and slow-release sodium fluoride. Biphosphonates bind to calcium-phosphate crystals and inhibit osteoclastic activity. Calcitonin inhibits bone breakdown, and sodium fluoride stimulates bone formation.

See Chapters 7A, 11, and 12 in RWNSG: *Pharmacology*

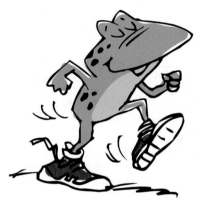

Nursing Responsibilities

For the patient with osteoporosis, the nurse should:
- Teach the patient about risk factors, the importance of exercise (walking or low-impact aerobics), adequate dietary calcium, vitamin D supplements, smoking cessation, and avoiding excess caffeine, alcohol, and soft drinks.

Do You UNDERSTAND?

DIRECTIONS: Circle the bone that may be affected by osteoporosis.

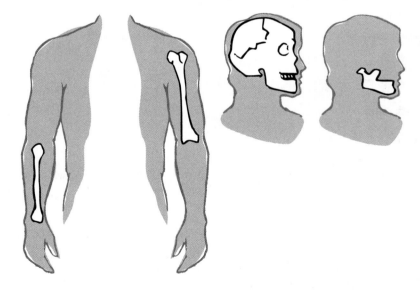

DIRECTIONS: Circle the beverages that are most likely to predispose an individual to osteoporosis.

Wine   Orange juice   Coffee   Milk

Answers: 1. radius; 2. wine, coffee.

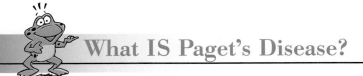

What IS Paget's Disease?

Pathogenesis

Paget's disease is the second most common bone disorder in the United States and usually affects the skull, spine, pelvis, and long bones. The cause of Paget's disease is unknown. Theories suggest that genetic predisposition leads to a dormant skeletal infection.

In the initial stages of the disease, rapid breakdown of bone occurs, followed by short periods of abnormal excessive bone formation. The rapid breakdown produces cavities in the bone that lead to frail bones. New bone that is formed is high in minerals but poorly constructed, which results in bone that is thick but soft and hypertrophic, structurally weak, and deformed. The affected bone develops a greater blood supply (increased vascularity) to support its high metabolic demands. The risk of pathologic fracture is increased.

At-Risk Populations

The population at highest risk for Paget's disease is men over the age of 50.

Persons of European descent are at high risk for Paget's disease.

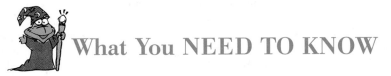

What You NEED TO KNOW

Clinical Manifestations

The clinical manifestations of Paget's disease include severe, persistent bone pain and pathologic fractures. Bowed-leg deformities lead to gait disturbances, such as a waddling gait. A thickening of cranial bones leads to skull enlargement, a change in the shape of the skull, and compression of cranial nerves. When the skull thickens and enlarges, the patient may complain that hats no longer fit properly. Cranial nerve compression can cause dizziness, headaches, blindness, facial paralysis, tinnitus, hearing loss, and mental deterioration. Bone deformity contributes to the complication of arthritis. The increased vascularity and high metabolic demands lead to complications of hypertension and cardiac failure.

Prognosis

The prognosis of a patient with Paget's disease depends on the degree of involvement. Because Paget's disease is gradual, most patients are unaware they have the disorder. Some patients have skeletal deformities but are asymptomatic and without pain. In the majority of patients, the deformities involve the skull or long bones, contributing to cranial damage or bowed legs.

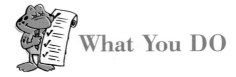

What You DO

Treatment

The treatment of Paget's disease includes preventing and treating fractures, pain, and deformities. Analgesics are used for the pain and nonsteroidal antiinflammatory drugs (NSAIDs) are used to decrease the inflammation associated with bone breakdown. Calcitonin is used to slow the rate of bone breakdown. Etidronate disodium (Didronel) produces rapid reduction in bone turnover and pain relief, thereby promoting disease remission. Mithramycin (Plicamycin) is a cytotoxic antineoplastic that is used in severe cases to control the disease and give remission for months after the drug is discontinued.

See Chapters 1D, 7A, 11, and 14 in RWNSG: *Pharmacology*

Nursing Responsibilities

For the patient with Paget's disease, the nurse should:
- Assess for and manage pain.
- Assess for fatigue; specific skeletal alterations, such as shortened stature, enlarged skull, and bowed legs; and pathologic fractures.
- Counsel the patient and family safety about precautions to prevent falls and fractures.
- Teach the basic first-aid measures as necessary should fractures or injuries occur.
- Monitor for complications of Paget's disease, such as cranial or spinal cord compression, hypertension, and cardiac failure.

Do You UNDERSTAND?

DIRECTIONS: Select the outcome(s) from the following list and fill in the blanks.

1. Bowed-leg deformity of Paget's disease leads to

   _____.

2. Increased vascularity of bone affected by Paget's disease leads to

   _____ and _____.

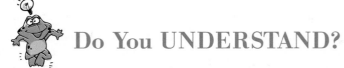

| Waddling gait disturbances | Hypertension | Cardiac failure |
| Diabetes | Sarcoidosis | Sore throat |

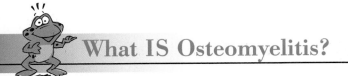

What IS Osteomyelitis?

Pathogenesis

Osteomyelitis is an infection of the bone with progressive inflammatory bone destruction, which results most frequently from *Staphylococcus aureus* invading bone tissue. The second most common invading bacteria are gram-negative bacteria. Fungi have also been implicated in osteomyelitis.

Bacteria may also travel through the blood from a distant body site, such as an abscessed tooth, sinuses or upper respiratory tract, middle ear, gastrointestinal or urinary tract, soft-tissue trauma, pressure sores, or burns.

Osteomyelitis begins with the introduction and adherence of bacteria to bone matrix. In the adherent state, bacteria are highly resistant to antibiotics. When bacteria invade the skeletal blood supply, an inflammatory response is triggered in the confined space. Drainage that results from the inflammation process enters the bone marrow, which forms abscess pockets. Because of the disruption in blood supply, the bone tissue becomes necrotic. Ordinarily, the rapidly growing long bones of the tibia, femur, and humerus are affected.

At-Risk Populations

Young children are most at risk for osteomyelitis.

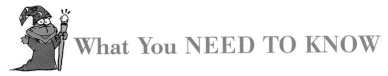

What You NEED TO KNOW

Clinical Manifestations

The clinical manifestations of osteomyelitis initially include vague pain in the affected extremity or back for 1 to 3 months. Later in the infection process, fever, chills, malaise, irritability, localized tenderness, redness, warmth in affected area, swelling, enlarged proximal lymph nodes, muscle spasm, and bone pain develop.

Prognosis

The prognosis is usually good. In severe cases, bone and joint deformity or a halt of bone growth can occur. Amputation is occasionally required to prevent the spread of bacteria throughout the body.

 TAKE HOME POINTS

In osteomyelitis, bacteria may enter the bone directly from a fracture, wound, surgery, or they may travel through blood from another infection in the body.

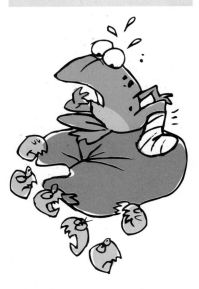

The population at highest risk for osteomyelitis is usually children under 12 years of age.

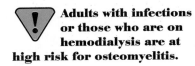 **Adults with infections or those who are on hemodialysis are at high risk for osteomyelitis.**

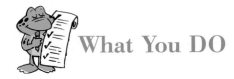

What You DO

Treatment

The treatment for osteomyelitis includes long-term antibiotics, surgical drainage and debridement of necrotic bone, and, in some cases, bone grafting. Amputation may be required if necrosis of the bone is extensive. The antibiotics used to treat *S. aureus* infections include nafcillin (Unipen) and cefazolin (Kefzol). Antibiotics that treat gram-negative bacteria include the third generation cephalosporins, the aminoglycosides, and ciprofloxacin (Cipro).

See Chapter 1A in RWNSG:
Pharmacology

Nursing Responsibilities

For patients with osteomyelitis, the nurse should:
- Encourage good hand-washing practices to prevent transferring the bacteria to others.
- Administer antibiotic therapy as prescribed.
- Assists with dressing changes as needed.
- Provide effective pain management and assistance with avoiding immobility complications.
- Teach the patient to perform exercises that help maintain strength and joint flexibility.

Do You UNDERSTAND?

DIRECTIONS: **Indicate in the space provided whether the statement is**
**   *true* or *false*.**

_____ 1. Osteomyelitis is usually found in elderly adults.
_____ 2. Osteomyelitis can be the result of bacteria entering an abscessed tooth.
_____ 3. Osteomyelitis is an infection of the bone resulting from food poisoning.
_____ 4. Vague pain is usually the initial symptom of osteomyelitis.

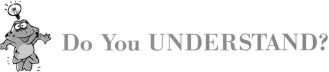

What IS Osteomalacia?

Pathogenesis

The pathogenesis of osteomalacia includes inadequate mineralization of bone matrix by calcium and phosphorous, leading to disorganized bone formation that lacks density. Osteomalacia results from impaired absorption of vitamin D, impaired renal or hepatic activation of vitamin D to an active hormone, dietary deficiency, lack of exposure to sunlight, and malabsorption of fat. Osteomalacia usually affects the ribs, spine, pelvis, and legs.

 In children, osteomalacia is known as rickets.

At-Risk Populations

Individuals in the northern hemisphere who endure long winters with inadequate exposure to sunlight are at risk. Other high-risk individuals include those with malabsorption syndromes and renal or hepatic disease.

The population at the highest risk for osteomalacia includes people in developing countries.

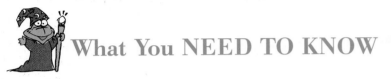

What You NEED TO KNOW

 In the United States, osteomalacia is most common in children, pregnant women, or elderly adults with dietary vitamin D deficiency.

Clinical Manifestations

The clinical manifestations of osteomalacia include bone pain, tenderness on palpation, muscle weakness, and skeletal abnormalities, such as short stature, pigeon-breast deformity of chest, squaring of the head, and swayback (lumbar lordosis). Pain usually increases with activity. Bone cysts and fractures of the wrists, ribs, vertebrae, and hips are common.

Prognosis

The prognosis of osteomalacia is fairly good when treatment is begun early. Skeletal deformities may improve or disappear. When osteomalacia is a result of malabsorption or renal or hepatic failure, the prognosis is poor.

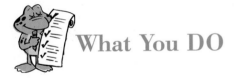

What You DO

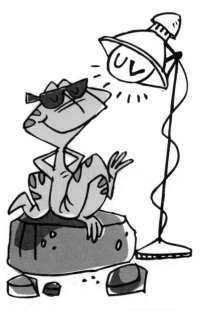

Treatment

The treatment for osteomalacia is exposure to ultraviolet light and the use of calcium and vitamin D supplements.

Nursing Responsibilities

For the patient with osteomalacia, the nurse should:
- Provide effective pain management and preventing injury.
- Assess the home environment for safety and fall risks.
- Teach the patient and family about a diet that is adequate in calcium and vitamin D, as well as the use of any needed ambulatory devices.

See Chapter 12 in **RWNSG:**
Pharmacology

Do You UNDERSTAND?

DIRECTIONS: **Indicate in the space provided whether the statement is** *true* **or** *false***. If false, then rewrite the statement in the margin space to the left to make it true.**

_____ 1. Osteomalacia is a result of a deficiency of vitamin C.

_____ 2. Bowed legs is the most common skeletal abnormality of osteomalacia.

What IS Osteoarthritis?

Pathogenesis

Osteoarthritis (OA), a degenerative joint disease (DJD), is a progressive, chronic, localized, noninflammatory deterioration that includes a loss of articular cartilage with a proliferation of new bone and soft-tissue growth in and around joints. OA involves the ends of long bones at the articular cartilage of weight-bearing joints and results from a breakdown of the articular cartilage, which cushions the bone ends.

The pathogenesis of OA initially involves enzymatic destruction of articular cartilage. The surface layers of articular cartilage flake off, and deep cracks develop. Later in the disease process, the articular cartilage erodes entirely, which allows bone ends to thin and become unprotected. Unprotected bone ends make contact and rub against each other. This stress on the bone leads to further density, hardness, and proliferation of new bone and soft-tissue growth. The new, but disorganized, bone growth leads to the formation of bone spurs (osteophyte), which alters the contour of the bone and joint. Osteophytes project outward from the bone. Microscopic fractures of the osteophytes result in free-floating fragments within the joint.

At-Risk Populations

Younger people and athletes or those with repeated joint trauma are at risk. Risk factors contributing to OA are repetitive or congenital abnormalities, trauma, instability, or disease of the joint.

The population most at risk for osteoarthritis includes individuals over the age of 65.

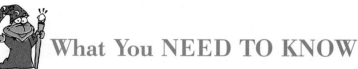

What You NEED TO KNOW

Clinical Manifestations

The signs and symptoms of OA include brief morning stiffness that lasts 15 to 30 minutes, joint pain and swelling that worsens late in the day, limited movement, and crepitus. The symptoms vary from mild to severe, depending on the amount

Answers: 1. false; vitamin D and calcium, lack of sunlight exposure, and malabsorption of fat cause osteomalacia; 2. false; short stature, squaring of the head, pigeon-breast, and lumbar lordosis or swayback are characteristics of osteomalacia.

of degeneration that has taken place. When severe OA involves the hand, Heberden's nodes (found on the distal interphalangeal joints) or Bouchard's nodes (found on the proximal interphalangeal joints) develop. As OA progresses, a loss of muscle strength and size occurs, along with an increase of muscle spasms.

Prognosis

The prognosis for OA is good. This disease is chronically progressive but the treatment is usually well tolerated and significantly improves mobility and the quality of life. Osteoarthritis is less crippling compared with rheumatoid arthritis, during which two bone surfaces may fuse, completely immobilizing the joint.

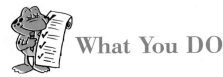

What You DO

Treatment

The treatment for OA involves weight loss, rest, and reduction of repetitive joint trauma. Surgical interventions include surgical fusion of the joint (arthrodesis), transection of the bone (osteotomy), and joint replacement. Heat applications provide comfort, and cold applications help to reduce pain. Range-of-motion and isometric exercises are used to strengthen muscles around the affected joints. Oral drug therapy includes NSAIDs and analgesics, as well as intraarticular glucocorticoids and hyaluronate. In some cases, glucosamine and chondroitin have been helpful in reducing discomfort.

See Chapters 7A, 11, and 14 in RWNSG: *Pharmacology*

Nursing Responsibilities

For the patient with OA, the patient should:
- Provide pain management and maintain joint function and mobility.
- Help the patient find a balance between rest and activity, while maintaining functional independence.
- Monitor the patient for depression, and facilitate a referral as needed.

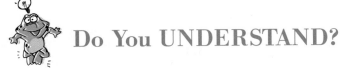

Do You UNDERSTAND?

DIRECTIONS: **Draw a finger with Bouchard's and Heberden's nodes at the site that they are most commonly found.**

Answers: Bouchard's nodes would be on the proximal interphalangeal joints; Heberden's nodes would be on the distal interphalangeal joints.

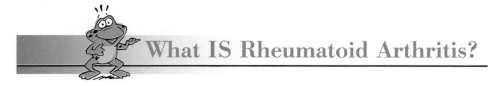

What IS Rheumatoid Arthritis?

Pathogenesis

Rheumatoid arthritis (RA) is a chronic, progressive, systemic, inflammatory disorder of connective tissue that affects symmetrical joints. The cause is unknown
but thought to be an autoimmune attack of the patient's own body tissue, a
genetic predisposition, or a dormant infection.

RA is characterized by progressive stages. In RA, the immune system mis-
takes normal tissues for foreign tissues and tries to neutralize and rid the body of
the perceived threat. Initially, the synovial membrane becomes inflamed. T cells
activate macrophages and B-cell–derived antibodies. These autoantibodies produce immune complexes that lead to inflammation. Inflammation of the synovium (synovitis) causes edema and excessive growth of the inflamed membrane. Exudate produced from the inflammatory process oozes into the articular
cartilage, forming a fibrous pannus layer. Harder bone tissue replaces the fibrous
material that eventually becomes completely immobile (ankylosis).

At-Risk Populations

RA that occurs before age 16 is known as juvenile arthritis. Juvenile arthritis usually resolves by adulthood.

The population at the highest risk for RA includes middle-age women, but all
age groups may be affected.

What You NEED TO KNOW

Clinical Manifestations

The initial manifestations of RA include low-grade fever, fatigue, malaise,
anorexia, and musculoskeletal pain. As the disease progresses, joint inflammation occurs with accompanying redness, swelling, warmth, pain, and the development of subcutaneous nodules over bony prominences. Morning stiffness usually lasts 30 minutes to 1 hour. In RA, symmetrical joints are affected.

Ordinarily, the hands and feet joints are affected first, with later involvement
of the wrist, elbow, knee, and ankle joints. Joint deformities such as ulnar deviation, hyperextension of the proximal interphalangeal joint (swan-neck deformity), and flexion of the proximal interphalangeal joint (boutonniere deformity) are characteristic findings of RA.

Prognosis

The prognosis of RA is rather poor because of the progressive joint destruction.
Patients with severe RA have a survival rate of less than 50%. Death from RA
is usually a result of cardiac, pulmonary, or vascular complications. Additionally,

deaths from RA may be related to the adverse effects of pharmacologic treatment, such as reduced resistance to infection or gastrointestinal (GI) bleeding. The destructive process can be disrupted with aggressive drug therapy started early in the disease.

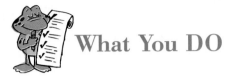

What You DO

Treatment

Treatment includes rest, hot and cold applications, braces, equipment to help with the activities of daily living, and physical therapy. Drug therapy includes NSAIDs, corticosteroids, immunosuppressives, and disease-modifying antirheumatic drugs (DMARDs).

> **See Chapters 7A, 11, and 14 in**
> **RWNSG: *Pharmacology***

Surgical techniques are also performed. A surgical synovectomy to remove the pannus layer and disrupt the inflammatory process is effective for some patients. Surgical total joint replacement is also successful in most patients.

Nursing Responsibilities

For the patient with RA, the nurse should:
- Provide effective pain management and maintain joint function.
- Help with frequent position changes to prevent muscle spasms and contractures, and to minimize stress on joints.
- Help the patient find a proper balance between rest and activity.
- Teach about the disease, weight reduction, proper nutrition, and appropriate exercises.
- When appropriate, provide postoperative care, with attention to maintaining existing system functioning.

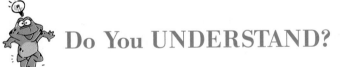

Do You UNDERSTAND?

DIRECTIONS: **Place a check mark next to each sign or symptom of RA.**

_____ 1. Low grade fever
_____ 2. Bad breath
_____ 3. Swelling of joints
_____ 4. Fatigue
_____ 5. Tongue thickening
_____ 6. Night blindness
_____ 7. Joint deformities

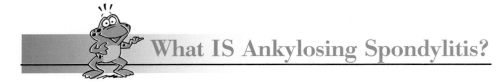

What IS Ankylosing Spondylitis?

Pathogenesis

Ankylosing spondylitis is a chronic, progressive disorder involving inflammation of the shoulders, spine, hips, sacroiliac joints, and stabilizing ligaments. The cause of this disease is unknown, but it is thought to have a strong genetic predisposition. Klebsiella infection or environmental triggers likely perpetuate the inflammatory response.

In ankylosing spondylitis, sacroiliac joint inflammation (sacroiliitis) occurs initially, followed by spinal joint involvement. The sacroiliitis and overgrowth of synovial tissues that is associated with the accumulation of lymphoid cells following inflammation leads to cartilage destruction and bony erosions. The inflammatory process destroys the articular cartilage on the ends of bones, replacing it with new bone formation. Later in the disease process, the entire spine becomes fused. The sacroiliitis progresses to fibrosis, calcification, and ossification of joints until ligaments are replaced by bone that becomes fixed.

At-Risk Population

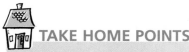
The population at risk for ankylosing spondylitis is usually Caucasian men between the ages of 20 and 40.

The population at risk for ankylosing spondylitis is usually Caucasian men between the ages of 20 and 40.

What You NEED TO KNOW

Clinical Manifestations

TAKE HOME POINTS

The pain of ankylosing spondylitis improves with exercise and is not relieved by rest.

Initially, the clinical manifestations of ankylosing spondylitis include early morning stiffness and chronic hip or low back pain. Later in the disease process, the low back pain progresses upward in the spine with a loss of spinal movement. Leg or buttock pain and leg weakness may also develop.

Systemic inflammatory effects such as fatigue, malaise, low-grade fever, and weight loss occur. Patients may experience chest pain resulting from thoracic compression. With spinal fusion, increased forward curvature of the spine (kyphosis), and thoracic compression, cardiac, pulmonary, and GI involvement usually occurs.

Prognosis

The prognosis for the patient with ankylosing spondylitis is poor. Over a 10- to 20-year period, the patient begins to flex the knees and hips in an effort to hold the head upright.

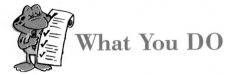

What You DO

Treatment

The treatment for ankylosing spondylitis includes the application of heat, resting joints, and physical therapy. Drug therapy includes NSAIDs and other analgesics, sulfasalazine (Azulfidine), and corticosteroids. Reconstructive surgery includes osteotomy, cervical spinal fusion, or total joint replacement.

See Chapters 1A, 11, and 14 in
RWNSG: *Pharmacology*

Nursing Responsibilities

For a patient with ankylosing spondylitis, the nurse should:
- Assist the patient in obtaining physical therapy services to help maintain proper posture.
- Encourage the patient and family to maintain an exercise regimen within the patient's abilities to maintain existing systems functioning.
- Encourage the patient to discontinue smoking to decrease pulmonary complications.
- Monitor heart rate and rhythm and respiratory status as kyphosis worsens.
- Monitor the functioning of the GI tract for evidence of worsening compression.

Do You UNDERSTAND?

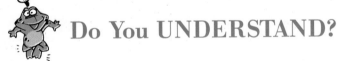

DIRECTIONS: Write the letter in the space provided that corresponds to the phrase that accurately completes each of the following statements.

_____ 1. In ankylosing spondylitis, pain is _____ at rest.
   a. better
   b. worse

_____ 2. Ankylosing spondylitis has _____.
   a. local effects
   b. systemic effects

_____ 3. After 20 years of ankylosing spondylitis, the patient has a
   _____.
   a. bowed-leg position
   b. stooped position

Answers: 1. b; 2. b; 3. b.

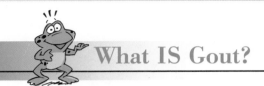

What IS Gout?

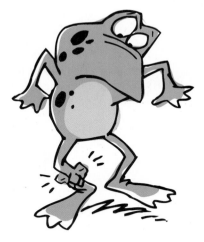

Pathogenesis

Gout is defined as a metabolic disorder resulting from an overproduction or under excretion of uric acid. A supersaturation of serum uric acid occurs, which precipitates and forms urate crystals. These crystals are deposited in connective tissue, particularly joints and surrounding tissue.

Gout moves through progressive stages. Initially, uric acid levels exceed 7 to 10 mg/dl without other significant signs and symptoms. The asymptomatic stage can last years with only 20% to 25% of patients progressing to the second stage. The next stage is called acute gouty arthritis, during which the serum uric acid level exceeds 10 mg/dl. Albuminuria is greater than 100 mg/24 hours. The supersaturation of uric acid in plasma and body fluids leads to urate crystal deposits in joints and surrounding tissue. Urate crystals tend to deposit in cooler body parts, such as fingers or toes. The metatarsophalangeal joint, also known as the great toe, is usually affected.

In the second stage of gout, the body's immune system attacks and treats the crystals as foreign substances. Polymorphonuclear leukocytes (PMNs) permeate the joint and phagocytize the urate crystals. Phagocytosis results in the death of PMNs and the release of lysosomal enzymes, as well as other inflammatory mediators into surrounding tissues. Ordinarily, at least a 1-year period exists between the first and second gouty attack. Recurrent attacks increase in frequency over a period of years.

The third stage of gout is the intercritical stage. With appropriate treatment, patients may be asymptomatic for months and up to 10 years. However, when the patient is not treated, the interval between attacks is usually less than 1 year.

The last phase is identified as chronic gout (chronic tophaceous gout) and may develop 10 years or more after the first attack. During this stage, chronic inflammation from urate crystals leads to the development of insoluble monosodium urate crystals (tophi). Tophi are commonly deposited in synovial membranes, cartilage, soft tissues, tendons, and other tissues that surround joints. Chronic gout attacks tend to have a rapid onset and may develop over a few hours. Without effective pharmacologic treatment, acute attacks may be observed every few weeks.

At-Risk Populations

Predisposing factors that lead to individual attacks include genetics, poor dietary and eating habits, dehydration, trauma, emotional stress, increased alcohol intake, and even several medications. A diet high in purines can lead to a gout attack if the patient has an inborn faulty metabolism; otherwise, no direct relationship exists.

Elevation of uric acid usually occurs in male adolescents; however, the male population at highest risk is over age 40. In women, gout is delayed until after menopause because estrogens tend to increase the renal excretion of uric acid.

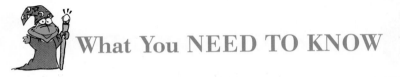

What You NEED TO KNOW

Clinical Manifestations

The clinical manifestations of gout include a localized inflammatory response that triggers excruciating pain, joint edema, warmth, redness, extreme sensitivity to the slightest touch, and limitation of joint movement. Fatigue, chills, fever, and an increased white blood cell count also accompany gout.

The first attack usually affects only one joint, but as the attacks occur more frequently, the attacks involve other joints and last longer. In later stages, tophi may be present in the helices of the ears, in the hands, feet, olecranon bursa, infrapatellar bursa, and Achilles' tendon. Tophi are generally not painful but may restrict joint movement and cause deformities.

Prognosis

The prognosis of gout is good when successfully managed with a reduction of precipitating factors and drug therapy. Early diagnosis and pharmacologic treatment can prevent tophi.

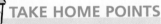

TAKE HOME POINTS

The great toe joint is most commonly affected, causing the patient to awaken at night with excruciating pain. The weight of the bed linens on the great toe is frequently intolerable.

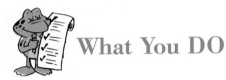

What You DO

Treatment

The treatment for gout includes rest, elevation, joint immobilization, cold applications, a low-purine diet, and high fluid intake. The NSAID indomethacin (Indocin) is typically used for an acute attack, followed by xanthine oxidase inhibitor or uricosuric drugs that help reduce uric acid levels. Corticosteroids and antimitotic drugs are used in some cases. Surgery is usually performed only to remove tophi deposits that have become extremely large and interfere with daily functioning or joint movement.

Nursing Responsibilities

For a patient with gout, the nurse should:
- Reduce precipitating factors such as stress and alcohol use.
- Assist the patient to remain as comfortable as possible during an acute attack.
- Encourage weight reduction because blood uric acid levels are higher in overweight people.
- Teach about the importance of diligent drug therapy.
- Periodically monitor uric acid levels and kidney function tests.

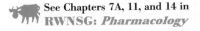

See Chapters 7A, 11, and 14 in
RWNSG: *Pharmacology*

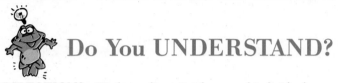

Do You UNDERSTAND?

DIRECTIONS: **Circle predisposing factors of individual gout attacks.**

Genetics	Poor eating habits	Dehydration	Trauma
Emotional stress	Excess alcohol intake	Living in the tropics	Allergies

12 Altered Nutritional States

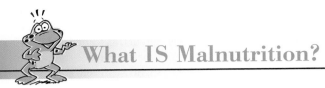

What IS Malnutrition?

Pathogenesis

Malnutrition is poor nourishment from improper intake or a defect in metabolism that prevents the body from using its food properly. Weight loss occurs when expended energy is greater than caloric intake and stored energy. Body proteins are used for energy, which causes a negative nitrogen balance. As malnutrition progresses to a state of starvation, fat cells become small, and accumulations of fat are depleted. The liver is reduced in size, the muscles shrivel (atrophy), and the lymphatic system, gonads, and blood deteriorate.

Vomiting and diarrhea cause nutrient loss from the gastrointestinal (GI) tract. Infection, surgery, bowel obstruction, cancer, burns, draining wounds, and chronic illnesses also contribute to malnutrition. People with chronic airway limitation (chronic obstructive pulmonary disease, COPD) can develop malnutrition when air hunger interferes with the ability to eat. The resulting malnutrition further complicates respiratory function and food consumption.

At-Risk Populations

Although poverty remains as the major cause of malnutrition, the condition is by no means confined to the underdeveloped areas of the world. Many risk factors for malnutrition exist.

Factors that increase the risk of malnutrition include inadequate nutrient intake resulting from poor availability of food, a knowledge deficit regarding the basic principles of nutrition, and substance abuse. Alcohol abuse frequently causes a person to rely on alcohol at the expense of food. Misplaced faith in vitamins as a substitute for food, for example, can cause malnourishment when carried to extremes. Overreliance on processed foods can occasionally result in a deficiency of valuable nutrients.

Kwashiorkor and marasmus are the two most common types of malnutrition in children. These disorders are known jointly as protein energy malnutrition (PEM). Kwashiorkor is a severe protein deficiency; marasmus is a severe deficiency of all nutrients. Kwashiorkor usually occurs in infants or children 1 to 4 years of age who have been weaned from breast milk to a high-carbohydrate, protein-deficient diet. Marasmus can occur at any age but is common in children under 1 year of age, particularly in areas in which food supplies are inadequate. Marasmus may also be found in children with failure to thrive, the cause of which is believed to be primarily emotional.

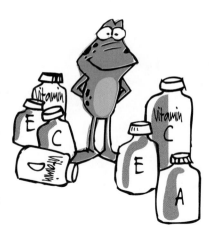

People at increased risk for malnutrition include infants and children, pregnant women, elderly adults, hospitalized patients, those who are cognitively impaired, substance abusers, minority populations, immigrants, and the homeless.

Patients with cultural differences who reside in long-term care facilities when the facility serves no ethnic food are also at risk for malnutrition.

High-fasting triglyceride and phospholipid concentrations are predictive of a poor prognosis for children with kwashiorkor.

In severe cases of malnutrition, death can result without nutritional intervention.

 See Chapter 12 in **RWNSG: Pharmacology**

 # What You NEED TO KNOW

Clinical Manifestations

The clinical manifestations of malnutrition are numerous. Each body system is affected by the lack of appropriate nutrients; however, generally, the symptoms of malnutrition are physical weakness, lethargy, and an increasing sense of detachment from the world. In severe cases, the patient may appear starved (emaciated), have intolerance to cold, have an increased number of infections, and experience poor wound healing. Loss of muscle mass, reduced vital capacity as a result of respiratory muscle atrophy, diminished cardiac output, ankle edema, and dry flaking skin are common. Laboratory testing may reveal low hemoglobin, serum albumin, and transferrin levels. Serum triglyceride and phospholipid levels increase with increasing severity of malnutrition; other serum values, however, such as cholesterol, are normal or slightly reduced.

Prognosis

Malnutrition may be mild or severe to the extent that damage done to the body is irreversible.

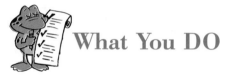 # What You DO

Treatment

High-calorie, high-protein foods are used most frequently to treat malnutrition. Oral feeding is the preferred method for nutritional intake. A fortified nutritional supplement (e.g., Ensure) may be added to the diet, and vitamin and mineral supplements may be given. When the patient is unable to eat, enteral feeding may be administered through a nasogastric, nasoduodenal, gastrostomy, or jejunostomy tube. Total parenteral nutrition (TPN) is a third option when the oral or enteral routes are inappropriate methods for feeding. TPN is a form of intravenous (IV) therapy that delivers all required nutrients to the patient.

Other treatment may be necessary, based on assessment findings. Some patients need financial help or assistance with eating. Lack of appetite, frequently related to depression or interaction of medications, may be identified and treated by the health care provider.

Nursing Responsibilities

The nursing responsibilities for the patient who is malnourished include the following:
- Identify patients at risk for malnutrition.
- Obtain a dietary history with attention to protein and calorie intake and availability and access to appropriate foods.
- Assess food preferences while ensuring a pleasant environment in which to eat.
- Administer oral, enteral, or parenteral nutrition, and vitamin and mineral supplements as ordered.
- Monitor electrolyte values and serum glucose and serum albumin levels.
- Accurately record intake and output.
- Obtain daily weights at the same time, on the same scale, and in the same type of clothing.
- 🍎 Provide age-appropriate and culturally appropriate patient and family teaching regarding the disorder and required treatment.
- Arrange with social services for financial and transportation assistance, when appropriate.

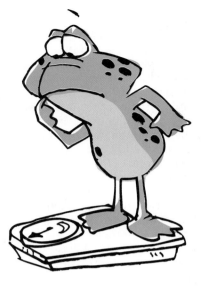

Do You UNDERSTAND?

DIRECTIONS: **Fill in the blanks by unscrambling the italicized words.**

1. A cause of increased loss of nutrients is _____.
   (*heardria*)
2. The _____ population is at increased risk of malnourishment. (*lydrele*)
3. _____ feeding is administered intravenously. (*rneaplarte*)
4. The nurse is responsible for obtaining _____ daily while the patient is receiving parenteral nutrition. (*htgiwe*)
5. _____ is a condition of severe protein deficiency. (*oorwasikhkr*)

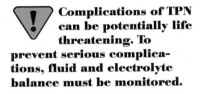

Complications of TPN can be potentially life threatening. To prevent serious complications, fluid and electrolyte balance must be monitored.

What IS Obesity?

Pathogenesis

Obesity is an imbalance between energy intake and expenditure, an increase in weight beyond that considered desirable with regard to age, height, and bone structure. Obesity can be classified as occurring from the ingestion of excess calories (exogenous) or resulting from inherent metabolic problems (endogenous). Physiologically, obesity is classified according to the structure and distribution of fat (adipose) tissue.

Answers: 1. diarrhea; 2. elderly; 3. parenteral; 4. weight; 5. kwashiorkor.

Child-onset obesity is related to a greater-than-normal number of fat cells (hyperplastic obesity) and larger-than-normal fat cells (hypertrophic obesity). In children, the fat tissue is located over the entire body, and few metabolic abnormalities exist. In contrast, adult-onset obesity is hypertrophic. The fat tissues are centrally located, and metabolic abnormalities are more common. However, abnormalities of metabolism are believed to be the result, rather than the cause, of obesity.

Non-Hispanic African-American women, Mexican-American women, and Native-American men and women are at greater risk than is the general population for obesity.

Although numerous theories of obesity exist, the leading cause of obesity is consumption of excess calories. Additionally, various neuroendocrine dysfunctions and some drugs, including corticosteroids, estrogens, and nonsteroidal antiinflammatory medications, are causes of obesity in some people.

Weight gained during certain periods in life leads to an increased number of fat cells. These periods are between 12 and 18 months, 12 and 16 years, and during pregnancy. Weight gain results from consuming foods, particularly calories and fat, in excess of body requirements. Furthermore, after a fat cell is formed, it is there to stay. When food intake equals metabolic needs, weight remains fairly constant throughout life.

At-Risk Populations

In the United States, 25% of adult women and 20% of adult men are obese.

Modifiable risk factors for obesity include a diet high in saturated fats, poor nutritional education, and minimal aerobic exercise. Nonmodifiable risk factors include heredity. When parents are overweight or obese as adults, particularly the biologic mother, a 75% chance exists that the children will be overweight or obese. Metabolism slows with advancing age thus contributing to the risk of obesity. The metabolic rate decreases significantly after menopause, which places women at risk for being overweight or obese.

Numerous diseases and complications are associated with obesity, including depression, sleep apnea, pulmonary disease, stroke, gallbladder disease, liver disease, and degenerative arthritis. The altered metabolism of obesity can lead to atherosclerosis and related ischemic heart diseases. Hypertension and left-sided heart failure (left ventricular hypertrophy) occur because blood must be pumped through an enlarged vascular system. Diabetes mellitus is four times more common in the obese patient compared with the person with average weight. Additionally, recent studies indicate a link between obesity and breast, endometrial, and ovarian cancer.

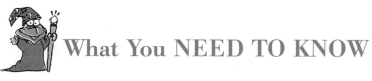

What You NEED TO KNOW

Clinical Manifestations

Height and weight tables, body mass indices (BMI), waist circumference, and a variety of other methods can be used to determine whether a person is overweight or obese. Generally, a person is considered as overweight when they weigh 10% more than optimal weight. Obese people are 15% above their optimal weight. Individuals who are 20% or more above their optimal weight are considered morbidly obese.

The BMI is used to predict problems associated with obesity. A BMI more than 30 is considered obese. The BMI is calculated as follows:

$$\text{Weight in kg} \div \text{height in meters}^2$$

Waist circumference is an indicator of obesity. Body fat that is distributed primarily in the abdominal area is of greater concern because of its association with other health problems (morbidity). Men with a waist circumference of 40 inches or more (102 cm) and women with a waist circumference of 35 inches or more (88 cm) are considered as obese.

Prognosis

Obesity is considered as a serious disease and has been linked to a shortened life span.

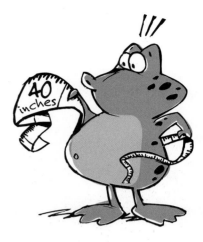

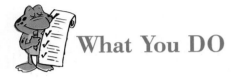

What You DO

Treatment

Treatment of obesity includes assisting the patient in establishing a healthy diet plan. The diet should be realistic for long-term success. A daily exercise routine should be incorporated with physical activity that is slowly increased and maintained. A support system for the obese patient is important to facilitate adherence to the diet and exercise plan.

Morbidly obese patients who do not respond to dietary management strategies to lose weight may require surgical procedures. Surgery is usually performed when patients are at high risk for complications associated with their obesity. The procedures involve removal of adipose tissue, jaw wiring, stapling the stomach, or banding the esophagus. The jejunal bypass (intestinal bypass) has been abandoned because of complications, particularly hepatic failure. All of the surgical procedures have advantages and disadvantages but are designed to reduce the body's ability to ingest or absorb nutrients. The procedures do not always cause permanent weight reduction.

> ⚠️ **Obesity is the second leading cause of preventable death in the United States.**

Nursing Responsibilities

For the obese patient, the nurse should:
- Obtain a health and dietary history before implementing treatment.
- Evaluate the patient's body image. Recognize that obese patients frequently have low self-esteem and poor body image. Patients frequently view self-control of dietary intake as a way to improve self-esteem. The patient's family must help find other ways to improve the patient's body image that are unrelated to food.
- Provide information to the patient and family on community resources for support with weight loss, such as Weight Watchers, Take Off Pounds Sensibly (TOPS), or Overeaters Anonymous (OA). Many support groups offer nutrition and weight loss programs.
- Encourage the patient and family to develop and use an exercise program that works for them and is maintained at least three times per week.
- Manage the procedure-specific perioperative care of the patient who is undergoing a surgical procedure to treat obesity.

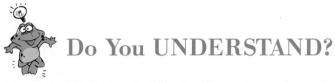

Do You UNDERSTAND?

DIRECTIONS: Using the following illustrations, color in the box on the graph provided that most accurately depicts the definition of obesity for each of the measurements.

1. Percentage over ideal body weight

5	10	15	20	25	30	35	40	45	50

2. BMI

5	10	15	20	25	30	35	40	45	50

3. Waist circumference in inches in men

5	10	15	20	25	30	35	40	45	50

4. Waist circumference in inches in women

5	10	15	20	25	30	35	40	45	50

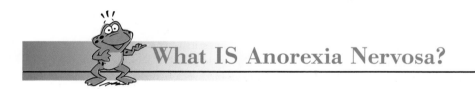

What IS Anorexia Nervosa?

Pathogenesis

Anorexia nervosa is a psychiatric disorder that is frequently misdiagnosed as a physical illness. The term anorexia means a loss of appetite. In anorexia nervosa, actual loss of appetite does not exist. Rather, a refusal to eat or an aberration in eating patterns and a loss of at least 15% to 25% of ideal body weight are present. Appetite is psychologic and is dependent on memory and associations, compared with hunger, which is physiologically aroused by the body's need for food. Two types of anorexia nervosa have been defined: the food-restricting type and the binge-eating–purging type. Most anorexia nervosa patients are women; men comprise 5% to 10% of anorexia nervosa patients.

The cause of anorexia nervosa is unknown but is associated with emotional states, such as anxiety, irritation, anger, and fear. One theory proposes that patients believe they have minimal control in other aspects of life, and the only part of life they can control is weight. The societal ideal of "beautiful" is also believed to be a factor in developing anorexia nervosa. Another theory proposes that because a patient with anorexia may not develop adult physical characteristics, excessive dieting may be a way of delaying maturity, thereby delaying sexual demands. Anorexia also appears to have a genetic basis, as evidenced by

Anorexia nervosa occurs primarily in girls after puberty. The prevalence of the disorder may be as high as 1 in 20.

Anorexia nervosa has been rapidly increasing throughout the world in developed countries as diverse as Russia, Japan, Australia, and the United States.

American Anorexia Bulimia Association, Inc.
http://www.aabainc.org/seweral/index.html.

the high incidence of anorexia found in identical twins. Additionally, some evidence suggests that anorexia nervosa is, in part, a disorder of the hypothalamus.

Although a person with anorexia has a normal appetite, the feeling of hunger is ignored. During the course of the disease, gonadotropins are not released from the anterior pituitary gland. The ovarian production of estrogens declines, and ovulation fails to occur. These conditions frequently persist long after nutritional status has improved. In some cases, menses cease before the actual weight loss becomes apparent. These factors indicate that the endocrine disturbance is not simply a consequence of malnutrition. In males who have anorexia nervosa, the level of gonadotropins and testosterone in the blood declines.

At-Risk Populations

The population at most risk for anorexia nervosa is young women, ages 12 to 18 years, who live in middle- to upper-class families. The risk for anorexia nervosa is also increased in members of professions that require low body weight, such as modeling, ballet, gymnastics, and wrestling.

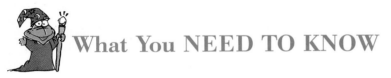 # What You NEED TO KNOW

Clinical Manifestations

The signs and symptoms of anorexia nervosa is usually that of a young person who is obsessed with the idea of being thin and an abnormal fear of becoming obese. Frequently, a prolonged refusal to eat to the point of danger occurs. Patients with anorexia nervosa can also have bulimia. For patients to be diagnosed with anorexia nervosa, five criteria identified by the American Psychiatric Association must be met. These criteria include:

1. An intense fear of becoming obese that does not diminish as weight loss progresses
2. Disturbance of body image, such as claiming to feel fat even when emaciated
3. Refusal to maintain body weight over a minimal normal weight for age and height
4. No known physical illnesses that would account for the weight loss
5. Amenorrhea in postmenarchal women

Self-induced vomiting, use of laxatives or diuretics or both, and compulsive vigorous exercise typically accompanies these criteria. Additionally, the patient may experience weakness or exhaustion, hypotension, slow heart rate (bradycardia), edema, dry skin, cold hands and feet, low body temperature, and endocrine disturbances. Laboratory examination will reveal low serum albumin and transferrin levels. A chronic state of anorexia causes decreased liver and renal function, anemia, osteoporosis from mineral loss, atrophy of the heart muscle, and cardiac arrest.

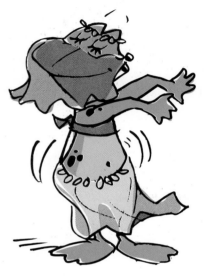

The population most at risk for anorexia nervosa is young women, ages 12 to 18 years, who live in middle- to upper-class families.

One in ten cases of anorexia leads to death from starvation, suicide, or cardiac arrest.

Prognosis

Outcome is greatly improved when anorexia is diagnosed and treated early. Lower weight and dysfunctional family relationships increase the likelihood of a poor outcome.

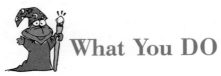

What You DO

Treatment

Treatment of anorexia nervosa is difficult and lengthy. The primary goals are to restore normal nutrition and resolve the underlying psychologic problems. Intervention begins with hospitalization and efforts to treat the patient for starvation. Vitamins and minerals and a diet of 1200 to 1600 kcal/day is typically prescribed and given in three meals and two snacks to prevent abdominal distention. The calorie count is gradually increased. The goal of weight gain is 2 to 4 pounds per week. Milk products and fats are slowly added to the diet to avoid cramping. When a patient refuses to eat, IV fluids are necessary. Fluids are slowly introduced and gradually increased to improve fluid volume deficit. Enteral or parenteral nutrition may be required. Various therapies help resolve the underlying psychologic problems. Treatment includes behavioral therapy, psychoanalysis, group therapy, insight-oriented therapy, and family therapy.

See Chapter 12 in **RWNSG:** *Pharmacology*

Nursing Responsibilities

The nurse is responsible for helping the anorexic patient to eat. Therefore the nurse should:
- Maintain a highly structured setting that includes precise meal times.
- Set firm limits regarding the selection of items from each category on the menu.
- Observe the patient during and after meals, and ensure that all food is eaten; purging is not practiced.
- Obtain daily weights each morning on the same scale and in the same type of clothing.
- Assist the patient in understanding that eating a healthy diet is a positive means for regaining control over behavior and activities.
- Assess blood pressure, urinary output, skin turgor, and mucous membranes to monitor fluid volume status.
- Provide emotional support and encouragement while allowing the patient opportunities to discuss feelings. The patient's strengths and positive coping skills are used as important parts of the care plan.
- Help the patient learn new methods of coping and achieve a sense of self-worth that is not exclusively based on appearance.

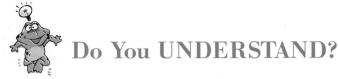

Do You UNDERSTAND?

DIRECTIONS: **Indicate in the space provided whether the statement is** *true* **or** *false*. **If false, then rewrite the statement in the margin space to the right to make it true.**

_____ 1. A clinical manifestation of anorexia nervosa is tachycardia.

_____ 2. Anorexia nervosa can result in death from suicide.

_____ 3. Females comprise an at-risk population for anorexia nervosa.

_____ 4. Amenorrhea is a criteria used in the diagnosis of anorexia nervosa.

_____ 5. Foods high in fat are immediately added to the diet plan for the anorexic patient to provide increased calories.

What IS Bulimia?

Pathogenesis

Bulimia is a compulsive eating disorder consisting of two types. Binge-purge disorder (bulimia nervosa) is characterized by recurrent episodes of binge eating (rapid consumption of a large quantity of food in 2 hours or less) and a sense of lack of control over eating. Purging in the form of self-induced vomiting or the use of laxatives or diuretics follows the episode of binge eating.

Binge-nonpurge disorder (binge eating disorder) involves uncontrolled eating that is usually kept secret. Patients engage in frequent binges but, dissimilar to the patient with bulimia nervosa, they do not purge afterward. Up to 40% of people who are obese may be binge eaters.

The cause of bulimia-binge disorder is unknown. A number of researchers believe that the eating disorder is a learned behavior that is associated with stress, anxiety, depression, loneliness, helplessness, and fear of becoming fat. The illness frequently occurs after a loss or the development of family problems. Another theory suggests that a disturbance in the appetite center of the hypothalamus contributes to bulimia-binge disorder. In some cases, the onset can be traced to the patient being physically or sexually abused. A strict weight-loss diet has also been associated with the onset of bulimia.

In bulimia-binge disorder, compulsive eating binges may occur as frequently as several times a day. The patient may consume thousands of calories at one sitting without hunger as a trigger. In other words, the amount of food consumed is out of proportion to the hunger that is felt. The patient is usually aware that the eating pattern is abnormal but has a preoccupying pathologic fear of becoming overweight. An unusually strong connection exists between feelings of self-worth and body shape and size. Poor impulse control results in overindulgence in other aspects of their life, such as substance abuse or sexual promiscuity.

Up to 5% of college-age women in the United States are bulimic.

Answers: 1. false; bradycardia may be a sign of anorexia nervosa; 2. true; 3. true; 4. true; 5. false; fats and milk products are slowly added to the diet to avoid cramping.

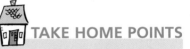

Young women between the ages of 15 and 30 years are at risk for bulimia and binge-eating disorder.

TAKE HOME POINTS

Bulimia is frequently a hidden disorder that remains unnoticed by family, friends, and other acquaintances. Recognition and treatment of the disorder may not occur until the patient reaches age 40.

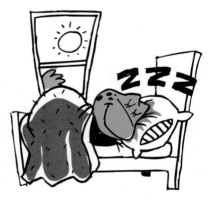

Bulimia can lead to death, usually as a result of cardiac arrest or suicide.

Patients with eating disorders tend to have a history of being overweight and weight gain on low-calorie diets. When intake is restricted, patients have difficulty losing weight. These young women soon come to learn that a large intake of food followed by purging controls the weight.

At-Risk Populations

The most common behavior that leads to anorexia, bulimia, or binge eating is dieting. Women with a history of poor family relationships, low self-esteem, and poor impulse control are most at risk.

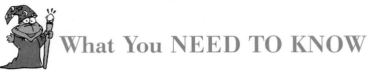

What You NEED TO KNOW

Clinical Manifestations

Similar to the patient with anorexia nervosa, the patient with bulimia-binge disorder uses self-destructive eating behaviors to deal with psychologic problems that may go much deeper than the obsession with food and weight.

Psychologic manifestations of bulimia include impaired impulse control, fear of obesity, and low self-esteem. Depression marked by feelings of gloom, suicidal ideation, irritability, and impaired concentration is common. Patients with long-term bulimia also report loneliness, boredom, and anger.

Other manifestations that frequently follow binge eating include abdominal pain and excessive sleeping. Frequent weight fluctuations of 10 pounds or more may be noted, although body weight is usually at or slightly below ideal. In patients suffering from the binge-purge type of bulimia, repeated vomiting can lead to blood-shot eyes, erosion of tooth enamel, swelling of the salivary glands that results from acid reflux and constant stimulation, and sore throat. The patient may complain of indigestion and heartburn from the vomiting, bloody emesis (hematemesis), constipation, hair loss, and irregular menses. Fistulas of the upper GI tract may form. The patient can experience an irregular heartbeat that may lead to cardiac arrest. Fluid and electrolyte imbalances also develop. Elevated blood urea nitrogen (BUN) and serum amylase levels are found on laboratory analysis.

Prognosis

The prognosis is poor because many people with bulimia do not seek help until they reach their 40s. By this time, eating behaviors are deeply ingrained and difficult to change. Drugs that are used to stimulate vomiting, bowel movements, or urination increase the risk of heart failure.

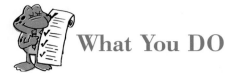

What You DO

Treatment

The treatment for bulimia has two goals: (1) to interrupt the binge-purge cycle by helping the patient gain control of eating habits and (2) to change attitudes toward food, eating, body size, and self. To accomplish these goals, a combination of diet management, drug therapy, and psychotherapy is used. When the patient also suffers from alcohol or drug dependency, the substance abuse is treated first.

Treatment begins with the patient being admitted to an inpatient eating disorders unit. A balanced diet is ordered that contains sufficient calories to meet the patient's basal metabolic needs. Drug therapy includes the use of selective serotonin reuptake inhibitors such as fluoxetine (Prozac) or other antidepressants. In some cases, a monoamine oxidase inhibitor (MAOI) drug such as tranylcypromine sulfate (Parnate) is used. Potassium supplements are ordered as needed.

See Chapters 2F and 12 in RWNSG: *Pharmacology*

Psychotherapy is started while the patient is hospitalized, focusing on helping the patient develop positive coping skills for dealing with stress, anxiety, and feelings of powerlessness. The patient is also educated in the importance of avoiding dieting and restricting caloric intake, which sets up the urge to binge eat and then to compensate by purging. Lengthy outpatient treatment is usually required.

Nursing Responsibilities

The nurse is responsible for assisting the patient in breaking the binge-purge cycle and avoiding the complications associated with psychologic and metabolic upset. Therefore the nurse should:

- Assist the patient in selecting the right portions of foods from all four food groups. The patient is usually allowed to refuse a specific number of foods (e.g., two or three) thus some sense of control is felt.
- Help the patient understand that only the foods provided by the dietary department must be eaten and that all of the meal must be consumed. Remain with the patient for at least 1 hour after eating to provide support and reduce the likelihood the patient will induce vomiting.
- Encourage the patient to eat slowly and develop a regular exercise program.
- Provide supervision and emotional support for the patient during stressful periods.
- Allow the patient to express feelings and assist in developing positive coping skills to deal with anxiety and stress.
- Assist the patient and family in identifying other areas of self-regard that are unrelated to food.

 Provide age-appropriate and culturally appropriate patient and family teaching regarding the disorder and treatment to help prevent the development of anorexia nervosa.

• Monitor potassium levels at regular intervals and administer potassium supplements as prescribed. In some cases, IV potassium replacement may be needed.

Do You UNDERSTAND?

DIRECTIONS: **Provide an answer to each of the following questions.**

1. Name at least three methods that bulimic patients use to prevent weight gain.

2. In what age decade do most people with bulimia usually seek help?

3. What are the two most common causes of death related to bulimia?

4. What are the three interventions used in the treatment of bulimia?

5. List six nursing responsibilities in caring for the bulimic patient.

Answers: 1. vomiting, laxatives, diuretics, fasting, excessive exercise; 2. 40s; 3. cardiac arrest, suicide; 4. diet management, drug therapy, psychotherapy; 5. assisting the patient in breaking the binge-purge cycle, helping the patient select the right portions of foods from all four food groups, observation of the patient during and after meals, allowing the patient to express feelings, providing emotional support to the patient during stressful periods, assisting the patient in developing positive coping skills, educating the patient regarding the long-term goal of improving self-esteem, monitoring potassium levels and administering potassium as ordered.

DIRECTIONS: **Complete the following crossword.**

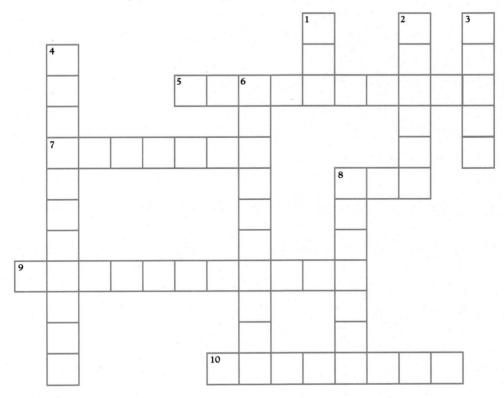

Down

1. This measurement is used to predict problems associated with obesity.
2. The nurse's responsibility is to obtain this measurement at regular intervals.
3. In a chronic state of anorexia nervosa, the function of this system is decreased.
4. Severe protein deficiency.
6. This clinical manifestation of anorexia nervosa involves the menstrual cycle.
8. This population is at risk for anorexia nervosa.

Across

5. A patient with anorexia nervosa has this physical appearance.
7. Anorexia nervosa may result in death from this cause.
8. Foods that are high in this nutrient are introduced slowly in the treatment of anorexia nervosa.
9. This clinical manifestation of anorexia nervosa involves the heart.
10. Protein-calorie malnutrition.

13 Sensory System

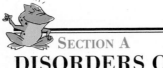

SECTION A
DISORDERS OF THE EYE

What IS Macular Degeneration?

Pathogenesis

Macular degeneration is a breakdown of cells in the macula and surrounding tissues of the eye. The result of the degeneration is loss of central vision in the affected eye. The exact cause of macular degeneration is unknown in approximately 75% of cases. Macular degeneration may be hereditary.

Two stages of macular degeneration have been identified: "dry" and "wet." Both stages are bilateral and progressive. The "dry" stage of macular degeneration is characterized by a decrease in the size of normally developed eye tissues (atrophy) with degeneration of the outer retina and underlying structures. Deposits of material from the pigmented epithelial cells produce yellowish spots on the retina. Eventually, these spots increase, enlarge, and may calcify.

The "wet" stage of macular degeneration involves the choroid, the layer immediately beneath the pigmented epithelial cell layer of the retina. When this layer is involved, a serous fluid leak with accompanying growth of choroidal blood vessels is noted. When the fovea is involved, central vision is lost.

At-Risk Populations

Exposure to sunlight without wearing sunglasses is a risk factor for macular degeneration.

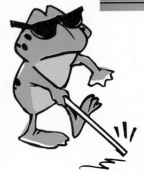

Most cases of macular degeneration appear in people 50 to 60 years of age (age-related macular degeneration) and is one of the most common causes of vision loss in older adults. Stargardt's macular degeneration is present at or existing at the time of birth (congenital).

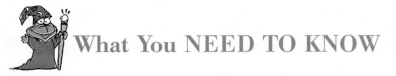

What You NEED TO KNOW

Clinical Manifestations

The clinical manifestation of macular degeneration is a loss of central vision. The patient may also note a blurred spot in the central field of vision and scotomas. Scotomas are areas of vision loss or depressed vision within the visual field that is surrounded by other areas of less depressed or normal vision. The leakage of serous fluid from the choroid produces a blurred, wavy distortion of vision.

Yellowish round spots (drusen) may be observed on the retina and macula using an ophthalmoscope. A dome-shaped deposit of retinal pigment epithelium may also be present.

Prognosis

Currently, nothing can be done to prevent, stop, or reverse the process of macular degeneration. However, the condition does not progress to total blindness and is usually self-limiting.

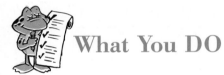

What You DO

Treatment

Because the majority of cases of macular degeneration cannot be stopped or treated, care involves making the most of the vision that the patient has. Occasionally, damage from "wet" macular degeneration can be stopped with the use of argon lasers, although laser treatment in this area results in a blind spot. The only helpful treatment when the fovea is involved is low-vision aids.

Nursing Responsibilities

Nursing responsibilities for the patient with macular degeneration include the following:
- Identify yourself to the patient with each contact.
- Assist the patient in coping with the fears and reality of vision loss and adapt to changes in vision.
- Teach the patient the proper way to use Amsler's grid at home for evaluating the progression of macular degeneration.
- Assist the patient in maximizing remaining vision by using low-vision aids (e.g., large-print books and newspapers, magnifying television screens, programmable telephone equipment).
- Provide the patient with information about community resources and low-vision support groups (e.g., American Association for the Blind, National Industries for the Blind).

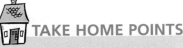

TAKE HOME POINTS

Macular degeneration is a progressive disorder resulting in loss of central vision. Patient safety becomes a primary consideration.

● Providing the patient and family information about the disorder and strategies to promote safety measures in the home (e.g., avoiding throw rugs; keeping furniture and belongings in the same place; removing unnecessary furniture; installing handrails in hallways, bathrooms, and on steps; obtaining pill organizers; "marking off" dials on stoves and microwaves with special tape or colors; obtaining special lighting).

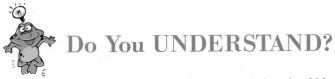

Do You UNDERSTAND?

DIRECTIONS: **Identify five nursing measures that should be implemented to increase a visually impaired patient's safety and comfort.**

1. _____
2. _____
3. _____
4. _____
5. _____

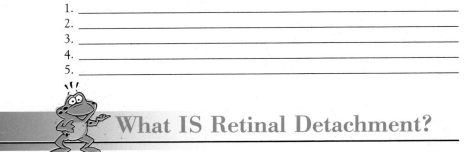

What IS Retinal Detachment?

Pathogenesis

Retinal detachment is characterized by a hole in the retina, liquid in the vitreous body with access to the hole, and subsequent fluid accumulation between the retina and the retinal pigment epithelium. Retinal holes and tears usually occur from spontaneous vitreous traction, but abnormal adhesions may be present between the retina and vitreous body secondary to diabetic retinopathy, injury, or other ocular disorders. Atrophy of the vitreous body may also result in a retinal tear.

The liquid seeps through the hole and separates the retina from its choroidal blood supply. Without intervention, the detachment continues to spread, and the detached retina loses the ability to function. The retina may become increasingly detached over a period of hours to years.

At-Risk Populations

Predisposing factors to a retinal detachment include aging, cataract extraction, degeneration of the retina, trauma, severe myopia, and a previous retinal detachment in the other eye. Patients with diabetes mellitus who have developed diabetic retinopathy are also at risk for retinal detachment. A family history of retinal detachment may also be a risk factor.

Answers: 1. identify yourself to the patient with each contact; 2. teach the patient the correct way to use a chart at home for evaluating macular degeneration (Amsler's grid); 3. help the patient maximize remaining vision with low-vision aids; 4. advise patient and family to examine the home for possible unsafe situations; 5. avoid raising your voice to the patient; vision-impaired patients are not hearing impaired.

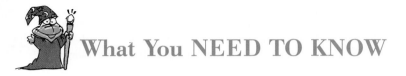

What You NEED TO KNOW

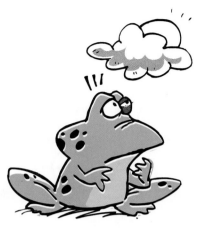

Clinical Manifestations

The clinical manifestations of retinal detachment are characteristic. Patients describe a shadow or curtain falling across the field of vision. No pain is present. The onset is usually sudden and may be accompanied by a burst of black spots or floaters, indicating that bleeding has occurred as a result of the detachment. The patient may also see flashes of light resulting from separation of the retina. Examination of the inner eye reveals the portion of the retina involved and the extent of the detachment. Without urgent care, the detachment may extend to involve the macula with subsequent loss of vision.

Prognosis

Involvement of the macula greatly compromises visual acuity.

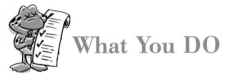

What You DO

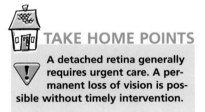

TAKE HOME POINTS

A detached retina generally requires urgent care. A permanent loss of vision is possible without timely intervention.

Treatment

In most cases, surgery is required to place the retina back in contact with the choroid and to seal the accompanying holes. A freezing probe or cold laser is used to seal the hole (cryotherapy) if the damage has not progressed to detachment. Both freezing and laser treatments cause an inflammatory response around the affected area that scars over and seals the hole.

A procedure known as scleral buckling may be used when a detachment has occurred. The sclera is depressed from the outside of the eye using special bands to position the choroid next to the retina. An air or gas bubble is then injected into the eye to create pressure on the retina from the inside. The gas bubble holds the retina in place next to the choroid during the healing phase.

Nursing Responsibilities

The nursing responsibilities for the patient with a detached retina include the following:

- Assess the patient for visual changes in both eyes. Explain to the patient that an extremely bright light may be noted when the eye is dilated for examination.
- Teach the patient about the clinical manifestations of further loss of vision and to avoid any activities that increase intraocular pressure (e.g., Valsalva maneuvers such as straining at stool, coughing, sneezing, lifting).
- Observe the eye patch postoperatively for any drainage. Only serous drainage is expected.

• Position the patient to maximize the benefits of pressure produced by the introduction of the gas or air bubble. The head of the bed is down, and the patient's head is turned to one side for a period lasting several days.

• Administer medications as ordered to reduce intraocular pressure and to reduce discomfort, nausea, and vomiting.

 Instruct the patient about the correct use of mydriatic and postoperative eye medications that help prevent infection and reduce inflammation.

• Apply warm or cold compresses to the affected eye several times daily for comfort.

 Instruct the patient to wear an eye shield or sunglasses during the day and an eye shield at night.

 Advise the patient to clean the eye with warm tap water using a clean washcloth.

 Instruct the patient to avoid vigorous activities and heavy lifting during the immediate postoperative period.

 Advise the patient to avoid air travel during the postoperative period because the air or gas bubble expands at high altitudes.

• Assess the home environment for safety hazards, such as throw rugs, electrical cords, stairs, and poor lighting.

 Advise the patient to contact the health care provider as soon as possible should severe pain develop.

See Chapter 13A in **RWNSG:**
Pharmacology

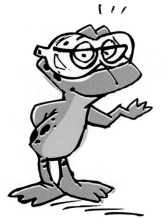

Do You UNDERSTAND?

DIRECTIONS: **Define the following terms.**
1. Scleral buckle: _____
2. Macula: _____
3. Cryotherapy: _____
4. Valsalva maneuver: _____

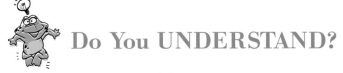

What IS a Cataract?

Pathogenesis

A cataract is a clouding (opacity) of the lens of the eye. The most common cataract is related to aging, although cataracts can have a variety of other causes. Cataracts may develop as a result of other eye disorders, such as retinal detachment, inflammation of the retina (retinitis), or an inflammation of the iris and ciliary body (iridocyclitis). Blunt trauma, lacerations, foreign bodies, radiation, exposure to infrared light, and chronic use of glucocorticosteroid medications may also result in cataract formation. Cataracts may be congenital and found in patients who have systemic disorders, such as diabetes or Down syndrome.

Answers: 1. a surgical technique used to repair a retinal detachment; 2. an irregular, yellowish depression on the retina, lateral to and slightly below the optic disc that receives and analyzes light only from the center of the visual field; 3. freezing of tissues to close the hole associated with retinal detachment; 4. any movement that increases pressure within the chest; occurs when the patient strains with bowel movement or urination, uses the arms and upper trunk muscles to move up in bed, or strains during coughing, sneezing, gagging, or vomiting; the maneuver increases not only pressure within the chest and the skull, but also intraocular pressure.

Cataracts develop because of alterations in the metabolism and transport of nutrients within the lens. Both a reduction in oxygen uptake and an initial increase in water content occur. Dehydration of the lens follows these two processes. Sodium and calcium content of the lens are increased. Potassium, ascorbic acid, and protein are decreased. The protein in the lens undergoes numerous age-related changes, including yellowing from formation of fluorescent compounds and molecular changes.

Cataracts progress through four stages. In the early stage, the cataract is not completely cloudy. Some light is transmitted through the lens, which allows for useful vision. In the second stage, the cataract is completely opaque, and vision is significantly reduced. Third-stage cataract lenses absorb water and increase in size, resulting in increased intraocular pressure (IOP). In the last stage of cataract formation, the proteins in the lens break down and leak out through the lens capsule. Macrophages swallow up the proteins, which, in turn, may obstruct the trabecular meshwork, causing additional increases in IOP.

At-Risk Populations

Patients who work in bright sunlight (e.g., lifeguards, commercial fisherman, construction workers) and those who live at high altitudes develop cataracts earlier in life. Glass blowers and welders are at risk for cataract formation if they do not use eye protection.

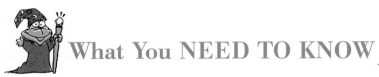

What You NEED TO KNOW

Clinical Manifestations

The clinical manifestations of cataracts include decreased visual acuity, blurred vision, occasionally, one-sided double vision, abnormal sensitivity to light (photophobia), and glare. Decreased color perception may also be present. Patients usually see "better" in low light when the pupil is dilated. The patient has no complaints of pain. A cloudy lens can be observed during examination of the eye. A cataract is suspected when the red reflex, which is normally observed with an ophthalmoscope, is distorted or absent.

Prognosis

In most cases of cataract, vision can be restored or improved by surgical intervention.

 Cataracts are the primary cause of reduced vision and blindness worldwide, beginning at the age of approximately 50.

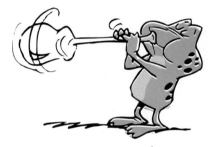

Cumulative exposure to ultraviolet light over the life span is the single most important risk factor in the development of cataracts. Some degree of cataract formation is to be expected in most persons over the age of 70.

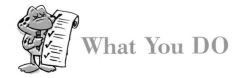

What You DO

Treatment

No known medical treatment is available to prevent or reduce cataract formation. Use of strong bifocals, magnification, appropriate lighting, and visual aids may be used as the cataract progresses. Surgical removal of the cataract is the most common intervention.

The most common procedure, an extracapsular cataract extraction (ECCE), consists of removing the lens and the anterior portion of the lens capsule. The posterior portion of the lens capsule is left intact. In some cases, the lens material can be broken down using ultrasonic vibration (phacoemulsification) and pieces of the anterior lens capsule can be removed by suction. This technique requires a much smaller incision in the eye. Intracapsular cataract extraction (ICCE) is performed less frequently. This procedure consists of removing the lens and the lens capsule.

After the removal of the cataract, the patient's lens may be removed (aphakia) or a new lens inserted in the posterior chamber of the eye. The newest implants fold during insertion, which allows for a small incision and does not require postoperative eye patching (except during sleep). Lens implants are permanent. Glasses may be needed after a lens implant.

Contact lens can be used for patients who have had the lens removed (aphakia). The simplest and least expensive way to help the patient see after the lens has been removed is to use eyeglasses with extremely thick lenses. The thick lenses magnify objects, but vertical lines appear curved, and distances can be difficult for the patient to judge. Contact lenses help correct vision with significantly less distortion compared with the thick eyeglasses.

Nursing Responsibilities

Pain following cataract surgery should be minimal. Acute pain, which is a signal of IOP, should be reported immediately. The nursing responsibilities for the patient who has a cataract extraction include the following:
- Document visual acuity in each eye.
- Evaluate the patient's lifestyle, environment, and ability to perform the activities of daily living.
- Advise the patient to leave the eye patch in place, wear glasses, take the prescribed eye drop, and avoid rubbing the eye.
- Advise the patient to avoid lifting more than 5 pounds (the weight of a gallon of milk), avoid straining or bearing down, and sleep on the side of the body on which the operation was performed.
- Use acetaminophen for discomfort. Aspirin or drugs that contain aspirin should be avoided to reduce the risk of bleeding.
- Advise the patient to report any pain that is unrelieved, redness around the eye, nausea, or vomiting.
- Instruct the patient to wear a metal or plastic eye shield at night to protect the eye from accidental injury.

- Assess the patient and family's ability to apply eye drops appropriately.
- Review the rationale and schedule for the administration of eye medications with the patient and family.
- Arrange for a home care referral, depending on the patient's age, ability, and support systems.
- Provide age-appropriate and culturally appropriate patient and family teaching regarding the disorder and postoperative care.
- Provide the patient and family information on the disorder and strategies to promote safety measures in the home.
- Advise the patient who has a permanent implant to carry identification regarding the implant at all times.

 Cataracts cause decreased visual acuity, blurred vision, double vision, and sensitivity to light and glare. Decreased color perception may also be present. Patient safety becomes a primary consideration.

Do You UNDERSTAND?

DIRECTIONS: **Match the terms in Column A to their definitions in Column B.**

Column A	Column B
_____ 1. Cataract	a. Abnormal intolerance to light
_____ 2. Visual acuity	b. Removal of the lens and the anterior
_____ 3. Diplopia	portion of the lens capsule
_____ 4. Photophobia	c. Clouding of the lens
_____ 5. Extracapsular	d. Clearness of visual perception of an image
cataract extraction	e. Double vision
_____ 6. Intracapsular	f. Removal of the lens including the entire
cataract extraction	lens capsule
_____ 7. Aphakia	g. Absence of the lens of the eye, occurring
	congenitally or as a result of surgery

What IS Glaucoma?

Pathogenesis

Glaucoma is a group of disorders characterized by IOP within the anterior chamber of the eye. IOP is controlled by the rate of aqueous humor production in the ciliary body and the resistance to outflow of aqueous humor from the eye. Normal pressure variations within the anterior chamber usually do not exceed 2 to 3 mm Hg. However, as aqueous fluid increases in the eye, the increased pressure interferes with blood supply to the optic nerve and the retina. These structures become ischemic and gradually lose function. IOP and arterial blood pressure are independent of each other, although changes in blood pressure can affect IOP.

The extent of pressure changes that cause ocular damage is not the same for each eye or in every person. Some people sustain damage with a relatively low pressure, while others sustain no damage from higher pressures. The disorder may occur alone or as a result of another condition. Glaucoma may be acute or chronic.

The angle between the cornea and the iris is used to describe glaucoma. Open-angle glaucoma (wide-angle glaucoma) is chronic, resulting from degenerative changes in the trabecular meshwork of the eye. Open-angle glaucoma results from multiple factors that are genetically determined but is usually bilateral, insidious in onset, and slow to progress. The angle between the cornea and the iris is wide, but the trabecular meshwork impairs drainage of aqueous humor. In closed-angle glaucoma (acute-angle glaucoma), the angle is narrow, acute obstruction to the outflow of aqueous humor is present, and a markedly elevated intraocular pressure occurs.

At-Risk Populations

Ninety percent of primary glaucoma occurs in people who have open angles. Persons with a narrow anterior chamber angle are predisposed to an acute onset of closed-angle glaucoma. Congenital glaucoma is rare and is the result of developmental abnormalities of eye structures.

Risk factors for the development of glaucoma include hypertension, cardiovascular disease, diabetes, and obesity. Smoking, caffeine or alcohol intake, use of illicit drugs or glucocorticosteroids, and altered hormone levels cause varying but transient elevations in IOP.

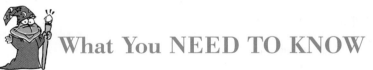

What You NEED TO KNOW

Clinical Manifestations

The signs and symptoms of glaucoma include IOP, indentation of the optic disc, and defects in the visual field. The manifestations are the same, regardless of the type of glaucoma. The difference in manifestations is in the speed of onset and the severity of pressure elevations.

No early signs and symptoms are present to alert the patient with open-angle glaucoma that vision is deteriorating. IOP readings are in the normal range, the angle is normal, and the optic nerves are normal. Subtle peripheral vision deficits may occur. A small crescent shape (scotoma) appears early in the disease. The signs and symptoms of closed-angle glaucoma appear suddenly, usually appearing in only one eye. Severe pain and blurred vision or vision loss is observed. Some patients see rainbow halos around lights and some will experience nausea and vomiting. Larger areas of significant vision loss are noted with narrow angle glaucoma. An eye examination may demonstrate a reddened conjunctiva and a cloudy cornea. The humor in the anterior chamber may appear cloudy (turbid) and the pupil nonreactive. Pressures exceeding 23 mm Hg require further evaluation of the eye.

Prognosis

In most cases, blindness can be prevented if treatment is started early.

Glaucoma is most common in African Americans between the ages of 45 and 65. The prevalence is five times that of Caucasians in the same age group.

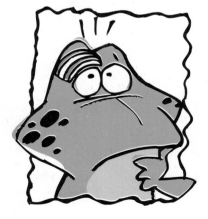

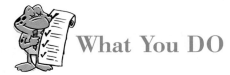

What You DO

Treatment

The treatment of glaucoma includes the use of ocular miotics to constrict the pupil and increase the outflow of humor. Beta-blockers or alpha-adrenergics are used to suppress the secretion of aqueous humor. Orally administered carbonic anhydrase inhibitors help reduce the production of aqueous humor. Mydriatic and cycloplegic agents inhibit the parasympathetic nervous system by blocking acetylcholine (ACH) and paralyzing the ciliary and dilator muscle of the iris, thus causing both dilation of the pupil and paralysis of accommodation. All of these drug classes are contraindicated in patients who have narrow-angle glaucoma, primarily because dilation of the pupil further restricts outflow of aqueous humor.

See Chapters 2A and 13A in
RWNSG: *Pharmacology*

Surgery may be required for patients in whom the progression of visual field loss and optic nerve damage cannot be halted. No single surgical procedure that is successful for all patients is available. The procedures that may be considered include the use of a laser to create an opening in the trabecular meshwork thus drainage of humor is enhanced. Channels may be surgically established to promote outflow of aqueous humor from the anterior chamber to the subconjunctival space. An iridectomy—the creation of a new route for the flow of aqueous humor to the trabecular meshwork—may also be performed. A laser is used to create the new opening. When other surgical procedures have failed, freezing of the ciliary body may be performed to decrease aqueous humor production.

Nursing Responsibilities

Nursing responsibilities for the patient with glaucoma include the following:

- Encourage the patient to stop smoking and to maintain body weight under 120% of ideal.
- Instruct patients to avoid alcohol and caffeine intake several hours before an eye examination.
- Teach patients to avoid activities that produce a Valsalva maneuver (e.g., straining at stool, bending over, lifting).
- Instruct the patient about what to expect at the time of surgery (e.g., popping sounds, flashing lights). A waiting period is required after surgery of approximately 1 to 2 hours to evaluate IOP.
- Position the postoperative patient on the nonoperative side to avoid pressure on the operative site.
- Review the signs and symptoms of infection: redness, swelling, drainage, blurred vision, and pain.
- Review the signs and symptoms of IOP: unrelieved pain, nausea, and decreased vision.
- Advise the patient that rubbing or applying pressure over the closed eye can damage healing tissue. Remind the patient of the importance of return visits, adherence with medication therapy, and rationale for eye protection after surgery, such as wearing an eye shield or eyeglasses at all times.

Do You UNDERSTAND?

DIRECTIONS: Indicate in the space provided whether the statement is *true* or *false*. If false, then use the margin space to the left to rewrite the statement to make it true.

_____ 1. Glaucoma usually results from the overproduction of aqueous humor.

_____ 2. Prolonged exposure to sunlight and heavy smoking has been associated with an increased risk of glaucoma.

_____ 3. In the most common type of glaucoma, the abnormality involves obstruction of the trabecular meshwork and the anterior chamber.

What IS an Ocular Infection?

Pathogenesis

Infections of the eye can involve numerous eye structures. For example, blepharitis is a common bilateral inflammation of the eyelid margins. Dacryocystitis is an inflammation and blockage of the tear duct. A hordeolum (stye) is an infection of the glands of the eyelids. Conjunctivitis is an inflammation of the conjunctiva. Keratitis is an infection of the cornea. Vasodilation of the conjunctival, episcleral, and scleral vessels produces the red eye present in eye infections. Invasion of eye structures by microorganisms contribute to eye discomfort, a reduction of visual acuity, and, in some cases, photophobia.

Eye infections are usually the result of bacteria such as *Staphylococcus aureus*, *Pseudomonas aeruginosa*, and *Streptococcus pneumoniae*. Fungi such as *Candida* or *Aspergillus*, viruses such as adenovirus, herpes simplex, or herpes zoster, protozoa such as *Acanthamoeba*, or chlamydia can also cause eye infections.

At-Risk Populations

Patients who have systemic connective tissue disorders such as rheumatoid arthritis are particularly susceptible to corneal infections and ulceration. Dry eyes, trauma, or ineffective eyelid closure predispose the eye to infection.

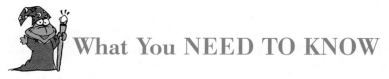

What You NEED TO KNOW

Clinical Manifestations

The signs and symptoms of eye infections are summarized in the table on page 377. Occasionally, the patient may experience a headache or blurred vision.

Signs and Symptoms of Eye Infections

INFECTION	EYE PAIN	DISCHARGE	VISUAL ACUITY	PHOTOPHOBIA
Viral conjunctivitis	Mild, burning	Watery	Normal	No
Bacterial conjunctivitis	Mild to moderate, burning	Purulent	Normal	No
Keratitis	Moderate aching	Clear	Decreased	Yes
Blepharitis	Mild	None	Normal	No
Hordeolum	Mild	Watery	Normal	Unusual
Dacryocystitis	Mild	Watery	Normal	Slight

Prognosis

The prognosis for the patient with an eye infection is generally good, providing that the infection is treated early. The patient usually remains at home but may need to be hospitalized if the infection progresses to the inside of the eye.

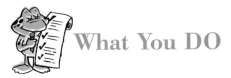 What You DO

Treatment

The goal of treatment is to prevent progression of the infection and to promote healing. Infections are commonly treated with warm compresses applied to the eye several times daily. Topical antibiotic, antifungal, or antiviral therapy is prescribed, with the frequency of instillation based on the severity of the infection. The infection usually disappears in 3 to 7 days.

See Chapters 1A, 1B, and 13 in RWNSG: *Pharmacology*

Nursing Responsibilities

The nursing responsibilities for the patient with an eye infection include the following:

- Assess the patient's level of discomfort and possible lack of sleep. In some cases, eye drops may be given as often as every 15 minutes around the clock, thus the schedule is a challenge not only for the patient, but also for the nurse.
- Practice diligent hand washing, even when gloves are worn to apply the eye drops.
- Adhere to the drug administration schedule to reduce the risk of complications. Adhering to the schedule also builds patient's trust and reduces anxiety.
- Advise the patient that some medications such as fortified bacitracin may cause stinging that lasts several minutes.
- Administer oral analgesics at regular intervals as indicated. Mild sleeping medications may be helpful at bedtime.
- Cleanse the eye using warm tap water and a clean washcloth. Teach the patient to avoid using the same washcloth on the other eye.
- Provide patient and family teaching regarding drug administration and the signs and symptoms of increasing infection.
- Assess the home environment if the patient's vision is greatly reduced.

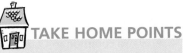 TAKE HOME POINTS

Recovery from most eye infections takes 3 to 7 days, providing the patient uses the eye medications as ordered.

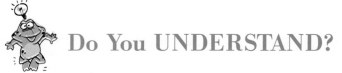

Do You UNDERSTAND?

DIRECTIONS: **Match the term in Column A with the definitions in Column B.**

Column A

_____ 1. Dacryocystitis
_____ 2. Hordeolum (stye)
_____ 3. Conjunctivitis
_____ 4. Keratitis
_____ 5. Blepharitis

Column B

a. Infection of the cornea
b. Infection of the glands of the eyelids
c. Inflammation of the lacrimal sac secondary to bacterial infection
d. Inflammation of the conjunctiva
e. Common bilateral inflammation of the eyelid margins

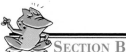

SECTION B

DISORDERS OF THE EAR

When sound strikes the ear, the eardrum (tympanic membrane) vibrates. The three small bones of the middle ear (hammer [malleus], anvil [incus], and stirrup [stapes]) function as levers, amplifying the motion of the eardrum and passing the vibrations on to the cochlea. The cochlea contains nerves that transmit sound. From this point, the eighth cranial nerve transmits the vibrations, translated into nerve impulses, to the hearing center in the brain. The inner ear also contains the semicircular canals that are essential to the sense of balance.

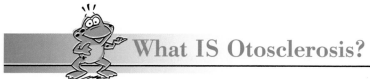

What IS Otosclerosis?

Pathogenesis

Otosclerosis is also known as "hardening of the ear." Approximately 10% of adults have otosclerosis. The cause is unknown. A formation of spongy bone occurs in the labyrinth of the ear. The formation of the spongy bone causes the stapes to become immobile. Immobility of the stapes prevents the transmission of sound vibration to the inner ear. The loss of vibration results in a conductive hearing loss.

At-Risk Populations

At one time, otosclerosis was thought to be a result of a vitamin deficiency or an infection of the middle ear (otitis media). Now, otosclerosis is known to be an autosomal dominant disorder, meaning transmission to children can occur when only one parent has the disorder. This middle ear disorder usually begins during adolescence or early 20s, affecting women approximately twice as frequently as it does men.

Otosclerosis may be worsened with pregnancy.

Otosclerosis is 10 times more common in Caucasians than it is in any other ethnic group.

Answers: 1. c; 2. b; 3. d; 4. a; 5. e.

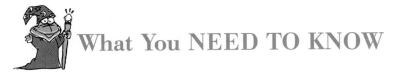

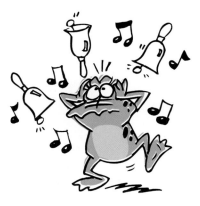

What You NEED TO KNOW

Clinical Manifestations

The signs and symptoms of otosclerosis include a slow, progressive hearing loss. Changes can be noted as early as adolescence. An early symptom of otosclerosis is ringing in the ears; however, the most noticeable symptom is progressive loss of hearing. The hearing loss usually affects both ears. The patient commonly speaks in a soft voice. Other symptoms include recurrent dizziness (vertigo) and postural imbalance.

The Rinne test compares air versus sensorineural conduction. A vibrating tuning fork is shifted between the mastoid bone (bone conduction) and the opening of the ear canal (air conduction). When the patient has otosclerosis, bone conduction is greater than air conduction. Normally air conduction exceeds bone conduction. The Weber test shows lateralization to the more affected ear when hearing loss is greater in one ear compared with the other. Audiometry testing confirms the hearing loss. A reddish blush from dilated blood vessels may be noted behind the eardrum (Schwartz's sign) using an otoscope to visualize ear structures.

Prognosis

The conductive hearing loss that results from otosclerosis is one of the most common correctable middle ear disorders that rarely progresses to deafness.

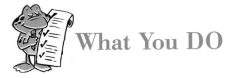

What You DO

Treatment

Because speech discrimination is usually unaffected, simple amplification of sound (with the use of hearing aid) is effective in treating otosclerosis. Although no cure is known for otosclerosis, surgical techniques frequently restore conductive hearing loss by freeing the damaged ossicle or replacing it with other tissues. In this operation, the damaged ossicle is removed and replaced with stainless steel or a plastic prosthesis (stapedectomy). However, the procedure is performed less frequently today because of the risk of profound deafness and persistent postoperative vertigo.

People who are at risk for otosclerosis or who are not candidates for surgery can be given medications to reduce the severity of bony fusion. Evidence suggests that sodium fluoride may help decrease the rate of hearing loss by replacing the hydroxyl ion in bone and decreasing resorption. Calcium gluconate and vitamin D can be used to retard bone resorption.

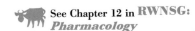

See Chapter 12 in *RWNSG: Pharmacology*

Nursing Responsibilities

The nursing responsibilities for a patient with otosclerosis include the following:

- Speak directly and clearly to (while facing) the patient.
- Recognize that hearing-impaired patients depend on visual clues for understanding, thus avoid showing annoyance with careless facial expressions.
- Use visual aids (e.g., pictures, diagrams, models) to help the patient understand medical terminology or procedures. An expert interpreter should be used when other attempts to communicate have failed or when speed and accuracy is important. The National Registry of Interpreters for the Deaf (NRID) has local chapters and can provide names of interpreters.
- Avoid the use of an intercom when caring for hospitalized patients. An intercom distorts sound and causes poor communication.
- Advise the patient to avoid aspirin or aspirin-containing products for 2 weeks before surgery to reduce the risk of bleeding.
- Have the patient lie on the nonoperative side, with the head of the bed elevated after surgery. This position reduces swelling (edema) and prevents dislodging of the prosthesis.
- Report any vertigo and nystagmus and advising the patient not to disturb packing in the ear canal.
- Advise the patient to avoid excessive exercise, straining, and activities that can lead to head trauma. Blow the nose gently, one nostril at a time. The nose should remain open when sneezing. Air travel should be avoided for up to 1 month after surgery.
- Encourage the patient to continue social involvement. Advocate the use of support groups for hearing impaired persons.
- Teach the patient the proper way to use and care for a hearing aid, when prescribed, and the procedure to use should the aid malfunction.
- Encourage the patient to keep follow-up appointments to determine the degree of hearing regained.

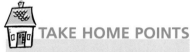

TAKE HOME POINTS

Speak to the patient who is hearing impaired in a normal voice. Occasionally, making the voice louder without shouting is helpful. Shouting exaggerates normal speaking movements, which causes sound distortion. Financial assistance may be available through vocational rehabilitation, Lions Clubs, and Medicaid in some states for the purchase of a hearing aid.

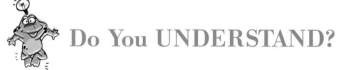

Do You UNDERSTAND?

DIRECTIONS: Indicate in the space provided whether the statement is *true* or *false*.

_____ 1. Otosclerosis is caused by vitamin deficiency or ear infection.
_____ 2. Otosclerosis is an autosomal dominant disorder.

Answers: 1. false; 2. true.

What IS Ménière's Disease?

Pathogenesis

Ménière's disease is an inner ear disorder that causes vertigo and hearing changes. Vertigo is a perception that the patient or the environment is moving with the patient remaining seated or supine to prevent falling. Vertigo is not synonymous with dizziness. Patients who are dizzy have a feeling of confusion (disorientation) in space.

Most cases of Ménière's disease have no known cause. Ménière's disease may develop after an injury to the head or a viral infection of the middle ear. A number of conditions are associated with Ménière's, including trauma, allergy, adrenal-pituitary insufficiency, and hypothyroidism. Anxiety appears to play an important role in triggering Ménière's attacks, as does abnormalities in the immune system.

The idiopathic form of Ménière's is thought to be a result of a single viral injury to the transport system of the inner ear. Ménière's disease is thought to result in dilation of the lymphatic channels in the cochlea and excess endolymphatic fluid in the vestibular and semicircular canals. Endolymph is a clear, intracellular fluid found in the labyrinth of the inner ear. Normal balance is dependent on the stability of fluid pressure.

The Ear and Balance Center of the University of Tennessee, Memphis: What Is Ménière's Disease?
http://www.ent.utmem.edu/vesti bulococh/menieres.html

At-Risk Populations

Patients who are at risk for Ménière's disease include those who have had a head injury or chronic infections of the middle ear. A relationship appears to exist between the number and severity of attacks of Ménière's disease and the degree of stress in a patient's life.

Ménière's disease is most common in men ages 40 to 60 years.

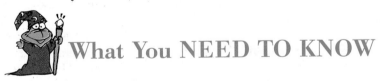

What You NEED TO KNOW

Clinical Manifestations

In approximately 90% of cases, only one ear is affected. Occasionally, Ménière's disease is referred to as a balance disorder, rather than a hearing disorder, because vertigo is frequently the most troublesome symptom in the early stages. Other clinical manifestations of Ménière's include ringing in the ears (tinnitus), a feeling of fullness, sensitivity to loud noises, progressive hearing loss, and headache. In the acute stage, severe nausea with vomiting, profuse sweating, disabling vertigo, and rapid, involuntary, rhythmic movement of the eyeball (rotary nystagmus) may occur. The accompanying sensorineural hearing loss is usually subtle, and the patient may not realize that hearing has been lost because of the ringing in the ears.

Ménière's disease is an unpredictable chronic disorder. Patients have symptoms that come in clusters. Some attacks last only minutes; other attacks may continue for hours, days, weeks, or months. Attacks may occur frequently or several weeks apart. Then, for some unknown reason, the episodes subside.

Prognosis

Control of Ménière's episodes is usually possible, although a cure is, to date, unavailable.

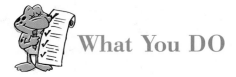

What You DO

Treatment

A low-salt diet has been the mainstay of treatment for Ménière's disease. A variety of medications have also been used in treatment. Although the scientific data supporting the use of diuretics in Ménière's is weak, many patients note an improvement in symptoms when taking the drug. Diuretics have been thought to reduce the fluid (endolymphatic fluid) volume within the cochlea. Drugs designed to suppress vertigo such as meclizine (Antivert), diazepam (Valium), and dimenhydrinate (Dramamine) may be useful in controlling the vertigo and alleviating acute symptoms. In severe cases, immunosuppressants such as prednisone may be used. Occasionally, sedatives may be ordered to promote sleep and rest. When the ringing sensation becomes too disturbing to the patient, it may be masked (for example by music piped in through headphones) to make sleeping easier.

Fortunately, the majority of patients with Ménière's require no surgery. In a small number of patients, vertigo will be persistent and incapacitating, thus they may benefit from surgical treatment. Resection of the vestibular nerve remains the gold standard for eliminating vertigo while preserving hearing. This operation involves cutting the balance nerve while leaving the hearing nerve intact. This operation offers a better than 95% chance of eliminating vertigo. Other surgical procedures may be directed toward relief of pressure by the bony structures surrounding the cochlea or diverting the flow of endolymphatic fluid by means of a shunt to the mastoid bone or to the subarachnoid space.

Nursing Responsibilities

Nursing responsibilities for the patient with Ménière's disease include the following:

 Advise the patient to rest quietly during an attack.
- Use nondrug therapies (e.g., meditation, imaging, deep breathing, quiet bedtime activities, among others) as much as possible to promote sleep and rest.
 Instruct patients to change position slowly to prevent injury.
 Teach the patient to reduce stress as much as possible and to avoid situations likely to trigger an attack.
- Assist the patient in identifying and avoiding food sources high in sodium.

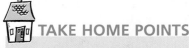

TAKE HOME POINTS

Few problems are more private than those involving the patient's balance. Balance problems, such as those found with Ménière's, may be debilitating and cause embarrassing gait problems. Patient safety can be jeopardized.

See Chapters 2B, 6B, and 7A in
RWNSG: *Pharmacology*

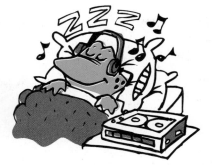

Do You UNDERSTAND?

DIRECTIONS: **Match the terms in Column A with the appropriate explanations in Column B.**

Column A

_____ 1. Protects auditory apparatus from intense vibration
_____ 2. Contains vestibule, cochlea, semicircular canals; organ for hearing and balance
_____ 3. Organ of hearing
_____ 4. Organs responsible for position sense and balance
_____ 5. Covers oval window of inner ear
_____ 6. Dense, fibrous rings surrounding the tympanic membrane

Column B

a. Tympanic membrane
b. External auditory canal
c. Inner ear
d. Malleus
e. Middle ear
f. Annulus
g. Cochlea
h. Footplate of stapes
i. Semicircular canals

What IS an Ear Infection?

Pathogenesis

The most common problems found in the ear are infections, primarily bacterial or fungal. Ear infections can be an acute or chronic problem. The most frequent infection, otitis externa, involves the external ear canal and is the most common cause of ear pain in an adult. Otitis externa begins as a result of excessive dryness or wetness, which damages the protective waxy lining of the external ear canal. The most common form is known as "swimmer's ear" because it occurs as a result of water remaining in the ear canal. *Pseudomonas* is the usual offending organism. Occasionally, otitis externa can involve the cartilage of the pinna with resultant loss of the distinctive shape of the external ear.

Otitis media is the most common middle ear infection and is common in children, although it can occur in adults as well. Otitis media may also result from air pressure trauma to the middle ear and may occur after air travel or scuba diving. When symptoms occur suddenly and are of short duration, the diagnosis is acute otitis media. *Pseudomonas*, *Staphylococcus*, *Klebsiella*, or *Bacteroides* may be the contributing causes of otitis media.

Between bouts of otitis media, fluid may form in the middle ear (serous otitis media). This fluid is formed when a vacuum develops because of a blocked eustachian tube in the middle ear. When the swelling subsides, the fluid may be too thick to drain. Occasionally, serous otitis media is found in conjunction with upper respiratory infections or allergies.

Chronic otitis media develops with repeated episodes of acute otitis media. Chronic otitis media can lead to retraction of the eardrum, scarring and

Answers: 1. a; 2. c; 3. g; 4. i; 5. c; 6. b.

Otitis media is a common problem in children but may persist in some adults. Infants who are bottle fed in a supine position may develop repeated bouts of otitis media as the milk traverses the eustachian tube to the middle ear.

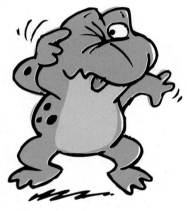

perforation of the eardrum, and death of the ossicles. The result of these disorders is a conductive hearing loss.

At-Risk Populations

The main predisposing factor for all forms of otitis media appears to be poor eustachian tube function. Failure of the eustachian tube to allow air to enter the middle ear impairs normal function and creates an environment in which bacteria can grow. Patients with debilitating systemic diseases such as diabetes are at risk for otitis externa.

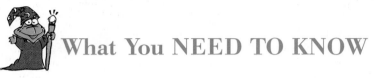

What You NEED TO KNOW

Clinical Manifestations

Acute external otitis is characterized by rapid onset of ear pain. The pain ranges from mild to severe and generally affects only one ear. The pain is more intense when the ear canal is edematous. An early symptom of otitis externa is itching in the ear canal. A tenderness that is present when the pinna is gently pulled is an early sign of external otitis. This finding is in contrast to otitis media in which touching the external ear causes no pain.

Inflammation is easily identified using an otoscope. In early infectious disorders, the drainage may be clear and not discolored by pus.

A patient with acute otitis media may report bubbling, crackling, or popping sensations in the ear, especially during swallowing. A sense of fullness in the ear and a fluctuating conductive hearing loss may be reported. The eardrum is immobile and is dull or red, rather than the normal pearly gray color. The eardrum may be infected, perforated, retracted or bulging, depending on the disease process involved.

Prognosis

Otitis is generally a self-limiting disorder. Although the problem may be recurrent in some people, when promptly treated, patients usually recover in less than 1 week.

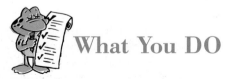

What You DO

Treatment

Acute otitis externa and media are best treated with a 1-week course of antibiotic-steroid drops. This treatment usually results in resolution of the symptoms. Analgesics such as regular- or extra-strength acetaminophen (Tylenol) are occasionally needed during the first 24 to 48 hours to control the pain . For some patients, decongestants may be used to help relieve the pressure within the ear.

See Chapters 1A, 6B, 11, and 13A in RWNSG: *Pharmacology*

Chronic otitis media is treated with a combination of eardrops and, occasionally, antibiotics by mouth. Ultimately, surgery (myringotomy) may be required to eradicate the infection and close the perforation of the eardrum resulting from the chronic infection. Systemic antibiotics may be needed for patients who have infection involving surrounding ear structures.

Nursing Responsibilities

The nursing responsibilities for the patient with otitis externa and otitis media include the following:

- Advise the patient with otitis externa to use either earplugs or cotton coated with petroleum jelly to avoid getting water in the ear while bathing, showering, or swimming.
- Meticulously clean the external to allow the local antibiotic to reach the affected area. Suction, irrigation, or manual removal of earwax can be used. Ear irrigation should not be used when the patient is suspected of having a perforated eardrum.
- Administer eardrops as scheduled with the patient lying on the unaffected side for 3 to 5 minutes to allow gravity to promote movement of the medication into the ear canal. Wait 15 minutes between medication administrations when the medication is needed in both ears.
- When the external ear canal is swollen, insert a wick to allow the drops to penetrate the canal. Eardrops are placed directly on the wick.
- Instruct the patient to chew gum, suck on something sour, and swallow frequently. Yawning and blowing air out against closed nostrils may help open a swollen eustachian tube.

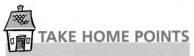

TAKE HOME POINTS

Otitis media is generally easy to treat when promptly diagnosed. Without prompt diagnosis and treatment, otitis media can lead to sinusitis, meningitis, and brain abscess because of the general anatomy of the ear and surrounding tissues.

Do You UNDERSTAND?

DIRECTIONS: **Compare the clinical manifestations of otitis externa with that of otitis media.**

Disorder	Acute otitis externa	Acute otitis media
Onset		
Offending organism(s)		
Location of pain		
Discharge		
Swelling		
Complications		

Answers: Acute otitis externa: rapid onset; *Pseudomonas*; external ear pain; discharge, swelling of external canal; loss of shape of pinna if external canal involved. Acute otitis media: rapid onset; *Pseudomonas*, *Staphylococcus*, *Klebsiella*, or *Bacteroides*; no external ear pain, no obvious discharge, no obvious swelling of external canal; perforation, scarring, hearing loss, chronic otitis media.

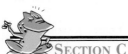

INFECTIOUS DISEASES OF THE SKIN

What IS Candidiasis?

Pathogenesis

Candida is a yeastlike fungus that can be found in the vagina, in the gastrointestinal tract, and on the skin and mucous membranes. *Candida* is normally kept in check by resident bacteria that inhibits growth. Favorable growth factors include a warm, moist environment, a change in pH, an increase in blood glucose, or a change in the immune system. Other possible contributing factors include food allergies, diet, endocrine disorders, tightly fitting clothing, hypothyroidism, and douching. Candidiasis, also known as a yeast infection, can be a result of antibiotic therapy, which suppresses the protective flora of the mucous membranes and skin surfaces.

At-Risk Populations

Individuals at risk for candidiasis include those with endocrine diseases, such as diabetes mellitus and Cushing's disease. Poor nutrition and debilitation can decrease resistance to infection. Patients with neoplastic diseases of the blood, who are immunocompromised, or who are receiving antineoplastic therapy are also at risk.

Candida can reside in the skin folds of the abdomen, the inguinal area, or under the breasts of those who are obese. Uncircumcised males are at risk for candidiasis only when he does not retract the foreskin and wash on a daily basis. Individuals whose hands are frequently in water, such as dishwashers and bartenders, may also be susceptible to candidiasis. Poorly fitting and poorly cleaned dentures have also been found to be a source of the infection.

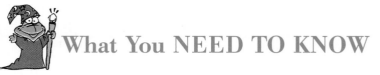

What You NEED TO KNOW

Clinical Manifestations

Skin problems result when *Candida* releases toxins that irritate the skin. Physical examination of the patient reveals a red, edematous area with well-defined borders. As the infection progresses, the individual may have white patchy areas with some scaling. When severe, pustules and vesiculopustules may develop. Itching and burning accompany the rash.

The areas of the skin that have folds, such as under the breasts, the axillae, groin, perianal area, and the scrotum, are prevalent sites. Candidiasis can also occur as a red, painful swelling around the nail beds.

Persons who are pregnant, on antibiotic therapy, or on birth control pills have an increased risk for candidiasis.

Children and adults with incontinence are at risk for candidiasis from constant moisture and irritation.

Candidiasis has also been found on the lower back, the intergluteal folds, and the buttocks, particularly in children. Diaper rash from *Candida* may appear as mild redness and inflammation to an extremely erythematosus area.

Vaginal manifestations of *Candida* include vulvar pruritus and irritation, dysuria, erythema, dyspareunia, and a thick, cheesy, odorless or foul-smelling, vaginal discharge. (Vulvovaginal candidiasis is discussed in Chapter 10.) A penile irritation (balanitis) that includes red lesions with defined borders and a white plaque with itching and burning may signal a *Candida* infection.

Oral candidiasis (thrush) is characterized by the formation of a creamy white coating, white plaques, or flaking on a red inflamed tongue or mucous membrane. The lesions may develop into shallow ulcers. The papillae on the tongue may appear large. The plaques on the tongue can be easily removed, but will cause bleeding. A slight fever or gastrointestinal irritation may accompany thrush. Denture wearers can also develop chronic candidiasis in areas under the dentures.

Prognosis

Candidiasis can be easily cleared with topical or oral antifungals that are available over the counter or by prescription. The infection is generally cleared in 3 to 7 days.

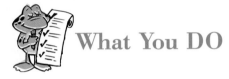

What You DO

Treatment

The patient with candidiasis should begin treatment as soon as symptoms develop. Antifungal drugs such as topical clotrimazole or miconazole are effective against *Candida*. Oral candidiasis can be treated with oral suspensions of nystatin in the form of a "swish and swallow" treatment. Severe inflammation can also be treated with a combination drug that includes antifungal and topical steroids.

Nursing Responsibilities

Nursing responsibilities for the patient with candidiasis include the following:
- Advise the patient to wear loose-fitting clothing and to keep the skin clean and dry. Dry cotton clothes can be effective in separating areas that remain moist, such as skin folds and skin under the breasts.
- Encourage the patient with candidiasis infections of the hands to wear gloves during dishwashing and to dry the hands thoroughly afterward.
- Instruct the patient about the proper administration of prescribed medications.

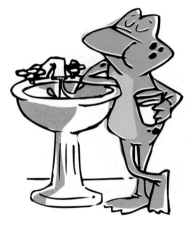

See Chapters 1A and 7A in RWNSG: *Pharmacology*

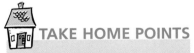

TAKE HOME POINTS

Candidiasis is generally cleared within 3 to 7 days by using topical or oral antifungals available over the counter or by prescription.

Do You UNDERSTAND?

DIRECTIONS: Indicate in the space provided whether the statement is *true* or *false*. If false, then use the margin space to the left to rewrite the statement to make it true.

_____ 1 Candidiasis can occur as a red, painful swelling around the nail beds.

_____ 2. The candidal lesion is usually nodular and tan colored with the center depressed and the borders rolled.

_____ 3. Skin on the chest and legs are the most common site of candidiasis.

_____ 4. Candidiasis, also called yeast infection, *Monilia*, and thrush, is caused by a yeastlike fungus.

What IS Folliculitis?

Pathogenesis

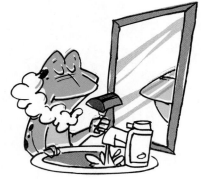

Folliculitis is an infection of hair follicles caused by microorganisms, injuries, or chemical irritation. The inflammation can be superficial or deep. Classification depends on the type of involvement. Folliculitis is a common skin disorder. The disorder usually develops with an infection that proliferates from another site into the hair follicles. Folliculitis is caused primarily by *Staphylococcus aureus*; but other organisms such as *Klebsiella, Enterobacter, Pseudomonas* or a dermatophyte such as a fungus can also cause an infection.

Predisposing factors to folliculitis include an abscess, a previous injury, abrasion, or a wound located near the hair follicle. Enzymatic and chemotactic factors that are produced from the bacteria cause the inflammation. Pseudofolliculitis (also called razor bumps) occurs primarily on skin surfaces that are shaved.

At-Risk Populations

Patients on long-term antibiotic therapy and those with existing injuries and infections are prone to folliculitis. An association also exists between folliculitis and persons who have poor hygiene. Patients with diabetes mellitus or who are taking corticosteroids are susceptible to the *Candida* form of folliculitis. *Pseudomonas aeruginosa* found in swimming pools and whirlpool tubs with inadequate chloride levels can cause folliculitis.

Answers: 1. true; 2. false; lesions are usually red and edematous with well-defined borders; 3. false; areas under the breasts, axillae, groin, perianal area, penis, scrotum are the most common sites; 4. true.

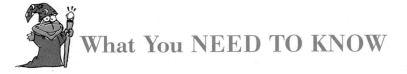

What You NEED TO KNOW

Clinical Manifestations

The hair follicle appears inflamed and tender. Some forms of folliculitis are painless. The patient may itch at the affected site. Small pustules, approximately 2 to 5 mm in size, form at the base of the hair follicle and may stay at the surface or go deeper, invading the entire follicle. The region becomes red, swollen, and tender, depending on the depth of infection. The hair shaft may not be visible in the center of the pustule. Lesions can appear singly or in masses. The most susceptible areas include the back, scalp, face, and extremities. *Pseudomonas* folliculitis can be found on the buttocks, hips, axillae, or external ear. *Candida* folliculitis can be found on the trunk, upper extremities, and the face.

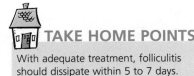

TAKE HOME POINTS

With adequate treatment, folliculitis should dissipate within 5 to 7 days.

Prognosis

Recurrent infections may require more than one treatment period.

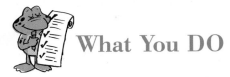

What You DO

Treatment

Pustules can be cultured to determine the organism present. Oral antimicrobial therapy is useful, depending on the type of bacteria. Topical erythromycin, mupirocin (Bactroban), or antifungals such as clotrimazole (Mycelex) are effective, depending on the type of infection. Saline compresses or Burrow's compresses can be used to decrease swelling. Treatment also consists of keeping the area clean and dry.

See Chapter 1A in RWNSG:
Pharmacology

Nursing Responsibilities

The nursing responsibilities for the patient with folliculitis include the following:
- Advise the patient to keep the area as clean and dry as possible and to improve hygiene when this area is a source of infection.
- Encourage patients to complete the prescribed course of antimicrobial therapy.
- Instruct the patient to postpone shaving when pseudofolliculitis develops.

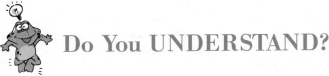

Do You UNDERSTAND?

DIRECTIONS: **Indicate in the space provided whether the statement is** *true* **or** *false*. **If false, then use the margin space to the right to rewrite the statement to make it true.**

_____ 1. Folliculitis can occur as a red, painful swelling around the nail beds.
_____ 2. Folliculitis is most commonly caused by *Staphylococcus aureus*.

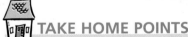

What IS a Furuncle or a Carbuncle?

Pathogenesis

Furuncles, also called boils, develop from folliculitis and are found primarily in skin areas that contain infected hair follicles. The infection spreads from another site and invades the hair follicle. The hair follicles become swollen, red, and firm. The lesion will frequently fester, rupture, and drain. The anterior nares may be the source of initial infection by *Staphylococcus aureus*.

Carbuncles are clusters of boils that begin in subcutaneous tissue, forming masses of painful, deep, swollen lesions. *Staphylococcus aureus* is the primary etiologic agent, but other aerobic and anaerobic organisms may also cause carbuncles.

At-Risk Populations

People at risk for furuncles and carbuncles include those who are obese, debilitated, or who have diabetes mellitus, alcoholism, malnutrition, or acne. Patients who are immunocompromised or who have blood disorders such as anemia are also prone to these infections. A relationship to corticosteroid use has been noted.

What You NEED TO KNOW

Clinical Manifestations

Furuncles and carbuncles occur primarily on the upper back, thigh, or neck regions but may also appear in areas prone to friction or trauma. A carbuncle begins with a firm, tender, red nodule that is 1 to 5 cm in size. In a few days, the nodule becomes larger, painful, and cystlike. Cellulitis may also form before or in conjunction with the infection. The lesions will drain pus. Carbuncles may invade deep tissue forming painful edematous masses with numerous open, draining sites. Systemic infection is possible and evidenced by fever, chills, and malaise and can result in endocarditis or osteomyelitis.

Prognosis

Carbuncles and furuncles should heal with adequate treatment. Some patients may resolve without any treatment. Furunculosis is a chronic, recurrent form of the disease that may last from months to years. Numerous treatments may be required to eliminate the infection.

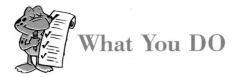

What You DO

Treatment

Treatment includes moist heat and antibiotics. Moist heat provides some relief from discomfort and promotes drainage. Antibiotic ointments may be applied to the lesions. With larger lesions, an incision with drainage may be necessary. When cellulitis is evident or more than one lesion is present, systemic cephalosporin or macrolide antibiotics are used. Treatment continues until the infection resolves but usually lasts 10 to 14 days.

Recurrent furunculosis is treated with longer episodes of antibiotics and general cleanliness. A culture should be obtained from patients with recurrent infection to determine the source of infection. Intranasal application of mupirocin calcium ointment (Bactroban) for 5 days is also effective for patients who carry S. *aureus* in their nasal passages.

See Chapter 1A in RWNSG: *Pharmacology*

Nursing Responsibilities

The nursing responsibilities for the patient with furuncles or carbuncles include the following:

🍎 Advise the patient of the importance of keeping the area clean and dry to prevent further infection.

• Encourage the patient to use sterile dressings while lesions are draining and that proper disposal of dressings is important.

• Isolate the hospitalized patient who has draining, methicillin-resistant S. *aureus* infections. Bed linens, towels, and clothing should be kept away from other individuals to prevent spread of the infection.

🍎 Instruct the patient about the proper administration of nasal antibiotic creams.

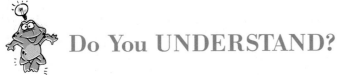

Do You UNDERSTAND?

DIRECTIONS: **Indicate in the space provided whether the statement is *true* or *false*. If false, then use the margin space to the right to rewrite the statement to make it true.**

_____ 1. Furuncles develop from carbuncles.

_____ 2. After a furuncle festers, it will rupture, drain, and the lesion will subside.

_____ 3. The staphylococcal organism frequently causes carbuncles.

_____ 4. Carbuncles are easily resolved in 3 to 4 days with local antibiotics.

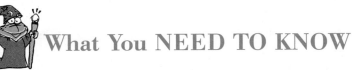

What IS Impetigo?

Pathogenesis

Impetigo, a bacterial infection of the skin caused by group A streptococcus or *S. aureus*, or both, is spread by skin contact with contaminated surfaces such as other skin areas, fingernails, and shared objects. Impetigo can appear as a secondary infection from minor trauma, such as abrasions, eczema, insect bites, or poison ivy. Approximately 10 days after exposure to the bacteria, honey-colored crusts appear on the skin. Impetigo is more common in hot, humid weather. Scratching the lesions contributes to spread of infection.

At-Risk Populations

Impetigo is a highly communicable disease that spreads quickly among family members, in nurseries, in schools, and in crowded areas.

What You NEED TO KNOW

Clinical Manifestations

Streptococcal impetigo appears as pustules, vesicles, or bulla on the skin. Inflammatory halos may appear around the lesion. As the lesions erupt, they leave a honey-colored serous liquid on the skin that forms a characteristic "stuck-on" crust. Clustered lesions create large crusts. Itching is common, although scratching excoriates the skin and spreads the infection. *S. aureus* also causes the bullous form of impetigo (bullous impetigo). These lesions begin as vesicles but enlarge to form bulla. The center may collapse with fluid located in the periphery of the lesion. The center contains a varnishlike crust with reddened skin underneath.

Prognosis

With adequate treatment and good hygiene practices, impetigo can be resolved in 2 weeks without any further problems. A type of streptococcal impetigo may progress to cause poststreptococcal glomerulonephritis without adequate treatment.

What You DO

Treatment

Interventions for impetigo include the application of topical mupirocin (Bactroban) or triple antibiotic ointments. Systemic antibiotics such as peni-

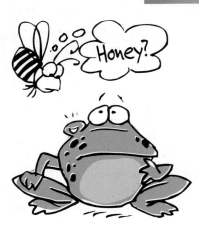

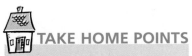 Impetigo commonly occurs in infants and children, but adults who are in poor health, malnourished, or have poor hygiene are also at risk.

TAKE HOME POINTS

Impetigo is more common in hot, humid weather. Scratching the lesions contributes to spread of the infection.

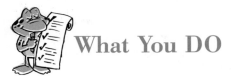

cillin or erythromycin are effective. For severe staphylococcal infections and bullous impetigo, intravenous (IV) therapy with penicillinase-resistant penicillin is necessary. Topical applications of cool saline compresses are helpful in relieving the itching and discomfort.

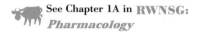

See Chapter 1A in **RWNSG:** *Pharmacology*

Nursing Responsibilities

The nursing responsibilities for the patient with impetigo include the following:

- Encourage the patient to keep the lesions clean and dry. The entire body can be cleaned with an antibacterial soap to prevent reoccurrence and spread to other areas. The crusts should be removed before the antibiotic cream is applied. To be effective, the cream is applied several times a day.
- Advise the caregiver to wear gloves to prevent spread of the infection.
- Advise the patient to avoid scratching.
- Encourage good hygienic measures to prevent spreading the infection to family members and others.

Do You UNDERSTAND?

DIRECTIONS: **Fill in the blanks.**

1. Impetigo is highly _____.
2. Streptococcal impetigo appears as small pustules, vesicles, or bulla that erupt on the _____.
3. Impetigo lesions can be found anywhere on the body, especially in _____ areas such as the face, hands, neck, and extremities.
4. _____ from impetigo is frequently a concern.

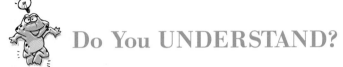

What IS Cellulitis?

Pathogenesis

Cellulitis is a bacterial infection of the dermis and subcutaneous tissue that is caused primarily by group A streptococcus or *S. aureus*, although many types of bacteria can cause cellulitis.

Erysipelas is an acute, inflammatory type of cellulitis that has lymphatic involvement. Paronychia is a cellulitis of the nail folds. Cellulitis can also develop around the eye. Group A streptococcus also causes perianal cellulitis, which is found in the anal area. The erysipeloid form of cellulitis is found in individuals that handle saltwater fish, shellfish, meat products, and poultry. Cellulitis can also appear in normally healthy skin.

Haemophilus influenzae may cause cellulitis in children between the ages of 6 months and 3 years. *H. influenzae* affects the head and neck areas and can lead to meningitis.

Children under the age of 5 have a higher rate of facial cellulitis, particularly in the presence of an insect bite, laceration, or eczema.

At-Risk Populations

People who are at risk for cellulitis include those with diabetes mellitus, human immunodeficiency virus, neoplasms, IV drug abusers, patients who are on antineoplastic therapy, and patients with poor circulation. Patients who have had previous trauma to the skin or existing skin ulcers are also at risk.

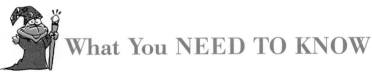

What You NEED TO KNOW

Clinical Manifestations

Cellulitis is usually found on the lower legs, ears, and face, appearing a few days after the infectious organism invades the skin. Local swelling, tenderness, warmth, and pain may occur. Bright red patches or plaques with indefinite borders begin to appear. Edema may be present at the site. The skin may be tender and warm with toxic striations. Regional lymphadenopathy may be present. In later stages, pustules, abscesses, and necrosis may develop. With repeated bouts of infection, lymphatic drainage becomes impaired, which can result in repeated infections, lymphedema, and epidermal thickening known as elephantiasis nostras. Secondary infections of the site can also occur.

Prognosis

With adequate treatment, cellulitis should resolve. Some individuals continue to have recurrent episodes that are difficult to treat.

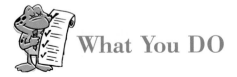

What You DO

Treatment

Treatment of cellulitis includes the use of systemic antibiotics, such as cephalosporins or macrolides. Resistant strains are treated with a penicillinase-resistant penicillin, such as nafcillin (Unipen) or vancomycin (Vancocin). Analgesics and soaking in Burrow's solution can be helpful in relieving discomfort. Lower extremities should be elevated to reduce swelling.

See Chapter 1A in RWNSG: *Pharmacology*

Nursing Responsibilities

The nursing responsibilities for the patient with cellulitis include the following:
- Encourage the patient to complete the course of antibiotic therapy.
- Remove any exudate and keep the area clean and dry. Dressings can be used when drainage is present.
- Elevate and immobilize the extremity when the involved area is edematous and encouraging the patient to wear support stockings
- Encourage good hygiene to prevent further occurrences.

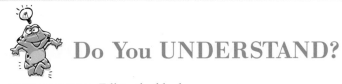

Do You UNDERSTAND?

DIRECTIONS: **Fill in the blanks.**

1. When _____ first occurs, it appears as small
_____, vesicles, or _____ on the skin.

2. Local _____, _____,
warmth, and pain may occur.

3. _____ borders and edema may be present
at the cellulite site.

What IS Herpes Simplex?

Pathogenesis

Primary herpes simplex virus (HSV) infections affect 200,000 to 700,000 people every year, with as many as 2 million new cases occurring each year. Recurrent infections can affect up to 30 million Americans annually. Two serotypes cause HSV infections: type 1 (HSV-1) or type 2 (HSV-2). HSV-1 is usually responsible for nongenital infections found on the mouth, face, and cornea. Common names for the infection include cold sores, fever blister, and canker sores. Previous exposure to one type does not prevent infection from the other type. Genital herpes is the most common infectious genital disease in industrialized countries.

HSV infection occurs in two stages: primary infection and recurrent infection. Primary infection develops 3 to 12 days after initial exposure to the virus. The virus begins replicating in the dermis and epidermis and then travels down nerve roots to the dorsal root where the virus lays dormant in the sensory ganglia until it is reactivated. During this latency period, the virus resides in the nuclei of host cells. After the virus is reactivated, it travels by way of the peripheral nerve root onto the skin or mucus membrane, creating lesions. Recurrent infections appear in the same manner as primary infections but may be less severe.

Triggers for recurrent infections include stress, lack of sleep, sunburn, ultraviolet light, overexertion, menstruation, fever, trauma, and systemic infections. Eczema herpeticum is a form of atopic dermatitis that develops into herpes lesions.

At-Risk Populations

The herpes virus is usually transmitted through intimate contact with another person who is shedding the virus from a mucosal surface or through body secretions. Seventy percent of transmission occurs when the individual has no symptoms. Oral transmission occurs through kissing, poor hand washing, and through oral intercourse. Genital herpes can be spread by sexual contact with an infected partner. Individuals who have multiple sexual partners are also at an increased risk. Other patients at risk for HSV infection include those who are immunocompromised, those with cancer, or patients receiving immunosuppressive drugs.

TAKE HOME POINTS

HSV-2 is usually responsible for genital infections, although both type 1 and type 2 can be found in either area.

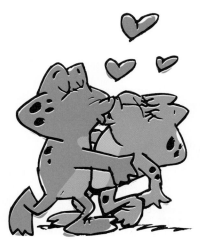

Answers: 1. cellulites, pustules, bulla; 2. swelling, tenderness; 3. indefinite.

The herpes virus can also be transmitted in utero, intrapartum, or postpartum. Neonatal rates have been estimated to be 1:2500 to 1:20,000 births. Perinatal herpes has a high morbidity and mortality rate, causing premature delivery, spontaneous abortions, and death after vaginal delivery. Transmission of the virus after vaginal delivery occurs in 20% to 50% of infants born of mothers with primary HSV and less than 8% in infants of mothers who have recurrent HSV.

Neonates who contract herpes during delivery have a 50% to 65% chance of death.

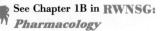

See Chapter 1B in RWNSG:
Pharmacology

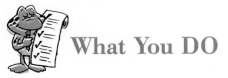

What You NEED TO KNOW

Clinical Manifestations

HSV can occur as a primary or recurrent infection. Patients with a primary HSV infection develop itching, burning, tingling, or pain in the affected area. A small cluster of vesicles appears on an erythematous base with vesicle rupture occurring in approximately 5 days. The vesicles may progress to pustules, ulcers, and crusts. The vesicles may be single or in groups on an erythematous base. A crust forms over the skin with lesions taking 1 to 3 weeks to resolve.

Lesions can be found on the face, lips, mouth, buttocks, or genital region. Patients with primary genital infections may experience prodromal symptoms, such as itching, tingling, and burning. The patient may also have influenza-like symptoms, such as fever, malaise, myalgias, and headaches. Lymph nodes may be tender in the region. In men, lesions may develop on the penis and scrotum, accompanied by urethritis. An increase in vaginal discharge may be noted in women with the genital form. Other symptoms include lower back pain, radiating pain, burning on urination, urinary retention, or lymphadenopathy. Herpetic infection of the eye may manifest as pain, irritation, watery eyes, or photophobia and can lead to blindness.

Prognosis

Because no cure for the herpes virus is available, treatment measures are aimed at symptoms. Herpetic infections may lay dormant for long periods. After a primary infection, antibodies to the virus develop, creating recurrences that are usually more localized and less severe. Some patients have no further occurrence of the infection.

What You DO

Treatment

A diagnosis of herpes infection is made based on the appearance of the lesions, a Tzanck smear, a viral culture, or serologic testing. Acyclovir (Zovirax), famciclovir (Famvir), and valacyclovir (Valtrex), when used early in an outbreak, have been found to be effective in most cases. A strain of acyclovir-resistant virus can develop in immunocompromised individuals. Penciclovir (Denavir) has also been found to be a possible treatment but must be applied every 2 hours while the patient is awake. A vaccine is currently in development for the prevention of genital herpes.

Therapy must be started early. When started within 48 hours of the beginning of prodromal symptoms, the effectiveness of treatment is increased. Therapy decreases viral shedding and promotes rapid healing. For individuals with frequent recurrences (e.g., six or more a year), oral acyclovir (Zovirax) may be given for longer periods. Drying agents such as benzoyl peroxide gel may be useful for facial lesions.

Nursing Responsibilities

Nursing responsibilities for the patient with HSV infection include the following:

- Support the patient during any needed adjustments in the patient's lifestyle. Taking care of the overall health is important, including getting adequate rest, eating well, and reducing stress.
- Encourage the patient to abstain from sexual activity during active herpes outbreaks. Although condoms provide some protection, they do not protect the external vaginal area or the base of the penis.
- 🍎 Teach patients that transmission of the virus may occur even when they are asymptomatic.
- Prevent secondary infections. Good hand washing and hygiene must be performed during times of outbreak.
- Encourage the female patient to have an annual Pap smear. HSV-2 infections are associated with an increased risk of cervical cancer.

The nurse should inform the pregnant woman who has an active HSV-2 infection that a cesarean delivery may be recommended.

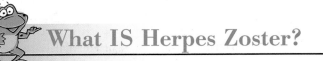

Do You UNDERSTAND?

DIRECTIONS: **Indicate in the space provided whether the statement is *true* or *false*. If false, then use the margin space to the right to rewrite the statement to make it true.**

_____ 1. Acyclovir, famciclovir, and valacyclovir have been found to be effective in most cases of herpes infections.

_____ 2. Getting adequate rest, eating well, and reducing stress has little effect on the development or recurrence of herpes simplex.

_____ 3. Abstinence from sexual activity is not indicated during active genital herpes outbreak.

_____ 4. Patients with HSV-2 are at greater risk for cervical cancer, thus an annual Pap smear is important.

What IS Herpes Zoster?

Pathogenesis

Herpes zoster is caused by the same virus—varicella-zoster—that produces chickenpox (varicella) and is characterized by acute inflammation along a dermatome of the skin. A decline in immunity, stress, or aging may be a cause of

Answers: **1.** true; **2.** false; these activities have a significant influence on the development or recurrence of HSV infections; **3.** false; abstinence is indicated during active outbreak of genital herpes; **4.** true.

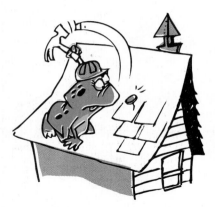

reactivation of latent varicella zoster virus. With initial exposure to chickenpox, the virus travels down the nerve fibers to the dorsal ganglion cells where it resides in a dormant state. After the varicella zoster virus is reactivated, it replicates in the affected sensory ganglion. The virus moves through the sensory nerve pathways to the skin where it creates pain, vesicles, and crusting. The inflammatory response along the nerve pathways and neuronal necrosis cause the intense pain. Reactivation is not completely understood, but it is believed to be a result of a decline in immunity.

At-Risk Populations

Individuals at risk for herpes zoster (shingles) include patients who are immunocompromised, who have leukemia, or who have conditions that require an organ transplant. The incidence of shingles also increases with age.

Adults over age 50 have an increased incidence of shingles. Older adults are particularly susceptible to this herpes virus because of a loss of large nerve fibers and a shift to smaller nerve fibers.

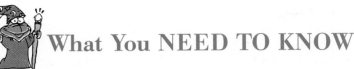

What You NEED TO KNOW

Clinical Manifestations

Before the eruption of the lesions, the patient with herpes zoster may experience itching, pain, or tenderness at the site. In 3 to 5 days, vesicles begin to erupt on the skin. The lesions may appear "bubbly" or like cobblestones in clusters. The underlying skin is red and swollen. Vesicles usually develop on the posterior surface of the body and move peripherally along unilateral dermatomes to the anterior body surface. In 1 to 2 weeks, the crusts fall off.

Primary eruption sites are the facial, thoracic, or cervical nerve roots. A few lesions may be observed outside the primary area, particularly in children and immunocompromised individuals. Associated pain and paresthesia accompany this illness. The pain of herpes zoster is intense and may last long after the vesicles have subsided. Postherpetic neuralgia may develop in 10% to 70% of the individuals who have this condition.

Permanent blindness can result when the herpes virus develops in the ophthalmic division of the trigeminal nerve. Rashes that resemble Herpes zoster have been noted after the varicella vaccine has been given. The vaccine itself can cause an outbreak of herpes in a few individuals. A second and third reoccurrence of herpes zoster may occur but usually involves dermatomes other than those involved in the original attack.

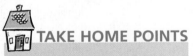
TAKE HOME POINTS

Postherpetic neuralgia can be described as the presence of pain at least 1 month or more after the lesions have disappeared.

Prognosis

No cure for herpes zoster is available. Treatment is aimed at alleviating symptoms. The virus may lay dormant for long periods and arise during periods of stress, immunosuppression, or during aging. After an initial episode, most patients never experience another episode. The varicella vaccine has been found to be effective in preventing chickenpox. The hope is that the vaccine may also prevent the occurrence of herpes zoster.

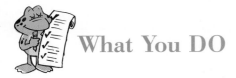

What You DO

Treatment

The drug of choice in the treatment of herpes zoster is acyclovir (Zovirax), although other antiviral drugs such as famciclovir (Famvir), valacyclovir (Valtrex), vidarabine (Vira-A), and sorivudine have been used. Treatment begins as soon as possible after appearance of symptoms. When given before or during the vesicular phase, lesion development and pain is lessened. Burrow's solution can be used to speed the drying of the lesions and remove crusts. Antibacterial sulfonamide cream can be applied to prevent secondary infections. Baking soda, aqueous alcohol lotions, or calamine lotion can also be used for itching at the affected site. Topical anesthetic agents may reduce pain at the site. Analgesics are frequently needed to relieve the pain. Opioid analgesics may be necessary when the pain is intense. Amitriptyline, an antidepressant, has been found useful because of its sedative effects. Corticosteroid use is controversial but may be helpful for some patients.

> See Chapters 1B, 2E, 7A, 11, and 14 in **RWNSG:** *Pharmacology*

Nursing Responsibilities

The nursing responsibilities for the patient with herpes zoster include the following:
- Prevent secondary infection of the lesions. The area should be kept free of contaminants. Covering the lesions is not recommended during treatment.
- Manage pain. When pain becomes too severe, the patient may need to be referred to a pain clinic.
- Advise the patient to notify the health care provider when the eye becomes involved, thus referral to an ophthalmologist can be made.
- Advise the patient with herpes zoster to avoid anyone who has not had chickenpox or who is immunocompromised. Herpes zoster can cause chicken pox in individuals who are susceptible.

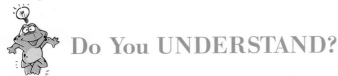

Do You UNDERSTAND?

DIRECTIONS: **Indicate in the space provided whether the statement is** *true* **or** *false***. If false, then use the margin space to the right to rewrite the statement to make it true.**

_____ 1. Herpes zoster is an acute inflammation along the dermatomes of the skin.

_____ 2. The incidence of herpes zoster is not influenced by age.

_____ 3. Pain always disappears when lesions disappear.

_____ 4. Herpes zoster is easily cured with antibiotics.

Answers: 1. true; 2. false; the incidence of herpes zoster is influenced by age; 3. false; pain does not always disappear when lesions disappear; 4. false; herpes zoster is incurable.

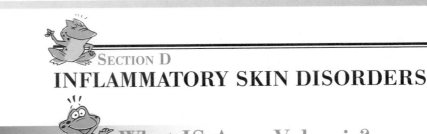

SECTION D
INFLAMMATORY SKIN DISORDERS

What IS Acne Vulgaris?

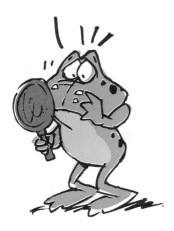

Pathogenesis

Acne vulgaris occurs when hormones called androgens overstimulate the skin's oil glands. The oil glands (sebaceous glands) secrete a substance called sebum, which normally travels up tiny hair follicles to the skin's pores where it lubricates and protects the skin. However, excessive sebum can get trapped within the follicle. Simultaneously, overworked oil glands enlarge, accelerating the normal shedding of skin cells inside the follicle. These skin cells mix with trapped sebum and clog the skin's pores. Clogged pores promote overgrowth of the bacterium that causes acne (Propionibacterium acnes). The bacteria produce further inflammation of hair follicles and surrounding skin resulting in acne.

At-Risk Populations

Acne affects men and women equally, but because males produce more androgen, they are more prone to develop more severe cases of acne than are females.

Acne usually occurs between the ages of 10 and 13 and lasts 5 to 10 years. The hormonal fluctuations of the menstrual cycle can make young women more sensitive to androgens that are already present, causing flare-ups immediately before menses.

A genetic predisposition to acne may be present. Approximately 85% of the population is affected by this disorder. Research studies have failed to find any relationship between diet and acne, although stress is thought to play an important part in the longer prevalence of the condition among women. Although the exact link between stress and acne is unknown, theories suggest that stress increases the secretion of androgen.

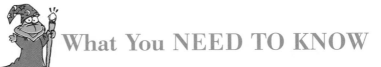

What You NEED TO KNOW

Clinical Manifestations

Acne typically occurs in areas where there are a large number of oil glands. The most common areas include the face, scalp, neck, chest, back, upper arms, and shoulders. Blackheads and whiteheads (open and closed comedones), occasionally filled with pus (pustules) and cysts, may be present.

Prognosis

Whiteheads and blackheads drain and heal over time. Pustules and deeper cysts can cause scarring, however, the scarring tends to lessen with time. The tendency to scar varies from patient to patient.

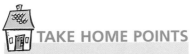

TAKE HOME POINTS

Overactivity of the skin's oil glands, not poor hygiene, poor character, or poor diet, is the cause of acne.

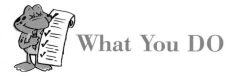

What You DO

Treatment

Many treatments for acne are available, including nonprescription medications, prescription medications, and surgery. Topical treatments include benzoyl peroxide, salicylic acid, and topical antibiotics. Benzoyl peroxide is an antimicrobial agent that is effective against the bacteria associated with acne. Salicylic acid reduces abnormal shedding of skin cells along the hair follicle. Topical (as well as orally administered) antibiotics such as clindamycin (Cleocin) and erythromycin kill acne bacteria on the skin's surface and reduce inflammation, but these antibiotics do not affect abnormal skin cell shedding or sebum production. For this reason, topical medications are frequently used together with other acne preparations such as vitamin A derivatives (retinoids). Retinoid and retinoid-like skin creams and lotions normalize skin cell shedding and growth and reduce inflammation, which combine to unclog pores. Retinoids are prescription medications. All of these medications have adverse effects thus limiting their use.

See Chapters 1A, 12, and 13B in RWNSG: *Pharmacology*

Acne treatment also includes the use of intralesional steroids and comedo extractions. In selected patients, cryosurgery is used. Dermabrasion is used for patients with severe scarring. A newer procedure, laser resurfacing (also called laser peel), removes the top layers of skin without bleeding, the use of chemical peels, or dermabrasion. Laser resurfacing is typically performed under local or general anesthesia.

Nursing Responsibilities

Responsibilities of the nurse include the following:
- Identify persons at risk for acne.
- Provide patient and family teaching about the disorder. Its treatment is important because many common misconceptions exist about the cause.
- Advise the patient to avoid any mechanical trauma to the lesions, such as squeezing, rubbing, or picking the comedones. Even resting the chin, forehead, or cheek on the hand can exacerbate the lesions. Hats, sweatbands, and shirt collars have contributed to acne.
- Encourage the patient to use medications as prescribed.

During the teenage years, appearance is important to the patient. Acne may damage the adolescent's self-esteem. The nurse must counsel the patient in this regard.

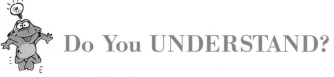

Do You UNDERSTAND?

DIRECTIONS: **Fill in the blanks.**

1. Acne vulgaris is an inflammation within the area of the
_____ _____.

2. A sebaceous follicle _____ the same as a pilo-sebaceous follicle.

3. _____ hormones do not contribute to the production of sebum.

4. Acne usually develops between the ages of _____ and _____.

5. The topical treatment of first choice for acne is _____ _____.

6. Two nursing responsibilities in reference to acne include _____ and _____.

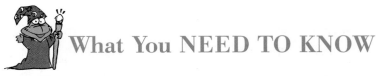

What IS Rosacea?

Pathogenesis

Rosacea, previously known as acne rosacea, is a chronic inflammatory process that is easily confused with acne vulgaris. In fact, rosacea may be present with acne. The cause of rosacea is unknown, although the pathogenesis is similar to that of acne vulgaris.

At-Risk Populations

Rosacea is more common in fair-skinned persons with an onset in middle-aged and older persons. The predisposing causes are unknown but a family history and ruddy complexion are common findings.

What You NEED TO KNOW

Clinical Manifestations

In the early stages of development (before the age of 20), repeated episodes of flushing occur. The flushing eventually becomes a permanent, redness (erythema) on the nose and cheeks that occasionally extends to the forehead and chin. The flushing is common in women. Erythema persists as the person ages, with the sebaceous follicles enlarging and the skin changing to a purple-red color. Eventually, vascular lesions form a group of small blood vessels (telangiectasia); an irregular, bulbous thickening of the nose (rhinophyma) develops. Rhinophyma is present more frequently in men than it is in women. Conjunctivitis and keratitis, which are rare, may accompany rosacea.

Prognosis

Rosacea is characterized by periods of exacerbation and remission. The disorder requires prolonged treatment.

Answers: ; 3. androgenic; 4. 10, 13; 5. benzoyl peroxide; 6. identifying patients at risk, patient and family teaching.

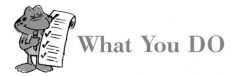

What You DO

Treatment

The treatment for rosacea is similar to those used for acne vulgaris. The antibiotic of choice is oral tetracycline. Topical metronidazole is an effective treatment, although it will make the affected area dry and red for a period. Telangiectases may be treated with electrodesiccation. Rhinophyma requires surgical removal of excess tissue through laser therapy.

See Chapter 1A in **RWNSG:**
Pharmacology

Nursing Responsibilities

The responsibilities of the nurse include the following:

- Identify patients who are at risk for rosacea.
- Advise patients that although alcohol intake is not related to the development of rosacea, persons with rosacea are heat sensitive. Patients should be taught to avoid vascular-stimulating agents, such as heat, cold, sunlight, hot liquids, highly seasoned foods, and alcohol.
- Provide patient and family teaching regarding the adverse effects of medications and risks associated with surgical intervention.
- Provide supportive understanding. The disorder frequently alters the patient's self-image.

Do You UNDERSTAND?

DIRECTIONS: Fill in the blanks.

1. Rosacea is characterized by periods of _____ and _____.
2. Telangiectasia is defined as _____.
3. The drugs commonly used in the treatment of rosacea include _____ and _____.
4. Rosacea is more common in _____, with an onset occurring in _____ and _____ persons.

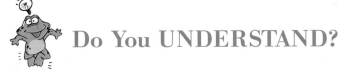

What IS Eczema?

Pathogenesis

The terms eczema and dermatitis are synonymous for the most common disorders (dermatoses) of the skin. Eczema is an inflammatory skin response to any injurious agent. Both endogenous and exogenous agents can cause an inflam-

Answers: 1. exacerbations, remission; 2. a lesion made up of a group of small blood vessels; 3. tetracycline, metronidazole; 4. fair-skinned persons, middle-age, older.

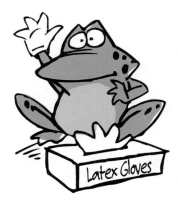

matory response. Several types of dermatoses have been identified, including allergic contact dermatitis, irritant contact dermatitis, and atopic dermatitis.

More than 2000 allergens produce the inflammatory skin response, including clothing, cosmetics, cleaning products, occupational exposure, plants and woods, metal alloys found in jewelry, additives such as perfumes and dyes, and soap ingredients. An example of allergic contact dermatitis is that caused by contact with latex products, specifically examination gloves and condoms. Allergic contact dermatitis is a cell-mediated response brought about by sensitization to an allergens and is a type IV hypersensitivity reaction.

Irritant contact dermatitis can occur in persons who are in sufficient contact with the irritant to cause a reaction. For example, a reaction can occur from mechanical means (e.g., rubbing), chemical irritants (e.g., household cleaning products), or environmental irritants (e.g., wool, fiberglass, urine, plants). Another example is the reaction caused from contact with cement products.

Atopic dermatitis (also known as atopic eczema) occurs in two clinical forms: infantile and adult. Atopic dermatitis is a subtype of a type I hypersensitivity reaction. A family history of asthma, hay fever, or atopic dermatitis is usually present.

At-Risk Populations

Eczema has no age boundaries. This group of skin conditions can affect all ages and cultural groups.

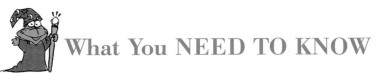

What You NEED TO KNOW

Clinical Manifestations

Vesicle formation, oozing, crusting, itching, erythema, and scaling characterize eczema, regardless of the specific form. The clinical manifestations can range from mild forms (e.g., itchy, hot, dry skin) to severe forms with raw, bleeding, and broken skin. The locations of the lesions are of great benefit in diagnosing the causative agent.

Prognosis

Eczema is a life-long problem characterized by periods of exacerbation and remission.

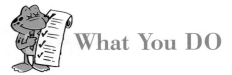

What You DO

Treatment

The treatment of the various types of eczema is aimed at removing the source of the irritant or allergen, which may mean that the patient modify behavior or even change employment to avoid the irritant or allergen. Modification mea-

Lesions of infantile atopic eczema usually begin in the cheeks and may progress to involve the scalp, arms, trunk, and legs. The skin of the cheeks may appear paler with extra creases under the eyes.

A marked follicle development exists in persons with dark skin. The lesions may be hypopigmented or hyperpigmented or both on a dark-skinned person.

The infantile form usually becomes milder as the child ages, frequently disappearing by the age of 15. Adolescents and adults have dry, leathery, hyperpigmented or hypopigmented lesions that are located in the antecubital and popliteal areas. The lesions may spread to the neck, hands, feet, eyelids, and behind the ears. Itching may be severe in both forms and secondary infections are common.

sures may include wearing protective clothing such as goggles or gloves. Another modification measure may be alerting persons who have irritant contact dermatitis and who work in heavy industrial areas to avoid strong hand cleansers. Grease and grime can be removed with inert oil, such as salad oil or mineral oil, before washing with soap and water.

Washing the affected areas to remove further contamination by the irritant or allergen can treat minor cases of eczematous dermatitis. Avoidance of temperature changes and stress helps to minimize abnormal and cutaneous vascular and sweat responses.

Apply antipruritic creams or lotions, and bandage exposed areas. Topical steroids may be helpful in some cases. Chronic dry lesions are usually treated with ointments and creams that contain lubricating, keratolytic, or antipruritic agents. Systemic interventions differ according to the type of irritant or allergen and the severity of the reaction. Extreme cases can be treated with oral antihistamines, systemic corticosteroids, and wet dressings.

Nursing Responsibilities

Care responsibilities for the person with eczematous dermatitis include primarily patient and family teaching about possible irritants, allergens, and avoidance behaviors.

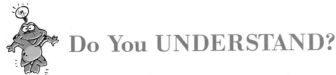

Do You UNDERSTAND?

DIRECTIONS: **Provide answers to the following questions.**

1. What is the synonymous term for eczema?

2. What is a severe form of eczema?

3. What is a treatment for eczema?

4. With chronic eczema, how does the skin appear?

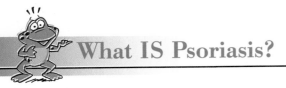

What IS Psoriasis?

Pathogenesis

Psoriasis is a common, but chronic, inflammatory skin disease. Although the cause of psoriasis is uncertain, the most accepted theory attributes the cause to a T-cell dermal immune response to an antigen. The activated T cells (primarily CD4-pos-

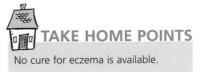

TAKE HOME POINTS

No cure for eczema is available.

See Chapters 6B, 7B, and 14B in RWNSG: *Pharmacology*

Answers: 1. dermatitis; 2. allergic contact dermatitis; 3. removal of the source of the irritant or allergen; 4. dry and leathery, with hyperpigmented or hypopigmented lesions.

In the United States, psoriasis affects approximately 1% of the population. The incidence is decreased in warmer, sunny climates.

All ages are affected, however, the onset of psoriasis usually occurs in the third decade of life. Childhood onset of psoriasis is associated with a familial history.

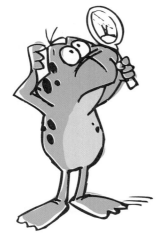

Psoriasis can persist throughout life and exacerbate at unpredictable times.

The pustular form of psoriasis may be fatal in individuals with suppressed immunity because of loss of fluid and electrolytes through the skin.

See Chapters 1A, 7B, 12, and 13B in **RWNSG:** *Pharmacology*

itive helper T cells) produce chemical messengers called cytokines, which stimulate keratinocyte proliferation from the basal layer of the epidermis. The migration time of the keratinocyte from the basal cell skin layer decreases from the normal 26 to 30 days to 4 to 7 days. Cell turnover and metabolism increase. Capillary blood flow increases to support the metabolic demands. Infiltration of neutrophils and monocytes causes the accompanying inflammatory changes. Skin trauma is a common precipitating factor in individuals predisposed to the disorder.

At-Risk Populations

An association appears to exist between psoriasis and arthritis. Psoriatic arthritis occurs in 5% to 7% of persons with psoriasis.

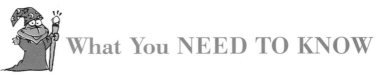

What You NEED TO KNOW

Clinical Manifestations

The areas of the body that are usually affected by this disorder include the scalp, hairline, elbows, knees, and sites of trauma. The severity of psoriasis may range from a life-threatening emergency to a minimal cosmetic problem. Psoriasis has a characteristic circular, patchy appearance of all sizes, covered with heavy, dry, silvery scales. The increased rate of cell proliferation, capillary dilation, and cell metabolism creates the red appearance of erythema. The extent of inflammation determines the size and distribution of the lesions.

Prognosis

Wide variations exist in the severity and extent of the condition, as well as with the development of arthritis. There is no known cure at this time.

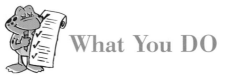

What You DO

Treatment

The goal of treatment is to suppress the clinical manifestations of the disorder. Treatment for psoriasis focuses on reducing epidermal cell proliferation and is used when less than 20% of the body surface is involved. Keratolytic medications, corticosteroids, and emollients are used in mild cases of psoriasis. Lesions of the genitalia, scalp, and nails are treated with shampoos and various lotions. Tar preparations and ultraviolet light or a combination of the two, as well as antimetabolites such as methotrexate and etretinate (vitamin A derivative), are used to treat moderate lesions. A combination of systemic corticosteroids, cyclosporin, topical agents, antimetabolites, and hospitalization may be used in severe cases.

Nursing Responsibilities

The nursing responsibilities for patients with psoriasis include the following:

- Instruct the patient to wear goggles to protect the eyes when ultraviolet light treatments are used.
- Teach the importance of hand washing before and after the application of medications.
- Teach the patient and family about the side effects of steroids and other medications used in treatment of psoriasis.

Do You UNDERSTAND?

DIRECTIONS: Indicate in the space provided whether the statement is *true* or *false*. If false, then use the margin space to the right to rewrite the statement to make it true.

_____ 1. Psoriasis can be life threatening.

_____ 2. A person diagnosed with psoriasis can develop arthritis.

SECTION E
MALIGNANCIES OF THE SKIN

What IS Basal Cell Carcinoma?

Pathogenesis

Basal cell carcinoma is a malignant lesion arising from epithelial cells. The most common sites of basal cell carcinoma are areas of the skin most exposed to the sun, such as the face and neck. Sun exposure and aging are the most common risk factors for basal cell carcinoma. Ultraviolet (UV) light exposure, particularly UVB rays, creates DNA mutations. The p53 gene normally halts uncontrolled cell growth. However, mutations in the p53 gene allow cancer cells to grow and to become more aggressive.

At-Risk Populations

The populations at risk for basal cell carcinoma are older adults and light-skinned individuals. Melanin in the skin has a protecting effect. Patients with preexisting skin conditions are also at risk for basal cell carcinoma.

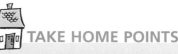

TAKE HOME POINTS

Support the body image of the patient with psoriasis. The disorder can be devastating to a patient's self-perception.

National Eczema Society
http://www.eczema.org/faqfile.htm

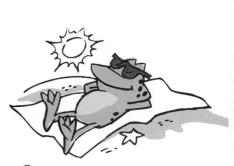

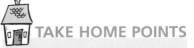

TAKE HOME POINTS

Basal cell carcinoma, squamous cell carcinoma, and malignant melanoma are the most common forms of skin cancer. Basal cell and squamous cell carcinoma are highly curable; malignant melanoma is the most deadly malignancy of the skin.

Answers: 1. true; 2. true.

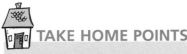 Light-skinned people produce less melanin and are therefore more susceptible to harmful rays of the sun.

TAKE HOME POINTS

The early warning signs of skin cancer include changes in the size or color of a mole and changes in the size or skin color of any spot or darkly pigmented growth. Early detection of unusual lesions is important.

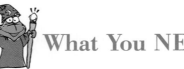# What You NEED TO KNOW

Clinical Manifestations

The clinical manifestations of basal cell carcinoma begin with a slightly elevated, pearl colored nodule. Skin cells are not shed in the normal keratinization process, thus the tumor arises. The growth rate is slow. As the lesion grows, it frequently ulcerates. Usually the center of the lesion is depressed and the borders are rolled.

Prognosis

The prognosis of basal cell carcinoma is good and with early diagnosis and treatment, a cure is expected. Metastatic spread is rare. Without treatment over months or years, basal cell carcinoma can destroy an ear lobe, eyelid, or other area by invading surrounding tissue.

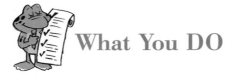# What You DO

Treatment

The treatment for basal cell carcinoma includes surgery, radiation therapy, cryosurgery, and electrodestruction.

Nursing Responsibilities

The nursing responsibilities for the patient with basal cell carcinoma are primarily preventative. The nurse should:

- Advise the patient to wear appropriate protective clothing and head covering when outdoors. Sunscreens with para-aminobenzoic acid (PABA) and a rating of at least 15 for UV protection should be used.
- Increase the patient's awareness of the potential harm to the skin from the increasing popularity of tanning booths.
- Teach the patient and family about the risk factors of skin cancer. The risk factors include a fair complexion, immunosuppression, and excessive UV exposure. The warning signs of skin cancer should also be included in the teaching.

TAKE HOME POINTS

The nurse should teach the patient to avoid excessive exposure to UV light and to avoid the sun, particularly between the hours of 10:00 AM and 3:00 PM when the ultraviolet light is strongest.

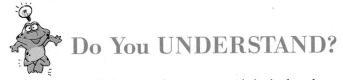

Do You UNDERSTAND?

DIRECTIONS: Indicate in the space provided whether the statement is *true* or *false*. If false, then use the margin space to the right to rewrite the statement to make it true.

_____ 1. No treatment is needed for basal cell carcinoma.

_____ 2. Change in size or color of any skin spot or dark pigmented growth are warning signs of skin malignancy.

_____ 3. As the basal cell lesion grows, it frequently ulcerates. The center of the lesion is usually depressed, and the borders are rolled.

_____ 4. Skin on the chest and legs are the most common sites for basal cell carcinoma.

What IS Squamous Cell Carcinoma?

Pathogenesis

Squamous cell carcinoma is a malignant tumor of the epidermis. These tumors grow more rapidly than basal cell tumors and can metastasize. Tumors can be limited to a localized area (in situ) or invasive and spread through to lymph. Squamous cell carcinoma tumors are firm. The surface is elevated with a granular quality that easily bleeds. Most squamous cell carcinomas arise from skin lesions, including chronic ulcerated areas, sun-damaged skin, or areas of horny growth, such as a wart, a callus, or scars.

The cause of squamous cell carcinoma is unknown, although sun exposure and aging are the most common risk factors. Mutation of p53 gene is considered part of the mechanism. Similar to basal cell carcinoma, UV exposure, particularly UVB rays, creates DNA mutations. The p53 gene normally halts uncontrolled cell growth. However, mutations in the p53 gene allow cancer cells to become more aggressive.

At-Risk Populations

Populations at risk for squamous cell carcinoma include older adults and light-skinned individuals.

Melanin in the skin has a protecting effect, thus light-skinned people are more susceptible to harmful rays of the sun. Immunosuppressed persons are also at increased risk.

Answers: 1. false; treatment is needed for basal cell carcinoma; 2. true; 3. true; 4. false; skin on the face and neck are the most common sites for basal cell carcinoma.

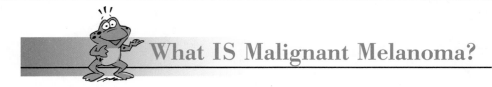

What IS Malignant Melanoma?

Pathogenesis

Malignant melanoma is a cancerous lesion arising from epidermal melanocyte cells. Melanocytes synthesize the pigment melanin. Malignant melanomas most commonly arise from an existing mole (nevus) but may also originate from normal skin surfaces. A nevus is a benign aggregation of melanocytes. When a nevus has a diameter of 6 mm or greater, it is considered highly suggestive for developing malignant melanoma.

Malignant melanoma is grouped into three varieties. Most malignant melanomas are the superficial spreading variety and occur in young and middle-age adults. The lentigo malignant melanoma occurs during adolescence, middle age, and in older adults. The pattern of tumor growth for both lentigo and superficial spreading is horizontally along the skin surface. Their potential for metastasis is less than that for the nodular variety of malignant melanoma. Nodular melanoma has a high potential of becoming metastatic because it grows vertically into deeper tissue. However, local invasion, regional lymph node metastasis, and distant metastasis are possible with all types of melanoma.

The cause of malignant melanoma is unknown. Sun exposure is the most common risk factor for malignant melanoma.

At-Risk Populations

 The populations that are most at risk for malignant melanoma are fair-skinned people and young to middle-age adults who live in the sunbelt states.

The populations most at risk for malignant melanoma are fair-skinned people and young to middle-age adults who live in the sunbelt states. Genetic predisposition, immunosuppression, exposure to radiation or sunlight also increases the risk.

What You NEED TO KNOW

Clinical Manifestations of Squamous Cell Carcinoma

Skin exposed to the sun such as on the face and neck is most commonly affected. Squamous cell carcinoma is observed less frequently on the hands or other parts of the body. The lesions are scaly or keratotic, slightly elevated with an irregular border, and usually have a shallow chronic ulcer. Later lesions grow outward, show large ulcerations, and have persistent crusts with raised, erythematous borders.

Prognosis for Squamous Cell Carcinoma

Squamous cell carcinoma remains confined at the epidermis for a long time. However, at some unpredictable time, the lesion may penetrate the basement membrane to the dermis and metastasize to regional lymph nodes. Invasive squamous cell carcinoma can be slow or fast growing with metastasis. Despite the unpredictable nature of the carcinoma, the prognosis of squamous cell carcinoma is good. A cure is expected with early diagnosis and treatment.

Clinical Manifestations of Malignant Melanoma

The manifestations of malignant melanoma vary. Most melanoma lesions are slightly raised and black or brown. The borders are irregular and the surfaces uneven. Periodically, melanomas ulcerate and bleed. Surrounding erythema, inflammation, and tenderness may occur. Dark melanomas are frequently mottled with red, blue, and white shades. The different colors represent three different concurrent processes: melanoma growth (blue), inflammation (red), and scar tissue formation (white).

Prognosis for Malignant Melanoma

The prognosis of malignant melanoma depends on several factors: the extent of metastasis, the initial lesion site and depth, lesion thickness, stage of the disease process, anatomic site, the patient's age, and the type of lesion. Initial lesions located on the extremities have the most favorable prognosis, and those located on the trunk, head, or neck have the poorest prognosis.

Lesions over 4 mm thick carry the poorest prognosis. Ten-year survival rates have increased steadily over the past 30 years but the mortality rate continues to increase. Five-year survival rates are best for nonmetastatic lesions that are diagnosed and treated early.

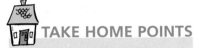
TAKE HOME POINTS

Nevi with a diameter of 6 mm or greater that bleed, itch, are deep brown, asymmetrical, or that have irregular borders are considered most susceptible to develop malignant melanoma.

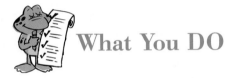
What You DO

Treatment for Squamous Cell Carcinoma

Treatment for squamous cell carcinoma is similar to that for basal cell carcinoma. These measures include surgery, radiation therapy, cryosurgery, and electrodestruction. Reconstructive surgery may be required for extensive tumors. For metastatic squamous cell carcinoma, a combination of radiation and antineoplastic therapy may be required.

See Chapter 1D in RWNSG: *Pharmacology*

Treatment for Premalignant Melanoma Lesions

Most nevi never become malignant; however, suspicious pigmented nevi should be removed. Indications for biopsy and removal of the lesion are changes in size or color of a mole, irregular notched margins, nodularity, and ulceration, scab formation, itching, oozing, or bleeding. Treatment includes surgical excision, cryosurgery, and electrodestruction.

Treatment for Malignant Melanoma Lesions

The treatment of first choice for known malignant melanoma is surgical excision. Dissection of regional lymph nodes may be required. Antineoplastic therapy is used for metastatic disease. Dacarbazine (DTIC) is the drug of choice. Immunotherapy, such as the drug interferon, is also used to treat metastatic dis-

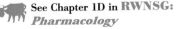
See Chapter 1D in RWNSG: *Pharmacology*

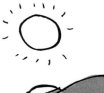

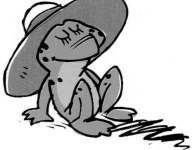

ease. Regional perfusion with antineoplastic drugs has been administered for melanomas located on the extremities.

Nursing Responsibilities

For patients with squamous cell carcinoma and malignant melanoma, the nurse should:

- Advise the patient to wear appropriate protective clothing and head covering when outdoors. Sunscreens with PABA and a rating of at least 15 for UV protection should be used.
- Increase the patient's awareness of the potential harm to the skin caused by the increasing popularity of tanning booths.
- Teach the patient and family about the risk factors of skin cancer. The risk factors include a fair complexion, immunosuppression, and excessive UV exposure. The warning signs of skin cancer should also be included in the teaching.
- Allow the patient to express fears related to the diagnosis of malignant melanoma. The disfiguring surgical procedures that are necessary with large tumors and reconstruction efforts can cause problems with self-esteem and body image. Be certain to include counseling or refer the patient to support groups to allow the patient to heal emotionally, as well as physically.

Do You UNDERSTAND?

DIRECTIONS: **Indicate in the space provided whether the statement is _true_ or _false_. If false, then use the margin space to the left to rewrite the statement to make it true.**

_____ 1. Treatment for squamous cell carcinoma includes surgery, radiation therapy, cryosurgery, and electrodestruction.

_____ 2. Teaching prevention includes using appropriate protective clothing and head coverings when outdoors.

_____ 3. Warning signs of squamous cell carcinoma include changes in the size or color of a mole.

_____ 4. As the squamous cell carcinoma grows, it frequently ulcerates.

DIRECTIONS: **Fill in the blanks with the words listed below.**

5. _____ is the preferred initial treatment for malignant melanoma.

6. An initial lesion located on the trunk, head, or neck has the poorest
_____.

7. Metastatic spread is common with _____ melanoma.

8. Change in size or color of any skin spot or dark pigmented growth are
_____ signs of malignancy.

excision	malignant	expulsion	nonmalignant
prognosis	extremities	herbal therapy	warning

14 Pain Syndromes

Pain is the most common symptom that prompts a person to seek professional help. Pain is also a complex phenomenon that is both personal and private. Failure to recognize and manage pain not only causes unnecessary suffering, but also can delay recovery and prolong hospitalization. When health care providers perform their duties using traditional methods, that is, simply calling for injections of pain killing medications such as morphine and codeine "as needed," the results are frequently undermedication and unnecessary pain.

The International Association for the Study of Pain (IASP) proposes that pain is an unpleasant sensory and emotional experience that is associated with actual or potential tissue damage, or it is described in terms of such damage. However, not all potentially tissue-damaging stimuli result in pain. For this reason, distinguishing pain from the ability to perceive pain and perception of pain as a result of suffering is important.

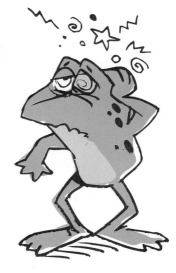

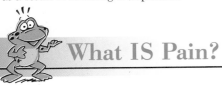

What IS Pain?

Pathogenesis

Nociceptors are free nerve endings that are present in almost all types of tissue; they act to sense and transmit pain signals (nociception). Suffering, conversely, is an emotion, a state of distress associated with events that threaten the intactness of the patient. Suffering evolves from the meaning attached to an event. Pain and suffering are not the same experiences. Suffering can occur in the presence or absence of pain and pain can occur in the presence or absence of suffering.

The mechanism by which pain is received is composed of four steps: transduction, transmission, perception, and modulation. *Transduction* involves nerve fibers that react to thermal, chemical, and mechanical stimuli. After the nerve fibers are activated, the information is transmitted to the central nervous system. The dorsal root of the spinal cord receives, transmits, and processes sensory

Undertreatment of pain occurs particularly in infants, children, and older adults who cannot always express their needs.

413

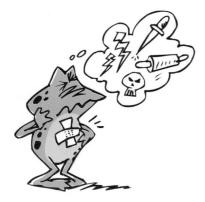

impulses (*transmission*). Afferent nerve fibers within the dorsal root then transmit the impulses through the brainstem and thalamus to the cortex of the brain, where the experience of pain is perceived. Pain *perception* does not depend exclusively on the degree of physical damage. Similarly, a lack of a behavioral response to the painful stimuli does not indicate that the patient lacks pain perception. *Modulation* is the process of altering the stimuli by either inhibiting or facilitating nociceptive signals. Modulation of the pain signals occurs at the peripheral, spinal cord, and brain levels. Descending fibers in the dorsal horn of the spinal cord release neurotransmitters that prevent afferent nociceptors from communicating with other ascending nociceptors. As a result, pain is blocked.

The causes of pain can be organized into two different types: nociceptive and neuropathic. Damage to somatic (i.e., the body as distinguished from the mind) or visceral tissue causes nociceptive pain. Acute nociceptive pain has an immediate onset with a limited and predictable duration. Anxiety or fear frequently intensifies acute nociceptive pain but persists until healing occurs. Examples of acute nociceptive pain include sprains and fractures, burns, tension headaches, and unstable angina. Without intervention, acute nociceptive pain can progress to acute neuropathic pain or a chronic nociceptive pain.

Additionally, patients may experience pain resulting from chronic or malignant circumstances. Chronic nociceptive pain is associated with prolonged pathologic factors that involves tissue or pain that persists beyond the normal healing period for acute injury or disease. The pain may be continuous or recurrent. Examples of chronic nociceptive pain include stable angina, gastritis, gout, tendonitis, and diverticulitis. In contrast, chronic neuropathic pain is associated with disorders in the peripheral or central nervous systems that result in pain long after the original injury has healed. Examples of chronic neuropathic pain include low back pain, diabetic neuropathy, and fibromyalgia.

Malignant pain is progressive and can be acute or chronic or both. The causes of this type of pain are frequently resistant to cure. Examples of malignant pain include cancer or tumors of the brachial or sacral nerve plexus.

At-Risk Populations

Pain is a common complaint. All people are at risk for pain at sometime in their lives.

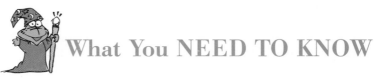

What You NEED TO KNOW

Clinical Manifestations

Pain consists of five components: affective, behavioral, cognitive, sensory, and physiologic. Emotions that are related to pain, the patient's behavioral responses to the pain, and the beliefs, attitudes, evaluations, and goals about pain influence the way in which the pain is modulated and perceived. The clinical manifestations vary with the type of pain but include behavioral, psychosocial, and nervous system responses. Pain threshold is the lowest intensity of painful stimuli that the patient perceives as pain. A patient's pain threshold varies depending on physiologic factors but is essentially the same for all people who have intact central and peripheral nervous systems.

Physiologic factors that influence pain perception include the patient's general state of health, the underlying cause of the pain, pain threshold and tolerance, intensity, frequency, quality, location, duration, radiation, aggravating and alleviating factors, the patient's prior experience with pain, level of anxiety, stressors at time of event, and the speed of onset.

Pain tolerance, conversely, is different for each patient and depends on subjective factors. Some patients tolerate a high level of pain without acute distress, while others have distress at a low level. Psychosocial factors that influence pain perception include family and occupational roles, spiritual belief systems, cultural or societal influences, sexual identity and stereotypes, communication skills, stage of growth and development, personality and motivation, the presence of fear, and the effect of the pain on the patient's activities of daily living. Patients who are told about the anticipated discomforts may actually experience decreased pain, less use of analgesics, and shorter hospitalizations.

Patients with acute pain can, in most cases, locate their pain to a single area; they describe their pain using descriptors such as throbbing, stabbing, intense, unbearable, gnawing, heavy, sharp, aching, nagging, exhausting, tiring, or shooting. Acute, unrelieved pain is manifested through sympathetic nervous system stimulation with increased cardiac output, peripheral resistance, pulse, and blood pressure. The increased cardiac workload and myocardial oxygen use and decreased oxygen delivery to the heart lead to increased risk of hypoxemia, ischemia, and myocardial infarction. Reflex muscle spasms and splinting leads to reduced respiratory capabilities and alveolar ventilation. Atelectasis and impaired oxygen and carbon dioxide exchange contributes to the hypoxia and increases the patient's risk for pneumonia. Muscle tightness and spasm lead to increased sympathetic activity, which, in turn, increases the sensitivity of nociceptors. The increased sympathetic tone leads to increased intestinal secretions and sphincter tone and decreased intestinal motility. Gastric stasis and paralytic ileus may result.

Chronic nociceptive pain is frequently described in affective terms (e.g., sickening, hateful). The clinical manifestations of chronic pain can be the same as that for acute pain, or no symptoms may be evident. Unlike acute pain, the patient may be unable to locate the pain to a single area. The patient with unrelieved malignant pain frequently describes the pain as all consuming and interfering with mood, family relationships, and quality of life.

Prognosis

The prognoses associated with pain usually depend on the cause of the pain and whether the pain is defined as acute, chronic, or malignant. Acute pain typically lasts less than 6 months. Chronic pain lasts 6 months or longer or 1 month after the normal end of the condition causing the pain. Malignant pain frequently has no foreseeable end in sight. However, all types of pain can be relieved with appropriate management.

Pain threshold does not vary by ethnic group. Persons from different racial or cultural backgrounds are consistent about the level of stimulus that is perceived as painful.

TAKE HOME POINTS

Vital signs that are used in isolation are unreliable indicators of the extent of a patient's pain. Pain reporting is the single best measure of pain for the person who is able to communicate.

Agency for HealthCare Research and Quality (formerly the Agency for Health Care Policy and Research): Clinical Practice Guidelines
http:www.ahrq.gov

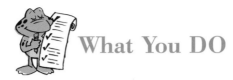

What You DO

Treatment

The principles of pain management center on establishing a therapeutic relationship, alleviating anxiety, providing distraction or diversion when appropriate, combatting anticipatory fears, and providing physical care. Treatment for the patient with pain includes nondrug and drug therapies. Nondrug therapies are always used as an adjunct to drug therapies, although cases may exist in which only nondrug therapies are required for pain relief.

Aggressive prevention of pain is better than treatment because pain is more difficult to suppress after it is established. The analgesic ladder proposed by the World Health Organization uses a stepwise approach in organizing drug therapy. For acute moderate to severe nociceptive pain, drug use starts with opioids (e.g., morphine, hydromorphone, methadone) stepping down to milder opioids (e.g., codeine, oxycodone) as the patient's pain becomes moderate to mild. As the pain level continues to improve, the patient may be given nonopioids (e.g., nonsteroidal antiinflammatory drugs, acetaminophen). For chronic or malignant pain, drug use starts with the nonopioids for mild pain, followed by mild opioids for mild-to-moderate pain, stepping up to the stronger opioids for moderate-to-severe pain.

Adjunctive drug therapies include the use of nonanalgesic pain relievers, such as antidepressants, anticonvulsants, antihistamines, phenothiazines, muscle relaxants, steroids, and anesthetics. Pain medications may be administered by mouth, through a patient-controlled analgesia (PCA) system, transmucosal (sublingual, transnasal, rectal), transdermal, or subcutaneous routes. Spinal analgesia, epidural analgesia, or nerve blocks may also be employed.

Noninvasive adjunctive therapies include positioning and range-of-motion and exercise programs to minimize joint and muscle stiffness. Cognitive-behavior therapies that may be used for the patient in pain include anticipatory guidance, distraction, imagery and hypnosis, conditioning, and relaxation strategies. Dermal stimulation, pressure, acupressure, massage, cutaneous vibration, transcutaneous electrical nerve stimulation (TENS), and heat and cold therapy may be used as adjunctive therapies. Invasive therapies include acupuncture, percutaneous electrical nerve stimulation (PENS), dorsal cord or deep brain stimulation, nerve blocks, and neurosurgical interventions. Each of the drug and nondrug therapies have benefits and risks, thus the patient's condition and willingness to accept therapy must be considered.

Nursing Responsibilities

Nursing responsibilities for the patient with pain include, first and foremost, adequate pain assessment. Ask the patient about the pain. Do not assume that the pain is being treated adequately because the patient has no complaint or appears to be sleeping. Only the patient can tell the health care provider about the pain experience. Pain is now considered as the fifth vital sign.

See Chapters 2D, 11, and 14 in RWNSG: *Pharmacology*

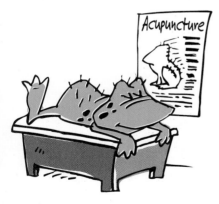

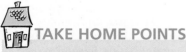
TAKE HOME POINTS

Pain is considered as the fifth vital sign and should be assessed in each patient.

The health care provider must remember that pain tolerance can vary from situation to situation. An accurate history is essential in assessing a patient's pain experience. The history should include each of the components identified in the following table.

ASSESSING PAIN: THE FIFTH VITAL SIGN

- Intensity (e.g., "On a scale of 1-10, how would you rate your pain?")
- Location (e.g., "Where is the pain?")
- Onset and pattern (e.g., "When did it start?" "Was it sudden or develop over time?" "Is it continuous or intermittent?")
- Extension or radiation (e.g., "Does the pain move to other areas?")
- Duration (e.g., "How long does the pain last?")
- Character or quality (e.g., sharp, dull, shooting, ache)
- Precipitating, aggravating, and alleviating factors (e.g., "What starts the pain?" "What makes it worse?" "What makes it better?")
- Associated manifestations (e.g., anorexia, nausea, restlessness, insomnia)
- Effects on activities of daily living (e.g., sleep, appetite, concentration, work, school, interpersonal relationships, marital relations, sex, home activities, driving, walking, leisure activities, emotional state)

The patient and health care provider can quantify the pain experience using pain assessment tools. Many specific assessment tools are available to assess pain in adults and children.

Be aware of the physiologic changes of aging when using pain medications in very young and in elderly patients. The physiologic changes alter drug absorption, distribution, metabolism, and elimination. Careful observation of the older patient is vital to effective and safe pain management.

Nursing responsibilities for the patient with pain include establishing and maintaining an effective relationship with the patient and the family or significant other. To do so, the nurse should:

- Act as planner, educator, patient advocate, interpreter, and supporter of the patient and the family or significant other.
- Listen and believe that which the patient has to say about the pain and be present to reassure or distract the patient as needed.
- Discuss the intentions of the health care provider and that which the patient and family or significant other is expected to do in relation to pain management.
- Accept the right of the patient to respond to the pain in the necessary manner; help may be needed to accept the response to pain.
- Explore the meaning of the pain to the patient and family or significant other.
- Teach the patient and family or significant other about pain management strategies, rather than simply treating the pain.

Tools that are appropriate for assessment of pain in children may also be useful with the older adult or patient who is cognitively impaired who has difficulty relating to a pain scale.

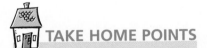

TAKE HOME POINTS

Remember that pain is a subjective and highly variable experience. Each patient defines pain differently based on values, culture, and physiologic experience. A patient's expression of pain is to be accepted as defined by the patient, not the health care provider.

- Use appropriate drug and nondrug therapies for pain management while continually evaluating patient response and making adjustments to the care plan as warranted.

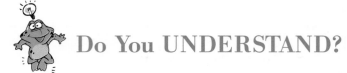

Do You UNDERSTAND?

DIRECTIONS: **Identify whether the pain is typically acute (A), chronic (C), or malignant (M) in nature.**

_____ 1. Sensations felt the first few weeks after a mastectomy
_____ 2. Migraine headache
_____ 3. Persistent low back pain
_____ 4. Chest pain from myocardial infarction
_____ 5. Osteoarthritis of the knee
_____ 6. Diabetic peripheral neuropathy
_____ 7. Postoperative incisional pain
_____ 8. Tumor of the sacral nerve plexus

References

Chapter 1

AIDS Knowledge Base. *Classification, staging and surveillance of HIV disease,* 1999, URL http://hivinsite.ucsf.edu/akb/current/01class index.html.

AIDS Knowledge Base. *Epidemiology of HIV/AIDS in the United States,* 1999, URL http://hivinsite.ucsf.edu/akb/current/01epius/index.html.

Bullock BA, Henze RL: *Focus on pathophysiology,* Philadelphia, 2000, Lippincott–Williams & Wilkins.

Burns MV: *Pathophysiology: a self-instructional program,* Stamford, CT, 1998, Appleton & Lange.

Copstead LC, Banasid JL: *Pathophysiology: biological and behavioral perspective,* ed 4, Philadelphia, 2000, WB Saunders.

Corey L, Handsfield HH: Genital herpes and public health: addressing a global problem, *JAMA* 283:791, 2000.

Cotran RS, Kumar V, Collins T: *Pathologic basis of disease,* ed 6, Philadelphia, 1999, WB Saunders.

Crowley L: *An introduction to human disease: pathology and pathophysiology correlations,* ed 5, Sudbury, MA, 2001, Jones and Bartlett.

Cunha M, Bullock BL: Altered immunity. In Bullock BA, Henze RL, editors: *Focus on pathophysiology,* Philadelphia, 2000, Lippincott.

Ellis P, Johnson DP: Dermatologic complications in HIV, *Nurse Pract Forum* 10(2):87, 1999.

Fox RL: Sjögren syndrome: new approaches to treatment, Medscape, 2000, URL http://www.medscape.com/Medscape/heumatology/TreatmentUpdate/2000/tu01/pnt-tu01.html.

Gamponia MJ, Graber MA: AIDS (acquired immunodeficiency syndrome). In *University of Iowa family practice handbook,* ed 3, 2000, URL http://www.vh.org/Providers/ClinRef/FPHandbook/Chapter16/01-16.html.

Guyton AC, Hall JE: *Human physiology and mechanisms of disease,* ed 6, Philadelphia, 1997, WB Saunders.

Guyton AC, Hall JE: *Textbook of medical physiology,* ed 9, Philadelphia, 1996, WB Saunders.

Halperin DT: Heterosexual anal intercourse: prevalence, cultural factors, and HIV infection and other health risks, Part I, *AIDS Patient Care STDS* 13(12):717, 1999.

Hansen M: *Pathophysiology: foundations of disease and clinical interventions,* Philadelphia, 1998, WB Saunders.

Porth CM: *Pathophysiology: concepts of altered health states,* ed 5, Philadelphia, 1998, Lippincott-Raven Publishers.

Rhodus NL: Sjögren's syndrome, *Quintessence Int* 30(10):689, 1999.

Rote NS, Huether SE, McCance KL: Hypersensitivities, infections, and immunodeficiences. In Huether SE, McCance KL: *Understanding pathophysiology,* ed 2, St Louis, 2000, Mosby.

US Public Health Service and Infectious Diseases Society of America: Guidelines for the prevention of opportunistic infections in persons infected with human immunodeficiency virus: a summary, *MMWR* 44(RR-8), 1999, URL http://www.ams-assn.org/special/hiv/ treatmnt/ guide/rr4810/rr4810/ref.htm.

Chapter 2

Banasik JL: Acute disorders of brain function. In Copstead LE, Banasik JL, editors: *Pathophysiology: biological and behavioral perspectives,* ed 2, Philadelphia, 2000, WB Saunders.

Cacchione PZ: Cognitive and neurologic function. In Lueckenotte AG, editor: *Gerontologic nursing,* ed 2, St Louis, 2000, Mosby.

Curtis SM, Porth CM: Disorders of brain function. In Porth CM: *Pathophysiology: concepts of altered health states,* Philadelphia, 1998, Lippincott.

Fahn S: Huntington disease. In Rowland LP, editor: *Merritt's neurology,* ed 10, Philadelphia, 2000, Lippincott–Williams & Wilkins.

Friedland R, Wilcock GK: Dementia. In Evans GJ et al: *Oxford textbook of geriatric medicine,* ed 2, Oxford, 2000, Oxford University Press.

Fulmer T et al: Providing care for elderly people who exhibit disturbing behavior. In Evans GJ et al, editors: *Oxford textbook of geriatric medicine,* ed 2, Oxford, 2000, Oxford University Press.

Ghajar J: Traumatic brain injury, *Lancet* 356(9233):923, 2000.

Hansen M: *Pathophysiology: foundations of disease and clinical interventions,* Philadelphia, 1998, WB Saunders.

Henze RL: Traumatic and vascular injuries of the central nervous system. In Bullock BA, Henze RL, editors: *Focus on pathophysiology,* Philadelphia, 2000, Lippincott–Williams & Wilkins.

Lundgren CL: Chronic sorrow in long-term illness across the life span. In Miller JF, editor: *Coping with chronic illness,* ed 3, Philadelphia, 2000, FA Davis.

Marks WJ: Management of seizures and epilepsy, American Family Physician, 1998, http:www.findarticles.com/df_0m3225/n7_v57/20545743/print.jhtml.

Morris GF, Marshall LF: Injury of the head and spinal cord. In Goldman L, Bennett JC, editors: *Cecil textbook of medicine,* Philadelphia, 2000, WB Saunders.

Pedley TA: The epilepsies. In Goldman L, Bennett JC, editors: *Cecil textbook of medicine,* Philadelphia, 2000, WB Saunders.

Small SA, Mayeux R: Alzheimer's disease and related dementias. In Rowland LP, editor: *Merritt's neurology,* ed 10, Philadelphia, 2000, Lippincott–Williams & Wilkins.

Tapper VJ: Parkinson's disease. In Buttaro TM et al: *Primary care: a collaborative process,* St Louis, 1999, Mosby.

Chapter 3

Aster RH, George JN: *Thrombocytopenia due to enhanced platelet destruction by immunologic mechanisms: hematology,* ed 4, New York, 1990, McGraw-Hill.

Barker LR, Burton JR, Zieve PD: *Principles of ambulatory medicine,* ed 5, Baltimore, 1999, Williams & Wilkins.

Carey CF, Lee HH, Woeltje KF: *The Washington manual of clinical therapeutics,* Philadelphia, 1998, Lippincott.

Carvalho AC: *Hemostasis and thrombosis: hematology*, New York, 1990, McGraw-Hill.

Casciato DA, Lowitz BB: *Manual of clinical oncology*, Boston, 1995, Little, Brown, and Company.

Dressler D: *Hemorrhagic disorders: diseases*, Springhouse PA, 1984, Springhouse.

Ewald GA: *Disorders of hemostasis. Manual of medical therapeutics*, ed 28, Boston, 1995, Little, Brown, and Company.

Gorroll AH, May LA, Mulley AG: *Primary care medicine*, Philadelphia, 1995, Lippincott.

Hillman RS, Ault KL: *Hematology in clinical practice*, New York, 1998, McGraw-Hill.

Kwaan HC, Soff GA: Management of thrombotic thrombocytopenic purpura and hemolytic uremic syndrome, *Semin Hematol* 34(2):159, 1997.

Moake JL: Thrombotic thrombocytopenia purpura today, *Hosp Pract* 34(7):53, 1999.

Muszkat M et al: Ticlopidine-inducted thrombotic thrombocytopenia purpura, *Pharmacotherapy* 18(6):1352, 1998.

Petersen KL: Diagnosing polycythemia vera, *J Am Acad Nurs Pract* 11(11):485, 1999.

Phipps WJ, Sands JK, Marek JF: *Medical-surgical nursing concepts & clinical practice*, St Louis, 1999, Mosby.

Ridolfi RL, Bell WR: Thrombotic thrombocytopenia purpura: report of 25 cases and review of literature, *Medicine* 60:413, 1981.

Rock GA: Comparison of plasma exchange and plasma infusion in the treatment of thrombotic: thrombocytopenia purpura, *N Engl J Med* 325:393, 1991.

Tezcan H et al: Bone marrow, *Transplant* 21(1):105, 1998.

Williams WJ et al: *Hematology*, New York, 1990, McGraw-Hill.

Chapter 4

Adult Treatment Panel II: Summary of the second report of the National Cholesterol Education Program expert panel on detection, evaluation, and treatment of high blood cholesterol in adults, *JAMA* 269:3015, 1993.

American College of Physicians: Guidelines for using serum cholesterol, high-density lipoprotein cholesterol, and triglycerides as screening tests for the prevention of coronary heart disease in adults, *Ann Intern Med* 124:515, 1996.

Black HR, Barkris GL, Elliott WJ: Hypertension: epidemiology, pathophysiology, diagnosis, and treatment. In Fuster V, Alexander RW, O'Rourke RA, editors: *Hurst's: the heart*, ed 10, New York, 2001, McGraw-Hill.

Dormandy JA : Circulation-enhancing drugs. In Rutherford RB, editor: *Vascular surgery*, ed 5, Philadelphia, 2000, WB Saunders.

Eaton L: Cardiovascular function. In Lueckenotte AG, editor: *Gerontologic nursing*, ed 2, St Louis, 2000, Mosby.

Fahey VA, McCarthy WJ: Arterial reconstruction of the lower extremity. In Fahey VA, editor: *Vascular nursing*, ed 3, Philadelphia, 1999, WB Saunders.

Graham LM, Ford MB: Arterial disease. In Fahey VA, editor: *Vascular nursing*, ed 3, Philadelphia, 1999, WB Saunders.

Hahn TL, Dalsing MC: Chronic venous disease. In Fahey VA, editor: *Vascular nursing*, ed 3, Philadelphia, 1999, WB Saunders.

Hiatt WR, Cooke JP: Atherogenesis and the medical management of atherosclerosis. In Rutherford RB, editor: *Vascular surgery*, ed 5, Philadelphia, 2000, WB Saunders.

Johnston KW: Upper extremity ischemia. In Rutherford RB, editor: *Vascular surgery*, ed 5, Philadelphia, 2000, WB Saunders.

Joint National Committee: The Sixth Report of the Joint National Committee on prevention, detection, evaluation, and treatment of high blood pressure, *Arch Intern Med* 157:2413, 1997.

Kaplan NM: *Primary hypertension*, Baltimore, 1998, Williams & Wilkins.

McCowen KC, Blackburn GL: Obesity, weight control, and cardiovascular disease. In Wong ND, Black HR, Gardin JM, editors: *Preventive cardiology*, New York, 2000, McGraw-Hill.

Monetta GL, Nehler MR, Porter JM: Pathophysiology of chronic venous insufficiency. In Rutherford RB, editor: *Vascular surgery*, ed 5, Philadelphia, 2000, WB Saunders.

Norris KC, Francis CK: African Americans. In Wong ND, Black HR, Gardin JM, editors: *Preventive cardiology*, New York, 2000, McGraw-Hill.

Ryan P: Facilitating behavior change in chronically ill persons. In Miller JF, editor: *Coping with chronic illness*, ed 3, Philadelphia, 2000, FA Davis.

Schroeder PS, Miller JF: Profiles of locus of control and coping in persons with peripheral vascular disease. In Miller JF, editor: *Coping with chronic illness*, ed 3, Philadelphia, 2000, FA Davis.

Smeltzer SC, Bare BG: Management of patients with coronary vascular disorders. In Brunner, Suddarth, editors: *Textbook of medical-surgical nursing*, ed 9, Philadelphia, 2000, Lippincott.

Sumner DS: Evaluation of acute and chronic ischemia of the upper extremity. In Rutherford RB, editor: *Vascular surgery*, ed 5, Philadelphia, 2000, WB Saunders.

Tripp TR: Laboratory and diagnostic tests. In Lueckenotte AG, editor: *Gerontologic nursing*, ed 2, St Louis, 2000, Mosby.

Walsh ME, Rice KL: Venous thrombosis and pulmonary embolism. In Fahey VA, editor: *Vascular nursing*, ed 3, Philadelphia, 1999, WB Saunders.

Wong, ND, Kashyap ML: Cholesterol and lipids. In Wong ND, Black HR, Gardin JM, editors: *Preventive cardiology*, New York, 2000, McGraw-Hill.

Wright JT, Hammonds VC: Hypertension: epidemiology and contemporary management strategies. In Wong ND, Black HR, Gardin JM, editors: *Preventive cardiology*, New York, 2000, McGraw-Hill.

Zierler RE, Sumner DS: Physiologic assessment of peripheral arterial occlusive disease. In Rutherford RB, editor: *Vascular surgery*, ed 5, Philadelphia, 2000, WB Saunders.

Chapter 5

Lewis SM, Heitkemper MM, Dirksen SR: *Medical-surgical nursing: assessment and management of clinical problems*, ed 5, St Louis, 2000, Mosby.

Manning WJ: Pericardial disease. In Goldman L, Bennett JC, editors: *Textbook of medicine*, ed 21, Philadelphia, 2000, WB Saunders.

Thelan LA et al: *Textbook of critical care nursing: diagnosis and management*, ed 2, St Louis, 1998, Mosby.

Wong DL et al: *Whaley & Wong's nursing care of infants and children*, ed 6, St Louis, 1998, Mosby.

Chapter 6

Bolgar PP: Pleural effusions. In Buttaro TM et al, editors: *Primary care: a collaborative approach*, St Louis, 1999, Mosby.

Bressler TR: Small cell lung cancer. In Miaskowski C, Buchsel, P, editors: *Oncology nursing: assessment and clinical care*, St Louis, 1999, Mosby.

Burns MV: *Pathophysiology: a self-instructional program*, Stanford, CT, 1998, Appleton & Lange.

Celli BR: Diseases of the diaphragm, chest wall, pleura, and mediastinum. In Goldman L, Bennett JC, editors: *Cecil textbook of medicine*, ed 21, Philadelphia, 2000, WB Saunders.

Colice GL, Rubins JB: Practical management of pleural effusions: when and how should fluid accumulations be drained? *Postgrad Med* 105(7):67, 1999, URL http://www.postgradmed.com/issues/1999/06_99/colice.htm.

Day MW: Caring for patients with pleural effusions, *Nursing* 28(10):56, 1998, URL http://www.findarticles.com/cf_0/m3231/n10_v28/21224629/print.jhtml.

Egan JJ: New treatments for pulmonary fibrosis? Lancet 354:1839, 1999, URL http://www.findarticles.com/cf_0/m0833/9193_354/58061352/print.jhtml.

Gapper KF: Nursing care of patients with lower respiratory disorders. In Monahan FD, Neighbors F, editors: *Medical-surgical nursing: foundations for clinical practice*, Philadelphia, 1998, WB Saunders.

Jenkins TW: Sarcoidosis. In Buttaro TM et al, editors: *Primary care: a collaborative approach*, St Louis, 1999, Mosby.

Judson MA: An approach to the treatment of pulmonary sarcoidosis with corticosteroids, *Chest* 115(4):1158, 1999, URL http://www.findarticles.com/cf_0/m0984/4_115/54514699/print.jhtml.

Lewis SM: Nursing management of lower respiratory disorders. In Lewis SM, Heitkemper MM, Dirksen SR, editors: *Medical-surgical nursing: assessment of clinical problems*, St Louis, 2000, Mosby.

Lind J: Nursing care of the client with lung cancer. In Itano J, Taoka KN, editors: *Core curriculum for oncology nursing*, Philadelphia, 1998, WB Saunders.

Lindsey LP, Thielvodt D: Non-small cell lung cancer. In Miaskowski C, Buchsel P, editors: *Oncology nursing: assessment and clinical care*, St Louis, 1999, Mosby.

Macklin LA, Bullock BL: Altered pulmonary function. In Bullock BA, Henze RL, editors: *Focus on pathophysiology*, Philadelphia, 1999, Lippincott–Williams and Wilkins.

Magaldi MC: Nursing care of patients with lower respiratory disorders. In Monahan FD, Neighbors M, editors: *Medical-surgical nursing: foundations for clinical practice*, Philadelphia, 1998, Lippincott.

Michaelson JE: Idiopathic pulmonary fibrosis, Chest, 2000, URL http://www.findarticles.com/cf_0/m0984/3_118/66188599/print.jhtml.

Toews GB: Interstitial lung disease. In Buttaro TM et al, editors: *Primary care: a collaborative approach*, St Louis, 1999, Mosby.

Turino GM: Respiratory diseases. In Goldman L, Bennett JC, editors: *Cecil textbook of medicine*, Philadelphia, 2000, WB Saunders.

Chapter 7

American Diabetes Association: Report of the expert committee on the diagnosis and classification of diabetes mellitus, *Clinical Practice Recommendations 2000* 23(Suppl 1), 2000, [On-Line], URL http://journal.diabetes.org/FullText/Supplements/DiabetesCare/Supplement100/.

Black J, Matassarin-Jacobs E: *Medical-surgical nursing: clinical management for continuity of care*, ed 5, Philadelphia, 1996, WB Saunders.

Copstead L, Banasik J: *Pathophysiology: biological and behavioral perspectives*, ed 2, Philadelphia, 2000, WB Saunders.

Huether S, McCance, K: *Understanding pathophysiology*, ed 2, St Louis, 2000, Mosby.

Lewis S, Heitkemper M, Dirksen S: *Medical-surgical nursing: assessment and management of clinical problems*, ed 5, St Louis, 2000, Mosby.

McCance K, Huether S: *The biologic basis for disease in adults and children*, St Louis, 1998, Mosby.

National Diabetes Information Clearinghouse: *Diabetes statistics*, Publication No. 99-3892, March 1999, NIH, URL http://star.aerie.com/health/diabetes/pubs/dmstats/dmstats.htm.

National Institute of Diabetes and Diseases of the Kidney: *Addison's disease*, 1998, URL http://www.niddk.nih.gov/health/endo/puds/addison/addison.htm.

National Institutes of Health: *Diabetes insipidus*, 1998, http://www.cc.nih.gov/ccc/patient_education/pepubs/di/pdf.

National Institutes of Health: *Secretion of inappropriate antidiuretic hormone*, 1998, http://www.cc.nih.gov/ccc/patient_education/pepubs/siadh/pdf.

Chapter 8

Black J, Matassarin-Jacobs E: *Medical-surgical nursing: clinical management for continuity of care*, ed 5, Philadelphia, 1997, WB Saunders.

Huerther SE, McCance KL: *Understanding pathophysiology*, St Louis, 1999, Mosby.

Chapter 9

Black J, Matassarin-Jacobs E: *Medical-surgical nursing: clinical management for continuity of care*, Philadelphia, 1998, WB Saunders.

Fujita K, Mizuno T et al: Complicating risk factors for pyelonephritis after extracorporeal shock wave lithotripsy, *Int J Urol* 7(6):224, 2000.

Gutierrez K: *Pharmacotherapeutics: clinical decision-making in nursing*, Philadelphia, 1999, WB Saunders.

Hansen M: *Pathophysiology: foundations of disease & clinical interventions*, Philadelphia, 1998, WB Saunders.

IgAN Foundation: *IgA nephropathy*, 2000, URL www.igan.org.

Lim CSet al: Bilateral emphysematous pyelonephritis with perirenal abscess cured by conservative therapy, *J Nephrol* 13(2):155, 2000.

McCance K, Huether S: Pathophysiology: *The biologic basis for disease in adults and children*, St Louis, 1999, Mosby.

Medline: *Goodpasture's syndrome*, 2000, URL http://medlineplus.nlm.nih.gov/medlineplus/kidneydiseasesgeneral.html.

National Institute of Diabetes and Diseases of the Kidneys: *Polycystic kidney disease*, 2000, URL http://www.niddk.nih.gov/health/kidney/pubs/polycyst/polycyst/htm.

National Institute of Diabetes and Kidney Disease: *Kidney disease*, 2000, URL http://www.niddk.nih.gov.

National Library of Medicine: *Bladder diseases*, 1999, URL http://www.nlm.nih.gov/medlineplus/bladderdiseases.html.

Porth C: Pathophysiology: *Concepts of altered health states*, ed 5, Philadelphia, 1998, Lippincott.

Wilson BA, Shannon MT, Stang CL: *Nurses drug guide*, New York, 2000, Appleton & Lange.

Chapter 10

American Cancer Society: *Cancer facts and figures: 1997*, Atlanta, 1997, The Society.

Applegate E: *The anatomy and physiology learning system*, Philadelphia, 2000, WB Saunders.

Baker DA: Diagnosis and treatment of viral STDs in women, *Int J Fert* 42(2):107, 1997.

Beckerman CR et al: *Obstetrics and gynecology*, Baltimore, 1998, Williams & Wilkins.

Black JM, Matassarin-Jacobs E: *Medical-surgical nursing: clinical management for continuity of care*, Philadelphia, 1998, WB Saunders.

Brenner P: Differential diagnosis of abnormal uterine bleeding, *Am J Obstet Gynecol* 175(3):766, 1996.

Centers for Disease Control and Prevention: 1998 guidelines for treatment of sexually transmitted disease, *MMWR Morb Mortal Wkly Rep* 47(RR-1), 1998.

Dull P, Miller KE: STDs in women: an update, *Fam Practice Recertification* 19(6):13, 1997.

Edmunds M, Mayhew M: *Pharmacology for the primary care provider*, St Louis, 2000, Mosby.

Junnila J, Lassen P: Testicular masses, *Am Fam Physician* 57:685, 1998.

McCance KL, Huether SE: *Pathophysiology: the biologic basis for disease in adults*, ed 3, St Louis, 1998, Mosby.

McConnell JD: Benign prostatic hyperplasia. In Rake RE: *Conn's current therapy*, Philadelphia, 2000, WB Saunders.

McMillan JA et al: *Oski's pediatrics: principles and practice*, ed 3, Philadelphia, 1998, Lippincott–Williams & Wilkins.

Meredith P, Horan N: *Adult primary care*, Philadelphia, 2000, WB Saunders.

Nickel JC: Prostatitis: myths and realities, *Urology* 51:362, 1998.

Porth CM: *Pathophysiology: concepts of altered health states*, ed 5, Philadelphia, 1998, Lippincott.

Rakel RE: *Conn's current therapy*, Philadelphia, 1999, WB Saunders.

Schwartz MW: *Clinical handbook of pediatrics*, ed 2, Baltimore, 1999, Williams & Wilkins.

Sherwood L: *Human physiology*, ed 3, Belmont, CA, 1999, West Publishing.

Singleton JK et al: *Primary care*, Philadelphia, 1999, Lippincott–Williams & Wilkins.

Uphold CR, Graham MV: *Clinical guidelines in family practice*, ed 3, Gainesville, FL, 1998, Barramarrae Books.

Chapter 11

Chen S, Gill M, Luu C, Takami S: Pain and rheumatoid arthritis: an update, *Drug Topics* 144(7):47, 2000.

Copstead LE: *Pathophysiology: biological and behavioral perspectives*, ed 2, Philadelphia, 2000, WB Saunders.

Fauci AS et al: *Harrison's principles of internal medicine*, ed 14, St Louis, 1998, McGraw-Hill.

Hansen M: *Pathophysiology: foundations of disease and clinical intervention*, Philadelphia, 1998, WB Saunders.

Huether SE, McCance K: *Understanding pathophysiology*, ed 2, St Louis, 2000, Mosby.

Ignatavicius DD, Workman ML, Mishler MA: *Medical-surgical nursing across the health care continuum*, ed 3, Philadelphia, 1999, WB Saunders.

Maher AB, Salmond SW, Pellino TA: *Orthopedic nursing*, ed 2, Philadelphia, 1998, WB Saunders.

Phipps WJ, Sands JK, Marek JF: *Medical-surgical nursing: concepts & clinical practice*, ed 6, St Louis, 1999, Mosby.

Porth CM: *Pathophysiology: concepts of altered health states*, ed 5, Philadelphia, 1998, Lippincott–Raven Publishers.

Reeves CJ, Roux G, Lockhart R: *Medical-surgical nursing*, St Louis, 1999, McGraw-Hill.

Smeltzer SC, Bare BG: *Brunner and Suddarth's textbook of medical-surgical nursing*, ed 9, Philadelphia, 2000, Lippincott.

Chapter 12

Intelihealth: Malnutrition, 2000, URL http://www.aradvocate.com/malnutrition.html.

Internet Mental Health: Eating disorders, 2000, URL http://www.mentalhealth.com/dis/p20-et02.html.

Medical Services Organization: About obesity, 2000, URL http://www.drrossfox.com/abotobs.html.

National Task Force on the Prevention and Treatment of Obesity: Overweight, obesity, and health risk, *JAMA–Arch Intern Med* 160(7):898, 2000.

Varcarolis E: *Foundations of psychiatric mental health nursing*, ed 3, Philadelphia, 1998, WB Saunders.

Chapter 13

American College of Preventive Medicine, Clinical Practice Guideline Committee: *Screening for skin cancer*, Washington, DC, 1998, American College of Preventive Medicine.

American College of Preventive Medicine, Clinical Practice Guideline Committee: *Skin protection from ultraviolet light exposure*, Washington, DC, 1998, American College of Preventive Medicine.

Barnhill RL: *Textbook of dermatopathology*, New York, 1998, McGraw-Hill.

Black J, Matassarin-Jacobs E: *Medical-surgical nursing: clinical management for continuity of care*, ed 5, Philadelphia, 1998, WB Saunders.

Braverman IM: *Skin signs of systemic disease*, ed 3, Philadelphia, 1998, WB Saunders.

Canadian Task Force on Preventive Health Care, Clinical Practice Guideline Committee: *Prevention of skin cancer*, Ottawa, 1999, Health Canada.

CancerNet: *Retinoblastoma*, 2000, URL http://cancernet.nci.nih.gov/young_people/yngconts.html.

Emmert DH: Treatment of common cutaneous herpes simplex virus infections, *Am Fam Physician* 61(6):1697, 2000.

Gutierrez K: *Pharmacotherapy: clinical decision-making in nursing*, Philadelphia, 1999, WB Saunders.

Hansen M: *Pathophysiology: foundations of disease & clinical interventions*, Philadelphia, 1998, WB Saunders.

Hay RJ: The management of superficial candidiasis, *J Am Acad Dermatol* 40(6):35, 1999.

McCance KL, Huether SE: *Pathophysiology: the biologic basis for disease in adults and children*, ed 3, St Louis, 1998, Mosby.

McCrary ML, Severson J, Tyring SK: Varicella zoster virus, *J Am Acad Dermatol* 41(1):1, 1999.

Porth C: *Pathophysiology: concepts of altered health states*, ed 5, Philadelphia, 1998, Lippincott.

Rhody C: Bacterial infections of the skin, *Primary Care Clinics in Office Practice* 27(2):459, 2000.

Rubin E, Farber JL: *Pathology*, ed 3, Philadelphia, 1999, Lippincott–Rubin.

Singleton JK et al: *Primary care*, Philadelphia, 1999, Lippincott–Williams & Wilkins.

Sorbel JD et al: Vulvovaginal candidiasis: epidemiologic, diagnostic, and therapeutic considerations, *Am J Obstet Gynecol* 178(2):203, 1998.

Wise RP et al: Post-licensure safety surveillance for varicella vaccine, *JAMA* 284(10):1271, 2000.

Chapter 14

Acute Pain Management Guideline Panel: *Acute pain management: operative or medical procedures and trauma*, Clinical Practice Guideline, AHCPR Pub no 92-0032, Rockville, MD, 1992, US Department of Health and Human Services.

Agency for HealthCare Research and Quality: Clinical practice guidelines, URL http:www.ahrq.gov.

Merskey H, Bogduk N: *Classification of chronic pain: descriptions of chronic pain syndromes and definitions of pain terms*, Seattle, 1994, International Association for the Study of Pain.

National Guideline Clearing House: Practice guidelines for acute pain in the perioperative setting, 1999, URL http://www.guideline.gov/index.asp.

Paster R: The spectrum of pain: the primary care physician's role in managing pain, *Intern Med World Rep* 15(Suppl):8, 2000.

Ready L: *International association for the study of pain task force on chronic pain*, Seattle, 1992, IASP Publications.

Illustration Credit Listing

Page 154: Redrawn from Cohn EG, Gilroy-Doohan M: *Flip and see EGC*, p 77, Philadelphia, 1996, WB Saunders.

Page 155 (*top*): Redrawn from Cohn EG, Gilroy-Doohan M: *Flip and see EGC*, p 75, Philadelphia, 1996, WB Saunders.

Page 155 (*bottom*): Redrawn from Paul S, Hebra J: *The nurse's guide to cardiac rhythm interpretation*, p 85, Philadelphia, 1996, WB Saunders.

Page 156: Redrawn from Chernecky C et al: Real-world nursing survival guide: ECG & the heart, p 140, Philadelphia, 2002, WB Saunders.

Page 272: Redrawn from Causer WG: *American Journal of Kidney Diseases* 11:449, 1998.

Page 275: Redrawn from McCance KL, Huether SE: *Pathophysiology: the biologic basis for disease in adults and children*, ed 3, p 1259, St Louis, 1998, Mosby.

Page 279: Redrawn from McCance KL, Huether SE: *Pathophysiology: the biologic basis for disease in adults and children*, ed 3, p 1260, St Louis, 1998, Mosby.

NCLEX Section

CHAPTER 1

Section A

1. Type II hypersensitivity reactions can be the result of
_____.

2. While monitoring a patient receiving a blood transfusion, the nurse notes that his blood pressure has fallen from 140/90 to 100/50, and his heart rate has increased from 84 to 118 beats per minute. He is also complaining of chills and low back pain. What should the nurse do first?
   1 Decrease the rate of the transfusion
   2 Increase the rate of the transfusion
   3 Stop the transfusion
   4 Notify the health care provider

3. While receiving an intravenous antibiotic for the first time, a patient complains of an itchy, runny nose and swollen lips. What should the nurse do?
   1 Continue the infusion
   2 Decrease the rate of the infusion
   3 Continue the infusion and notify the patient's health care provider
   4 Stop the infusion and notify the health care provider

4. Which symptom indicates a possible allergic reaction?
   1 Fever
   2 Diaphoresis
   3 Rash
   4 Chills

5. Which drug would be most useful in treating a severe allergic reaction?
   1 Hydromorphone
   2 Cortisone
   3 Methylprednisolone
   4 Furosemide

6. When treating hypersensitivity reactions, epinephrine can be given to:
   1 Decrease smooth muscle constriction.
   2 Decrease the heart rate.
   3 Control HTN.
   4 Maintain the inflammatory response.

Section B

7. RhoGAM is given after childbirth to:
   1 Treat jaundice in the neonate.
   2 Decrease hemolysis of red blood cells in the neonate.
   3 Treat hyperbilirubinemia in the mother.
   4 Prevent sensitization of the mother to Rh factor.

8. Bronchospasm associated with hypersensitivity reactions is the result of:
   1 Histamine release.
   2 Pulmonary vasodilation.
   3 Dilation of the alveoli.
   4 Inadequate antibody production.

9. Allergic reactions and allergies should be documented in multiple places including the _____, _____, and _____.

10. Antibodies do *not* participate in type _____ hypersensitivity reactions.
   1 I
   2 II
   3 III
   4 IV

Section C

11. Which group is most likely to develop systemic lupus erythematosus?
   1 Teenage girls of any race
   2 Caucasian men
   3 African-American women
   4 African-American men

12. People with lupus are most at risk for which of the following disorders?
    1 Cardiac abnormalities
    2 Liver failure
    3 Decreased coagulation
    4 Psychiatric problems

13. Signs and symptoms associated with sclerosis (scleroderma) include which of the following?
    1 Taut, shiny skin
    2 Small, white lumps under the skin
    3 Hyperactive bowel sounds
    4 Large wheals on the skin

CHAPTER 2

Section A

1. A patient mentions that he experienced transient slurred speech and numbness in one arm that lasted for approximately 2 hours and then subsided spontaneously. What did this patient likely experience?
   1 Stroke
   2 Brain attack
   3 Transient ischemic attack
   4 Hypotensive episode

2. An arteriovenous malformation is best defined as a(an):
   1 Ballooning of the arterial wall.
   2 Nest of abnormally shaped twisted vessels.
   3 Abnormally shaped vessel that forms because of atherosclerosis.
   4 Stroke.

3. The wife of a patient who has had a stroke reports that her husband woke up with slurred speech and was unable to get out of bed without assistance. Two days later, the patient is still experiencing neurologic deficits. What did this patient experience?
   1 Hemorrhagic stroke
   2 Thrombotic stroke
   3 Syncopal event
   4 Transient ischemic attack

4. The highest rate of mortality is encountered in patients who experience a _____ stroke.

5. Which of the following measures would be contraindicated for a patient with a recent stroke?
   1 Keeping the head of the bed elevated at all times
   2 Keeping the patient's hips relaxed
   3 Grouping the patient's care together to facilitate undisturbed rest for the remainder of the day
   4 Widely spacing procedures that increase intracranial pressure, such as bathing

Section B

6. Meningitis means that infection is present in
   _____.

7. Viral meningitis can enter the body as a result of:
   1 Mumps infection.
   2 Hand washing.
   3 Chicken pox infection.
   4 Eating undercooked meats.

8. Which of the following factors is *not* a typical symptom associated with meningitis?
   1 Decreased level of consciousness
   2 Headache
   3 Agitation
   4 Rash

9. Patients with which of the following disorders are likely to make a complete recovery within 10 to 14 days?
   1 Fungal encephalitis
   2 Bacterial meningitis
   3 Viral meningitis
   4 Bacterial encephalitis

10. The nurse notes that a patient with bacterial meningitis is oozing blood from old venipuncture sites. What should the nurse do first?
    1 Apply a pressure bandage
    2 Avoid invasive procedures whenever possible
    3 Evaluate the patient for other sources of infection
    4 Notify the primary care provider immediately

Section C

11. Which of the following is a potential complication of injury to the occipital lobe?
    1 Seizure activity
    2 Left-sided paralysis
    3 Loss of vision
    4 Aphasia

CHAPTER **2**—cont'd

12. Epidural hematomas are usually the indirect result a:
    1 Venous leak.
    2 Skull fracture.
    3 Capillary leak.
    4 Coagulation defect.

13. Headache, irritability, and the decreased ability to concentrate are thought to be symptoms:
    1 Cerebral hypoxia.
    2 Postconcussion syndrome.
    3 Subdural hematoma.
    4 Autonomic dysfunction.

14. Which type of intracranial hematomas can occur several weeks after the injury?
    1 Acute subdural hematomas
    2 Epidural hematomas
    3 Chronic subdural hematomas
    4 Subarachnoid

15. Which of the following signs are suggestive of skull fracture?
    1 Clear, thin fluid coming from the nose and ears
    2 Bruising around the jaw
    3 Areas of local edema in the scalp
    4 Bloody drainage from the ears

Section D

16. Which of the follow is the cause of Parkinson's disease?
    1 Loss of acetylcholine
    2 Excess secretion of acetylcholine
    3 Loss of dopamine
    4 Excess secretion of dopamine

17. Which of the following is *not* a symptom associated with Parkinson's disease?
    1 Cogwheel rigidity
    2 Broad-based gait
    3 Tremors
    4 Bradykinesia

18. Which of the following disorders is primarily treated with medical therapy only?
    1 Parkinson's disease
    2 Multiple sclerosis
    3 Myasthenia gravis
    4 Epilepsy

19. Which of the following signs and symptoms is uncharacteristic of multiple sclerosis?
    1 Blurred vision or diplopia
    2 Weakness in the extremities
    3 History of falls
    4 Muscle rigidity

20. What is an early symptom of myasthenia gravis?
    1 Blurred vision
    2 Dropping eyelids
    3 Loss of coordination
    4 Dementia

21. Which of the following interventions is most appropriate for a patient experiencing a seizure?
    1 Restrain the patient's arms and legs to ensure that they are not injured
    2 Using a gloved hand to clear the patient's airway
    3 Rolling the patient on their side.
    4 Moving the patient to a hospital bed

Section E

22. Symptoms associated with Alzheimer's disease are thought to be a result of:
    1 Genetic defects
    2 Deficits in neurotransmitters
    3 Trauma
    4 Excess acetylcholine

23. Which class of medication can have a negative effect on the patient with Alzheimer's disease?
    1 Anticholinergics
    2 Calcium channel blockers
    3 ACE inhibitors
    4 Diuretics

24. Multiinfarct dementia is *not* commonly associated with:
    1 Carotid emboli.
    2 Vasculitis.
    3 Arterial thrombosis.
    4 Head trauma.

25. Pharmacologic therapies to prevent multiinfarct dementia include which of the following?
    1 Aspirin
    2 Lasix
    3 Haldol
    4 Ibuprofen

26. The characteristics of Huntington's disease in the early stage is _____.

CHAPTER *3*

Section A

1. ITP is more common in what population?
   1 Children
   2 Young adults
   3 Pregnant women
   4 Older adults

2. Which of the following factors may adversely affect the clotting process?
   1 Liver disease
   2 Renal failure
   3 H2 blockers
   4 Antibiotic therapy

3. Which of the following drugs should patients with bleeding disorders avoid?
   1 Antibiotics
   2 Antacids
   3 Nonsteroidal antiinflammatory drugs
   4 Antifungal medications

4. Which organ system can be adversely affected by thrombotic thrombocytopenia purpura?
   1 Pulmonary
   2 Cardiac
   3 Renal
   4 Liver

Section B

5. Which of the following vitamins are required for synthesis of erythrocyte precursors?
   1 B12
   2 Vitamin A
   3 Vitamin D
   4 Folic acid and vitamin C

6. Pallor in the dark-skinned individual can be detected:
   1 On the palms of the hands.
   2 On the chest.
   3 In the whites of the eyes.
   4 On the lips.

7. Vitamin B12 deficiency usually results from a lack:
   1 Calcium
   2 Iron
   3 Intrinsic factor
   4 Sunlight

8. Folate deficiency anemia is frequently observed in what group?
   1 Older adults
   2 Alcoholics
   3 Menstruating women
   4 Infants

CHAPTER *4*

Section A

1. High-density lipoproteins benefit the circulation because they:
   1 Increase the diameter of blood vessels.
   2 Improve elasticity of the vessels.
   3 Carry fat away from arteries.
   4 Inhibit platelet activity.

2. Which of the following diseases can contribute to the development of hyperlipidemia?
   1 Hyperthyroidism
   2 Diabetes mellitus
   3 Pancreatitis
   4 Malnutrition

3. Patients who have two risk factors for cardiovascular disease but do not have actual cardiac disease should ideally have a low-density lipoprotein at what level?
   1 100 mg/dl or less
   2 Less than 130 mg/dl
   3 Less than 160 mg/dl
   4 Less than 190 mg/dl

4. The patient with vascular disease should be instructed to avoid:
   1 Caffeine.
   2 Excessive heat.
   3 NSAIDs.
   4 Sunlight.

5. Initial signs and symptoms of Raynaud's phenomenon include:
   1 Persistent erythema and swelling of the hands.
   2 Poor capillary refill in the toes.
   3 Blanching of the fingers.
   4 Pain and itching of the fingertips.

CHAPTER 4—cont'd

Section B

6. Venous stasis can be a consequence of all of the following *except*:
   1 Congestive heart failure
   2 Compression of veins by masses
   3 Increased arterial flow
   4 Severe hypotension

7. Pneumatic compression devices are used in hospitals to prevent:
   1 Venous dilation.
   2 Venous stasis.
   3 Venous ulcers.
   4 Venous distention.

8. What lifestyle changes do *not* help minimize the effect of venous stasis?
   1 Engaging in regular structured exercise
   2 Maintaining ideal body weight
   3 Preventing injury to the lower extremities
   4 Avoiding salt in the diet

9. Why is compression therapy helpful in the treatment of venous ulcers?
   1 It protects the area from further injury.
   2 It prevents infection.
   3 It improves tissue perfusion and prevents further swelling.
   4 It dissolves blood clots.

10. Risk factors that can contribute to the development of venous stasis include all of the following *except*:
    1 Obesity
    2 Sedentary lifestyle
    3 Coagulation defects
    4 Abdominal mass

Section C

11. Antihypertensive drugs should never be discontinued suddenly because of the risk for:
    1 Renal damage.
    2 Angina.
    3 Malignant hypertension.
    4 Severe hypotension.

12. Which of the following factors can contribute to the development of hypertension?
    1 Inadequate intake of calcium
    2 Excess intake of alcohol
    3 Depression
    4 Inadequate intake of potassium

13. Poorly controlled hypertension contributes to the development:
    1 Embolic strokes
    2 Coronary artery disease
    3 Migraine headaches
    4 Peripheral vascular disease

14. Measures to reduce blood pressure to healthy levels include which of the following?
    1 Eating foods high in protein
    2 Avoiding sources of stress
    3 Minimizing tobacco use
    4 Reducing body weight

15. The best diet for a person with hypertension includes:
    1 Low sodium, low potassium, and with liberal fluids
    2 Low sodium, fresh fruits, and vegetables
    3 Foods that are high in saturated fat and low in cholesterol
    4 Foods that are low in fat and moderate amounts of alcohol

CHAPTER 5

Section A

1. Which of the following conditions carries no increased risk for aneurysms?
   1 Viral pneumonia
   2 Marfan's syndrome
   3 Atherosclerosis
   4 Hypertension

2. Which symptom can suggest a thoracic aneurysm?
   1 Hoarseness
   2 Substernal pain
   3 Pulsating abdominal mass
   4 Epigastric pain

3. Signs and symptoms of a dissecting aneurysm include all of the following *except:*
   1 Pallor
   2 Falling blood pressure
   3 Rapid, bounding pulse
   4 Decreased capillary refill

4. Causes of secondary cardiomyopathy include which of the following?
   1 Alcohol
   2 Hypotension
   3 Renal failure
   4 Pericardial effusion

5. The type of cardiomyopathy that involves abnormal thickening of the interventricular septum is _____ cardiomyopathy.
   1 Dilated
   2 Hypertrophic
   3 Restrictive
   4 Ischemic

6. Which medications should be avoided in patients with IHSS?
   1 Beta-adrenergic blockers
   2 Atropine
   3 Nitroglycerin
   4 Epinephrine

Section B

7. Which infectious organism contributes to the development of valvular heart disease?
   1 *Staphylococcus aureus*
   2 Group A beta-hemolytic streptococcus
   3 *Pneumocystis carinii*
   4 *Pseudomonas aureus*

8. Which of the following describes an incompetent valve?
   1 Fails to open appropriately during the cardiac cycle.
   2 Fails to close appropriately during the cardiac cycle.
   3 Leaves too little blood in the chamber behind the valve.
   4 Causes increased cardiac output.

9. Stenosis of the mitral valve may result in:
   1 Decreased cardiac output and atrophy of the left atrium.
   2 Pulmonary hypertension only.
   3 Atrophy of the left atrium only.
   4 Decreased cardiac output and pulmonary hypertension.

Section C

10. Chronic pericarditis is the result of repeated inflammation that:
    1 Damages the myocardium
    2 Causes stenosis of the valves
    3 Causes scar tissue in the pericardium
    4 Leads to thinning of the pericardial sac

11. Which complication may be observed first as a consequence of pericarditis?
    1 Ventricular bradycardia
    2 Decreased cardiac output
    3 Hypertension
    4 Bounding peripheral pulses

12. Pulsus paradoxus associated with pericardial effusion occurs as a result of:
    1 Increased filling of the ventricles.
    2 An irregular heart beat.
    3 Decreased filling of the ventricles.
    4 Stenosis of the coronary vessels.

Section D

13. Nitroglycerin is used for ischemic heart disease because it:
    1 Increases afterload and decreases preload.
    2 Decreases afterload and increases preload.
    3 Dilates coronary arteries, decreases preload and afterload.
    4 Dilates coronary arteries, increases preload and afterload.

CHAPTER 5—cont'd

14. A patient with a myocardial infarction 2 days ago is NPO for a coronary angiogram. The patient is scheduled to receive nitroglycerin and a beta-adrenergic agent. Which of the following should the nurse do?
    1 Hold the drugs until the patient returns from the procedure
    2 Call the health care provider to determine whether the medications can be given with sips of water
    3 Maintain the patient NPO
    4 Administer one half of the medications

15. Which symptom would suggest that a patient is experiencing angina rather than a myocardial infarction?
    1 Pain in the chest that does not respond to nitroglycerin
    2 Diaphoresis
    3 Abnormal cardiac rhythms
    4 Pain in the chest that is relieved by nitroglycerin

16. What diet should be provided for a patient who is experiencing an acute myocardial infarction?
    1 Clear liquid
    2 Low sodium
    3 Bland
    4 Regular

Section E

17. Medications that primarily dilate veins will decrease:
    1 Preload.
    2 Tissue oxygenation.
    3 Contractility.
    4 Afterload and contractility.

18. With heart failure, left ventricular preload is:
    1 Decreased.
    2 Increased.
    3 Unchanged.
    4 Decreased, then increased.

19. Signs and symptoms of compensation for acute heart failure include a(an):
    1 Decrease in pulse rate.
    2 Strong and bounding pulse.
    3 Increase in urine output.
    4 Increase in pulse rate.

20. The nurse is caring for a patient diagnosed with heart failure. During the initial assessment, the nurse auscultated crackles in the bases of the lungs. Three hours later, the nurse auscultates crackles in the apices and bases of the lungs. The nurse knows that the change in assessment indicates:
    1 Improvement in left ventricular failure.
    2 Worsening of left ventricular failure.
    3 No change in left ventricular failure.
    4 A need for fluids.

Section F

21. A patient is vomiting and suddenly develops sinus bradycardia with a heart rate of 40 beats per minute. The cause of the bradycardia is most likely related:
    1 Hypoxemia.
    2 Vagal stimulation.
    3 Myocardial ischemia.
    4 Dehydration.

22. A patient with atrial fibrillation complains of abdominal pain, and the abdomen is distended and firm. The nurse suspects:
    1 Congestive heart failure.
    2 Appendicitis.
    3 A bowel infarct.
    4 Pulmonary embolus.

23. A patient develops sinus bradycardia with a heart rate of 45 beats per minute. The nurse should first perform which of the following?
    1 Administer atropine
    2 Notify the health care provider
    3 Prepare for a pacemaker
    4 Assess blood pressure

24. Which statement regarding premature ventricular contractions (PVCs) is *true*?
    1 PVCs may or may not produce a pulse.
    2 PVCs always produce a pulse.
    3 PVCs never produce a pulse.
    4 PVCs are always treated.

25. Anticoagulants are frequently administered for patients with:
    1 Sinus bradycardia.
    2 Sinus tachycardia.
    3 Atrial fibrillation.
    4 Premature ventricular contractions (PVCs).

CHAPTER *6*

Section A

1. The interstitium is:
   1 Lining of the thoracic cavity.
   2 Outermost covering of the lungs.
   3 Wall between the alveoli.
   4 Outer membrane of the heart.

2. Signs and symptoms of pulmonary fibrosis include which of the following findings?
   1 Productive cough
   2 Slow, labored respirations
   3 Tachypnea
   4 Pallor

3. Corticosteroids are given to treat lung disease in an attempt to:
   1 Support the immune response.
   2 Decrease scarring of lung tissue.
   3 Increases the inflammatory response.
   4 Increase scarring of lung tissue.

4. Which individual has the highest risk for pulmonary disease?
   1 Nonsmoker who works on a farm
   2 Nonsmoking housewife
   3 Smoker who works in a boutique
   4 Smoker who works in a steel mill

Section B

5. Identify the statement that is *not* true.
   1 Bronchitis is always a result of an infectious organism.
   2 Chronic bronchitis can lead to the development of COPD.
   3 Bronchitis usually subsides in 10 days.
   4 Bronchitis patients can benefit from inhaling warm moist air.

6. Which drug should *not* be given to treat a common cold?
   1 Antitussives
   2 Antihistamines
   3 Antibiotics
   4 Expectorants

7. Which topic would *not* be appropriate to teach the patient with chronic bronchitis?
   1 Avoidance of people with upper respiratory infections
   2 Avoidance of smoke and respiratory irritants
   3 Signs and symptoms of respiratory infection
   4 Decreasing fluid intake

8. Which of the following conditions is a risk factor for infectious respiratory disease?
   1 Obesity
   2 Dermatitis
   3 Immunocompromise
   4 Allergies

9. Which of the following is *not* a risk factor for pneumonia?
   1 Impaired level of consciousness
   2 Sedentary lifestyle
   3 Diabetes mellitus
   4 Cystic fibrosis

Section C

10. Which symptom is typically observed with chronic bronchitis?
    1 Severe prolonged nonproductive cough lasting 3 months or more
    2 Prolonged productive cough lasting 3 months or more for 2 consecutive years
    3 Chest pain
    4 Weight gain

11. In children, asthma is usually a result of which of the following?
    1 Exposure to temperature extremes
    2 Blockages in distal airways
    3 Allergies
    4 Dilation of distal airways   ·

12. Chronic bronchitis is *not* a result of:
    1 Stress.
    2 Exposure to a respiratory irritant.
    3 Smoking.
    4 Virus.

13. Which dose of oxygen would be safest for a patient with emphysema?
    1 35% by face mask
    2 2 L per minute by nasal cannula
    3 100% by nonrebreather face mask
    4 10 L per minute by nasal cannula

CHAPTER **6**—cont'd

Section D

14. The most curative treatment for single lesion lung cancer is which of the following?
    1 Radiation therapy
    2 Surgery
    3 Chemotherapy
    4 Antineoplastics

15. Which individual has the greatest risk for developing lung cancer?
    1 Nonsmoking spouse of a smoker
    2 65-year-old person who has smoked for 50 years
    3 Nonsmoker with a family history of lung cancer
    4 60-year-old person who has smoked for 20 years

16. Which symptom is *not* suggestive of lung cancer?
    1 Thick, tenacious yellow sputum
    2 Bloody sputum
    3 Localized chest pain
    4 Persistent cough

17. A patient with lung cancer presents with swelling of the face, arms, and hands. This is probably a result of which of the following?
    1 Fluid retention
    2 Vascular damage
    3 Compression of the superior vena cava
    4 Compression of the inferior vena cava

CHAPTER **7**

Section A

1. Which of the following is the most common cause of pituitary dysfunction?
    1 Congenital defects
    2 Drug overdose
    3 Head injury
    4 Tumor

2. The nurse is explaining diabetes insipidus to a patient with the disorder. The nurse should explain that the signs and symptoms are related to a deficiency in which hormone?
    1 ADH
    2 FSH
    3 HGH
    4 Oxytocin

3. Which laboratory values would be expected in a patient with SIADH?
    1 Serum sodium of 150 mEq/l and a dilute urine
    2 Serum potassium of 5 mEq/l and dilute serum
    3 Serum sodium of 120 mEq/l and dilute urine
    4 Serum potassium of 3 mEq/l and concentrated urine

4. The nurse is caring for a 25-year-old woman admitted for diagnostic workup for acromegaly. Physical assessment would identify which of the following symptoms?
    1 Alopecia
    2 Growth spurt of inches in the last year
    3 Increased forehead and jaw size
    4 Orthostatic hypotension

Section B

5. Which of the following can prevent endemic goiters?
    1 Avoiding the use of harsh mouthwashes
    2 Encouraging the intake of calcium supplements with vitamin D
    3 Encouraging the use of iodized salt
    4 Restricting the intake of caffeine

6. The clinical manifestations of primary hypothyroidism are all a result of which of the following?
    1 Absence of thyroid hormones
    2 Congenital absence of the thyroid
    3 Excessive intake of iodine
    4 Thyroid enlargement

7. A patient with primary hypothyroidism asks the nurse how long the levothyroxine medication should be taken. Which of the following is the nurse's best response?
    1 For approximately 2 to 3 years
    2 For the remainder of your life
    3 Until all symptoms are under control
    4 Until the health care provider decides that the medication is no longer required

8. Hypoparathyroidism is most frequently treated with:
    1 Biphosphates
    2 Antihypercalcemic medications
    3 Calcium preparations and vitamin D
    4 Normal saline administered intravenously

9. Hyperparathyroidism is most frequently treated with:
   1 Formulations of vitamin D
   2 Calcium preparations
   3 Biphosphates
   4 Thiazide diuretics

Section C

10. Mr. Wong has been diagnosed with adrenal insufficiency and is taking a daily dose of glucocorticosteroids. You have told him to contact his health care provider if a minor illness develops. "That's silly!" he snorts. "Why should I call the doctor when I get a cough and runny nose? I can handle that myself!" What does Mr. Wong need to know?
    1 A minor illness increases the body's need for glucocorticoids. He should consult the health care provider about a temporary increase in medication dosage.
    2 A minor illness increases the body's need for mineralocorticoids. He should consult the local pharmacist for recommendations of an over-the-counter product.
    3 A minor illness decreases the body's need for mineralocorticoids. He should consult the health care provider about a temporary decrease in medication dosage.
    4 A minor illness decreases the body's need for glucocorticoids. He should consult the local pharmacist for instructions on the ways to reduce the medication dosage.

11. Patients at risk for Cushing's syndrome include those who have which of the following?
    1 Increased secretion of mineralocorticoids
    2 A history of receiving glucocorticoids
    3 Bilateral adrenal atrophy
    4 A reduced quantity of cortisol in the hypothalamus

Section D

12. What percentage of Americans are affected by type 2 diabetes?
    1 10%
    2 50%
    3 70%
    4 90%

13. Which of the following characterizes type 1 diabetes?
    1 Inadequate insulin production
    2 Insulin resistance
    3 Lack of any insulin production
    4 Obesity

14. Women who are at high risk for developing GDM include all of the following *except* those who have which of the following?
    1 First degree-relative with diabetes
    2 History of GDM
    3 Given birth to an infant whose birth weight was 6 pounds
    4 Native-American heritage

CHAPTER 8

Section A

1. Risk factors for GERD do *not* include which of the following?
   1 Asthma
   2 Smoking
   3 Alcohol
   4 Genetics

2. The treatment for hiatal hernia does *not* include advising the patient to:
   1 Avoid alcohol.
   2 Avoid restrictive clothing.
   3 Elevate the head of the bed.
   4 Eat three large meals each day.

Section B

3. Curling's ulcers are stress ulcers that occur in patients:
   1 With burns.
   2 With preexisting ulcers.
   3 With severe head injuries.
   4 Who are bedridden.

Section C

4. The major clinical manifestation of acute pancreatitis is which of the following?
   1 Cardiovascular hypotension
   2 Disseminated intravascular coagulation
   3 Mild to severe abdominal pain
   4 Serum amylase of 100 units

5. The major therapy for acute pancreatitis is:
   1 Control of alcohol intake.
   2 Meperidine (Demerol) for pain management.
   3 Peritoneal lavage.
   4 Placement of an NG tube and making the patient NPO.

CHAPTER *8*—cont'd

6. For which condition should the patient with pancreatitis be monitored?
   1 Hypercalcemia
   2 Hyperkalemia
   3 Hypocalcemia
   4 Hypoglycemia

7. Following recovery from acute pancreatitis, the pancreas should do which of the following?
   1 Cease to produce insulin
   2 Appear normal, except for alcohol-induced pancreatitis
   3 Continue to be inflamed and become necrotic
   4 Will atrophy when the inflammatory process is gone

Section D

8. Which of the following characteristics is common to both ulcerative colitis and Crohn's disease?
   1 Involves mucosal layer of intestinal wall
   2 Frequent fatty stools
   3 Malabsorption of small intestine
   4 Nutritional deficit

Section E

9. The primary clinical manifestation of cholecystitis is which of the following:
   1 Jaundice
   2 Decreased bilirubin levels
   3 Constipation
   4 Intolerance to fatty foods

10. Hepatic encephalopathy is manifested by which of the following?
    1 Ascites
    2 Cerebral dysfunction
    3 Dark urine
    4 Splenomegaly

11. Medical management of the patient with cirrhosis is primarily directed toward _____.

Section F

12. Which of the following is *not* considered a predisposing factor in the development of colon cancer?
    1 Low-fiber, high-fat diet
    2 High-fiber diet
    3 High-refined carbohydrate diet
    4 Ulcerative colitis

CHAPTER *9*

Section A

1. The health care provider teaches a patient with cystitis about proper fluid intake. What is the recommended fluid intake per 24 hours?
   1 1000 ml
   2 1500 ml
   3 2000 ml
   4 3000 ml

2. Hypertension may be a sign of which of the following UTIs?
   1 Acute cystitis
   2 Chronic cystitis
   3 Acute pyelonephritis
   4 Chronic pyelonephritis

3. The most common organism that causes cystitis or pyelonephritis is:
   1 *Escherichia coli.*
   2 *Staphylococcus aureus.*
   3 *Klebsiella pneumoniae.*
   4 *Proteus.*

4. Which of the following are the most prominent clinical manifestations of cystitis?
   1 Urgency and dysuria
   2 Nocturia and incontinence
   3 Hematuria and bladder spasms
   4 Hesitancy and cloudy urine

5. Which of the following menus would *not* be most appropriate for the patient with chronic cystitis?
   1 Tossed vegetable salad, milk, apple
   2 Grilled cheese, prunes, tea
   3 Egg salad, ham, milk
   4 Hamburger on whole wheat bread, milk, tea

6. Your 15-year-old patient has been diagnosed with cystitis. To prevent recurrence of the infection, you would teach her to modify which of the following behaviors?
   1 Increasing her fluid intake
   2 Wiping front to back after a bowel movement
   3 Adhering to an alkaline-ash diet
   4 Taking showers rather than baths

7. Which of the following findings on a urinalysis most likely indicates a UTI?
   1 Four to five red blood cells; high power field
   2 Bacteria count of 1000 to 10,000/ml
   3 Glucose level of 3+
   4 4+ ketones

8. Which of the following drugs is commonly used as a urinary tract analgesic?
   1 Nitrofurantoin (Macrodantin)
   2 Sulfamethoxazole/trimethoprim (Bactrim)
   3 Phenazopyridine (Pyridium)
   4 Ciprofloxacin (Cipro)

Section B

9. Which of the following is *not* a risk factor in calculi formation?
   1 Excessive calcium intake
   2 High production of mucoproteins
   3 High concentrations of struvite
   4 Excessive production of inhibitors

Section C

10. Which renal condition usually has a history of recent infection with beta hemolytic streptococcus?
    1 Chronic renal failure
    2 Glomerulonephritis
    3 Nephrosis
    4 Pyelonephritis

Section D

11. An individual has an elevated blood level of urea and creatinine because of complete calculi blockage of one ureter. This condition is referred to as:
    1 Prerenal disease.
    2 Intrarenal disease.
    3 Postrenal disease.
    4 Hypercalcemia.

12. What is the earliest symptom of chronic renal failure?
    1 Increased BUN
    2 Oliguria
    3 Polyuria
    4 Pruritus

Section E

13. What is the most common cause of IgA nephropathy?
    1 Increased production or reduced clearance of IgA in the kidneys
    2 Poststreptococcal glomerulonephritis
    3 Decreased production or increased clearance of IgA in the kidneys
    4 Genetic, autosomal dominant disorder

Section F

14. Wilms' tumors are most common in children in which of the following age groups?
    1 Under the age of 5 years
    2 Ages 5 to 10
    3 Ages 10 to 15
    4 Ages 15 to 21

CHAPTER *10*

Section A

1. The most common symptom of cryptorchidism is:
   1 Swelling of the scrotal sac.
   2 Perianal pain.
   3 Undescended testis.
   4 Infertility.

2. Signs of orchitis do *not* include:
   1 Severe pain.
   2 High fever.
   3 Infertility.
   4 Edema.

3. Patients at risk for epididymitis include:
   1 Men over the age of 50.
   2 Prepubescent males.
   3 Newborn males.
   4 Males between the ages of 12 and 35.

CHAPTER *10*—cont'd

4. The four common forms of prostatitis are:
   1 Acute bacterial, chronic bacterial, bacterial, and prostatodynia.
   2 Chronic bacterial, nonbacterial, prostatodynia, and viral.
   3 Acute bacterial, chronic bacterial, nonbacterial, and prostatodynia.
   4 Acute bacterial, chronic viral, nonbacterial, and prostatodynia.

5. The pathophysiologic factors of benign prostatic hyperplasia include:
   1 Hypertrophy of the prostatic cells.
   2 Atrophy of prostatic cells.
   3 Stricture of the vas deferens.
   4 Inflammation of the epididymis.

6. The risk of developing benign prostatic hyperplasia _____ as men age.
   1 Decreases
   2 Increases
   3 Stays the same
   4 Increases tenfold

7. The cause of BPH is *not* related to which of the following factors?
   1 Increased testosterone and estrogen levels
   2 Stimulation of alpha-adrenergic nerve endings interfering with opening of the bladder sphincter
   3 Smoking
   4 Alcohol consumption

8. Testicular carcinoma metastasizes most frequently to which organ?
   1 Lung
   2 Brain
   3 Bladder
   4 Liver

9. Risk factors for prostatic carcinoma do *not* include:
   1 African-American men.
   2 Men who have undergone vasectomy.
   3 Men who work with fertilizer.
   4 Alcoholic men.

Section B

10. Primary dysmenorrhea is defined as:
    1 Increased menstruation.
    2 The absence of menstruation.
    3 Painful menstruation.
    4 A symptom of pregnancy.

11. Secondary dysmenorrhea is *not* be a result of:
    1 Pelvic inflammatory disease.
    2 Adhesions or fibroids.
    3 Endometriosis.
    4 Urinary tract infections.

Section C

12. Recurrent genital herpes infections result from:
    1 Reactivation of the virus from sacral dorsal root ganglia.
    2 Activation of virus from genital tissues.
    3 An immune response arising from repeated exposure to the virus.
    4 Reinfection with herpes simplex type I virus.

13. A patient with syphilis who complains of a maculopapular rash on the trunk, palms of the hands, and soles of the feet is most likely in which stage of the disease?
    1 Primary
    2 Secondary
    3 Latent
    4 Tertiary

14. The typical site of chlamydia infection in women is the:
    1 Transition zone of the endocervix.
    2 Intrauterine tissue.
    3 Ovaries.
    4 Vulva region.

CHAPTER *11*

1. The stage of bone healing when the hematoma becomes strong granulation tissue is in the:
   1 Callus ossification stage.
   2 Cellular proliferation stage.
   3 Callus formation stage.
   4 Cellular consolidation stage.

2. In rheumatoid arthritis, the changes begin in the joint:
   1 Tophi.
   2 Bursa.
   3 Cartilage.
   4 Synovium.

3. The pathophysiologic changes in osteoarthritis involve:
   1 Faulty purine metabolism.
   2 Uric acid crystals that trigger a phagocytic response by leukocytes.
   3 A thick layer of granulation pannus tissue that covers and invades articular cartilage.
   4 Joint ends repeatedly hitting together, leading to a loss of joint matrix and erosion of cartilage.

4. The pathophysiologic factors of gout involves:
   1 Autoimmune lesions of collagen tissue.
   2 Uric acid level increase in the blood.
   3 Inflammation of the synovial membrane in a joint.
   4 Cartilage and bone eroding the narrow joint spaces.

CHAPTER 12

1. The nurse is preparing to administer a feeding to the patient receiving enteral nutrition through a nasogastric tube. What is the priority nursing action?
   1 Measuring intake and output
   2 Weighing the patient
   3 Assessing the patient for diarrhea
   4 Determining tube placement

2. A patient with an eating disorder is attending group meetings with Overeaters Anonymous. Which of the following is *not* a characteristic of this form of self-help group?
   1 People with similar problems are able to help others.
   2 The group is designed to serve people who have a common problem.
   3 The group members provide support to each other.
   4 The leader is a nurse or psychiatrist.

3. A 17-year-old patient diagnosed with anorexia nervosa is a member of a predischarge support group. When she verbalizes her financial inability to buy new clothes, other group members offer to provide her with some of their used clothes. The patient accepted the clothes but believed that they were too tight and she reduced her caloric intake. The nurse recognizes this behavior as:
   1 Normal behavior.
   2 Evidence of the patient's altered or distorted body image.
   3 Regression because the patient is approaching discharge.
   4 Indicative of the patient's ambivalence about moving towards outpatient treatment.

4. The nurse is evaluating the progress of a 28-year-old woman admitted to the psychiatric unit with a diagnosis of bulimia nervosa. Which of the following behaviors would indicate that the patient had progressed?
   1 Her conversations focus on food.
   2 She identifies healthy ways of coping with anxiety.
   3 She spends time alone in her room after each meal.
   4 She engages in rigorous exercise.

5. The nurse is caring for a 2-year-old patient who is diagnosed with a form of malnutrition known as kwashiorkor. The nurse knows this patient is deficient in which nutrient?

CHAPTER 13

Section A

1. Which statement about macular degeneration is true?
   1 Adequate intake of vitamin A can prevent macular degeneration.
   2 Peripheral vision remains intact.
   3 Laser therapy is used to successfully cure both the "wet" and "dry" types.
   4 Macular degeneration can be easily diagnosed using a slit-lamp.

2. Which of the following surgical procedures is used to correct a retinal detachment?
   1 Iridectomy
   2 Keratoplasty
   3 Scleral buckling
   4 Trabeculectomy

CHAPTER *13*—cont'd

3. Postoperative care of the patient with a detached retina includes:
   1 Administering miotic eye drops.
   2 Allowing the patient to ambulate.
   3 Covering only the affected eye with a pressure dressing.
   4 Encouraging the patient to remain in a head-down, lateral position.

4. Your next-door neighbor is complaining of a sudden severe pain in the eye and a "curtain" closing in the field of vision. This person should be immediately referred to an:
   1 Oculist.
   2 Ophthalmologist.
   3 Optician.
   4 Optometrist.

Section B

5. Conductive hearing loss is most commonly a result of:
   1 A disease or trauma to the inner ear.
   2 Anything that blocks the external ear.
   3 Disease or trauma to the external ear.
   4 Nerve pathways leading to the brainstem.

6. The most common problem found in the external ear is(are):
   1 Invasion by insects and foreign bodies.
   2 Injury or trauma.
   3 Allergic reactions.
   4 Infection.

7. The technique used to administer eardrops to a child is to pull the pinna:
   1 Up and back.
   2 Down and back.
   3 Forward and down.
   4 Forward and up.

Section C

8. The usual transmission mode for type 2 herpes simplex is through:
   1 Kissing and touching.
   2 Sexual encounters.
   3 Contaminated food or water.
   4 Coughing.

Section D

9. The skin lesions of psoriasis are:
   1 Nonscaling, violet-colored, pruritic papules.
   2 Black comedones.
   3 Pruritic vesicles.
   4 Thick, scaly, erythematous plaques.

10. Acne vulgaris is a result of:
    1 Oily skin.
    2 Poor diet.
    3 Poor hygiene.
    4 Excessive melanocytes.

11. The health care provider instructs patients with rosacea to use caution with alcohol and hot drinks because they can cause:
    1 Vasoconstriction.
    2 Vasodilation.
    3 Hypothermia.
    4 Hyperthermia.

Section E

12. What are the characteristic findings of the lesion of malignant melanoma?

13. Squamous cell carcinoma of the skin is manifested as:
    1 Irregular pigmentation.
    2 An ulcerated, hyperkeratotic nodule with dermal invasion.
    3 A slightly elevated, pearl-colored nodule.
    4 Multifocal brown macules.

14. Which malignant skin lesion metastasizes the earliest?
    1 Basal cell carcinoma
    2 Kaposi sarcoma
    3 Malignant melanoma
    4 Squamous cell carcinoma

15. An untreated basal cell carcinoma:
    1 Metastasizes frequently.
    2 Frequently involves regional lymphatic tissues.
    3 Ulcerates and involves local tissues.
    4 Grows rapidly.

CHAPTER *14*

1. Endorphins are found in the brain stem and will:
   1 Increase pain perception.
   2 Decrease pain sensations.
   3 May increase or decrease pain transmission.
   4 Have no effect on pain sensation.

2. Acute pain is primarily characterized by which of the following sympathetic nervous system responses?
   1 Increased blood pressure and pulse
   2 Pink skin and skeletal muscle tension
   3 Constricted pupils and dry skin
   4 Decreased or normal blood pressure and pulse

3. Chronic pain is characterized by which of the following parasympathetic nervous system responses?
   1 Increased blood pressure and pulse
   2 Pallor and skeletal muscle tension
   3 Dilated pupils and diaphoresis
   4 Decreased or normal blood pressure and pulse

4. List at least five factors that influence a patient's response to pain.

5. A 19-year-old patient experienced a traumatic amputation of the left foot in a motorcycle accident. The patient complains of a burning sensation in the left foot. What is this sensation called and how would you explain it to the patient?

NCLEX CHAPTER *1* ANSWERS

Section A

1. Type II hypersensitivity reactions occur when antibodies interact with antigens. These antigens can be foreign, such as a drug, or in transfused blood. In certain conditions, autoantibodies can bind with red blood cells, ultimately resulting in hemolysis.

2. 3 The symptoms cited reflect a possible hemolytic reaction to the transfusion. The transfusion must be stopped immediately, and then the health care provider notified thus appropriate treatment can begin. Continuing the transfusion at any rate places the patient at risk for renal failure and even death.

3. 4 Itching and swelling are signs of an allergic reaction. The infusion must be stopped and the health care provider notified. If the infusion continues, then the patient's airway may begin to swell, placing the individual at risk for respiratory arrest.

4. 3 Rash may be present with hypersensitive allergic reactions. Fever, diaphoresis (sweating), and chills are symptoms of infection.

5. 3 Methylprednisolone, a corticosteroid, has a stronger, more immediate effect than has cortisone and prevents tissue response to inflammatory mediators and lysosomal enzyme release. Hydromorphone is a narcotic analgesic, cortisone is a corticosteroid used in treatment of inflammatory disorders, and furosemide is a loop diuretic.

6. 1 Epinephrine results in the stimulation of beta$_1$-receptors, which lead to an increased heart rate and relaxation of smooth muscles. Epinephrine causes vasoconstriction, which would then lead to elevated, not decreased blood pressure. Epinephrine does not affect the inflammatory response.

Section B

7. 4 RhoGAM is given as a preventive agent. It is an immune serum given to prevent an Rh-mother from becoming sensitized to the blood cells of her Rh+ fetus. RhoGAM will not treat or decrease jaundice in the neonate, but it might prevent it from occurring if given to the mother appropriately during pregnancy.

8. 1 Histamine constricts smooth muscle, resulting in bronchiolar constriction, and causes increased permeability of the vessels, resulting in vascular congestion and edema. Histamine has no direct action on the alveoli and antibody production but is responsible for mediating the immune response.

NCLEX CHAPTER *1* ANSWERS—cont'd

9. 4 Patient's record; current chart; on the patient's (armband)

10. 4 Type IV reactions are the result of sensitized T lymphocytes. Also called delayed reactions, type IV reactions tend to occur 24 to 72 hours after exposure to an antigen. Type I, II, and III reactions involve antibody formation.

Section C

11. 3 African-American women have three times the incidence of lupus than do Caucasian women. This disease can, however, develop in any race and at any age, although it is more common between the ages of 20 and 40.

12. 1 Most patients with lupus die of cardiovascular complications. Vascular abnormalities can also lead to renal and liver damage and/or renal or liver failure. These patients tend to experience hypercoagulable states and are at increased risk for venous and arterial thromboses. The stress of a serious chronic illness can lead to psychiatric problems, but lupus does not, in and of itself, cause psychiatric problems.

13. 4 Excess collagen accumulates in the tissues and causes taut, shiny skin that eventually becomes thick and hard. Abnormal calcium deposits in the skin form small lumps that can leak and drain. Patients with sclerosis tend to experience decreased peristalsis, which can cause symptoms similar to a bowel obstruction.

NCLEX CHAPTER *2* ANSWERS

Section A

1. 3 Transient ischemic attacks are typically brief in duration and leave no permanent deficit. A true stroke or brain attack is likely to leave permanent neurologic deficits. Changes in level of consciousness-associated hypotensive episode resolves after the blood pressure returns to normal levels.

2. 2 An arteriovenous malformation is best defined as a nest of abnormally shaped twisted blood vessels. A dilation (ballooning) of a vessel wall is more consistent with an aneurysm; however, these can form in any vessel, not in arteries alone. Atherosclerosis does not change the shape of a blood vessel. A stroke or brain attack is an interruption of blood flow to the brain.

3. 2 Thrombotic strokes tend to occur at night, during sleep. A hemorrhagic stroke is characterized by sudden onset of symptoms. A syncopal event, also known as fainting, does not result in neurologic deficits. A transient ischemic attack is a neurologic deficit lasting for less than 24 hours.

4. Hemorrhagic strokes tend to have the highest rate of mortality, regardless of the age in which they occur.

5. 3 The recent stroke patient must be evaluated regularly, thus care should not be grouped together, leaving the patient without nursing contact for extended periods. All of the other measures listed—elevating the head of the bed, keeping the patient's hips unflexed, and spacing out procedures likely to cause increased intracranial pressure—are appropriate nursing responsibilities for patient care.

Section B

6. The term *meningitis* refers to infection that is limited to the meninges.

7. 1 Viral meningitis can be caused by the mumps virus. Frequent hand washing is a good precaution against the spread of viral meningitis. Chicken pox does not cause viral meningitis. Eating undercooked meats can lead to several conditions, including salmonella poisoning, *E. coli* virus infection, and tuberculosis.

8. 3 Agitation is not typically observed with a central nervous system infection. More commonly present are headache, rash, and altered levels of consciousness.

9. 3 Viral syndromes (e.g., viral meningitis) are typically self-limiting and resolve within 10 to 14 days. Bacterial and fungal central nervous system infections, such as fungal encephalitis, bacterial meningitis, and bacterial encephalitis, require intensive therapy in the acute-care setting.

10. 1 The nurse should first attempt to control bleeding with a pressure bandage and then notify the primary care provider immediately, because oozing from old puncture sites can be a symptom of disseminated intravascular coagulation, a potentially life-threatening complication. Avoidance of invasive procedures and evaluation of the patient for sources of infection occur later in care.

Section C

11. 3 Loss of vision can result when the injury is to the occipital lobe. Seizures can result from any type of head injury. Injury to the right hemisphere causes left-sided paralysis. Injury to Broca's area results in aphasia.

12.2 In most cases, epidural hematomas result from damage to cerebral arteries caused by a skull fracture. Subdural hematomas are usually observed with torn cerebral veins. A coagulation defect or capillary leak is an incidental finding, not directly related to the epidural hematoma.

13.1 Many people who are recovering from concussions can experience persistent headaches, irritability, and impaired concentration for up to 2 months after the initial injury. Autonomic dysfunction, cerebral hypoxia, and subdural hematomas typically cause more severe symptoms, including changes in vital signs.

14.3 Chronic subdural hematomas are usually the result of a slow leak of venous origin; symptom may not be present for up to 3 weeks after the initial injury. Acute subdural hematomas accumulate more rapidly and cause a sudden change in neurologic status soon after the injury. Epidural hematomas are the result of arterial bleeding in the skull and result in the rapid accumulation of blood in the epidural space. Subarachnoid hemorrhage causes sudden changes in neurologic status and occurs shortly after the initial injury.

15.1 Clear, thin fluid draining from the nose and ears is a symptom of a cerebrospinal fluid leak resulting from a skull fracture. Bruising around the jaw and local edema in the scalp are suggestive of head injury but do not necessarily indicate a fracture. Bloody drainage from the ears indicates a possible infection or penetration of the ear by a foreign body.

Section D

16.3 Parkinson's disease is the result of a loss of dopamine. A rise or fall in actylcholine levels does not cause Parkinson's disease.

17.2 Bradykinesia is not characteristic of Parkinson's disease. Cogwheel rigidity; small, shuffing steps; and tremors are associated with Parkinson's disease.

18.2 The only therapy available for multiple sclerosis is medical in nature. Epilepsy, myasthenia gravis and Parkinson's disease have surgical and pharmacologic interventions.

19.4 Muscle rigidity is a sign of Parkinson's disease, not multiple sclerosis. Although symptoms may vary among individuals, visual changes, weakness, and a history of falls are commonly seen in the early stages of multiple sclerosis.

20.2 Weakness of the ocular muscles causes ptosis or drooping eyelids, an early sign of myasthenia gravis. Dementia may be observed with Parkinson's disease, loss of coordination and blurred vision may be evident in patients with multiple sclerosis.

21.3 Rolling the patient to his or her side is the only appropriate intervention for the patient experiencing a seizure. Trying to restrain the patient during a seizure may result in fractures and other serious injuries. Individuals attempting to help a convulsing person by manually clearing his or her airway have lost fingers! Attempting to pry open the mouth of a patient experiencing a seizure may also cause serious injury to the patient.

Section E

22.2 Symptoms associated with Alzheimer's disease are thought to be a result of deficits in neurotransmitters. Genetic defects can lead to the development of a disease but are not responsible for the development of symptoms. Trauma to the head can cause neurologic damage but does not cause the progressive decline observed with Alzheimer's disease. Excess acetylcholine does not cause gradual neurologic decline.

23.1 Medications with anticholinergic properties can adversely affect acetylcholine levels and can cause further decline in cognitive function. Calcium channel blockers, ACE inhibitors, and diuretics can be given to patients with Alzheimer's disease when necessary to treat other medical conditions.

24.4 Trauma can cause neurologic damage but will not necessarily interrupt blood flow and cause multiinfarct dementia. Carotid and cardiac emboli, cerebral arterial and venous thrombosis, and vasculitis can cause multiinfarct dementia.

25.1 Aspirin will inhibit platelet activity and thereby decrease the risk of embolic formations that cause multiinfarct dementia. Lasix, Haldol, and ibuprofen do not improve cerebral blood flow or decrease the risk for clot formation.

26. In the early stages of the disease, Huntington's disease is characterized by hostile outbursts and depression.

NCLEX CHAPTER *3* ANSWERS

Section A

1. 1 Idiopathic thrombocytopenia purpura is most commonly observed in children, although it may occur in any age group. In contrast, thrombotic thrombocytopenia purpura is occasionally present in pregnant women.

2. 1 Liver disease can adversely affect the clotting process, because it is ordinarily responsible for synthesis of clotting factors. Renal failure can cause anemia, but does not adversely affect platelet count or clotting components. Antibiotic therapy does not usually adversely affect clotting function.

3. 3 Nonsteroidal antiinflammatory drugs can decrease platelet aggregation, therefore they should be avoided by people with clotting disorders. Some antacids include copious amounts of aspirin and these should be avoided as well. However, normally, antacids, antibiotics, and antifungal medications are safe for people with clotting disorders.

4. 3 Renal failure can be present in patients with thrombotic thrombocytopenia purpura. Problems with the liver, pulmonary system, and cardiac system are not directly caused by thrombotic thrombocytopenia purpura.

Section B

5. 4 Folic acid and vitamin C are necessary for synthesis of erythrocyte precursors. B_{12} is needed for DNA synthesis. Vitamin A is needed for visual acuity. Vitamin D is needed for creation of strong bones and teeth.

6. 1 Pallor may be detected on the palms of the hands of dark-skinned individuals. The chest, lips and whites of the eyes will not show pallor in a dark-skinned person.

7. 3 B_{12} deficiency results from a lack of intrinsic factor. Osteoporosis is caused by a calcium deficiency. A lack of iron causes iron deficiency anemia. Rickets results from a lack of exposure to sunlight.

8. 2 Folate deficiency is most frequently observed with alcoholics who do not maintain an adequate diet. Older adults are at most risk for vitamin B_{12} anemia. Menstruating women most frequently have iron deficiency anemia. Infants are not at risk for anemia. Infants breast-feed and absorb folate from their mothers. For infants who are bottle-fed, most formulas are fortified with folate.

NCLEX CHAPTER *4* ANSWERS

Section A

1. 3 High-density lipoproteins carry fat away from arteries. High-density lipoproteins have no effect on the diameter or elasticity of blood vessels. Drugs can inhibit platelet activity, but lipoproteins do not.

2. 2 People with diabetes tend to experience problems with lipid metabolism, which can contribute to hyperlipidemia. Hypothyroidism contributes to hyperlipidemia, not hyperthyroidism. Pancreatitis can occur as an indirect consequence of hyperlipidemia but does not, in and of itself, elevate lipid levels. Patients who are malnourished tend to have low, not elevated, lipid levels.

3. 2 Patients who have risk factors should keep their low-density lipoprotein level at 130 mg/dl or less. Patients who have already had cardiovascular disease should strive to keep their low-density lipoprotein level at 100 mg/dl or lower. Patients with low-density lipoprotein levels over 130 mg/dl are considered to be at increased risk for cardiovascular disease.

4. 4 Heat causes vasodilation, thus it is not a contraindication. Caffeine causes vasoconstriction, thus is contraindicated for the patient with vascular disease. Sunlight does not affect vascular disease, unless excessive exposure to sunlight is involved, which causes vasodilation. NSAIDs are not contraindicated in patients with vascular disease.

5. 3 A classic symptom of Raynaud's phenomenon is bluish-white blanching of one or more fingers. Raynaud's phenomenon does not initially cause redness or swelling. Burning pain typically occurs after circulation has been restored, but the fingertips do not itch.

Section B

6. 3 Increased arterial flow does not contribute to venous stasis. Congestive heart failure, compression of veins by masses, and severe hypotension contribute to venous stasis.

7. 2 Pneumatic compression devices are used to prevent venous pooling in the hospitalized, immobilized patient. Pneumatic compression devices do not help venous dilation, venous ulcers, or venous distention.

8. 4 Avoiding salt in daily diet does not affect venous stasis. Engaging in regular structured exercise, maintaining ideal body weight, and preventing injury to the lower extremities can decrease the effect of venous stasis and should be a part of routine patient teaching.

9.3 Compression therapy reduces swelling and improves oxygenation of tissue, which promotes healing. Occlusive dressings are used to protect venous ulcers from further damage or infection. Compression therapy does not dissolve blood clots; medication is required.

10.3 Coagulation defects do not contribute to the development of venous stasis. Obesity, a sedentary lifestyle, and abdominal masses contribute to venous stasis.

Section C

11.3 Suddenly discontinuing antihypertensive drugs can result in a malignant hypertension, not hypotension. Renal damage and angina can be an indirect consequence of the malignant hypertension, but does not ensue as a result of stopping drug therapy.

12.2 Excess consumption of alcohol in conjunction with other risk factors is most likely to cause hypertension. Electrolyte (e.g., calcium, potassium) imbalances do not generally affect blood pressure. Depression can indirectly cause a stress response, which can then elevate blood pressure.

13.2 Poorly controlled hypertension causes damage to the vascular endothelium and increases the workload of the heart, both of which contribute to coronary artery disease.

14.4 Weight reduction is the most efficient way to reduce blood pressure. Eating foods high in protein increases the consumption of animal fat, which is known to contribute to the development of hypertension. For most patients, stress cannot be avoided, but they can learn techniques and strategies for coping with stress. Tobacco use should be eliminated to decrease blood pressure; merely reducing consumption does not lower blood pressure.

15.2 A diet that is low in sodium, with liberal amounts of fresh fruits and vegetables, is most desirable for the patient with hypertensive disease. Patients with hypertension may need to avoid excess fluids, particularly when they have cardiac disease in conjunction with hypertension. Diets high in saturated fat and even moderate alcohol consumption have both been shown to contribute to hypertension.

NCLEX CHAPTER 5 ANSWERS

Section A

1.1 Viral pneumonia does not affect the integrity of the vessel wall thus the risk of aneurysm is not increased. Marfan's syndrome, hypertension, and atherosclerosis affect the integrity of the vessel walls and cause decreased elasticity, tearing, and eventual rupture in some cases.

2.1 Hoarseness can occur when a large thoracic aneurysm presses on the trachea. Substernal pain is associated more frequently with angina or esophagitis. An abdominal aortic aneurysm can cause a pulsating mass that can be seen or felt. Epigastric pain may be a result of angina, gastric ulcers, or gastroesophageal reflux disease.

3.3 A dissecting aneurysm will cause loss of intravascular volume, which would cause a weak, thready pulse or loss of palpable peripheral pulses. Pallor, falling blood pressure, and decreased capillary refill are reflective of loss of perfusion as a result of declining intravascular volume.

4.1 Chronic alcohol abuse causes damage to the myocardial fibers. Hypotension has no direct adverse affect on the heart. Renal failure can cause dysrhythmias but does not damage the myocardium. Pericardial effusions interferes with the pumping action of the heart.

5.2 Hypertrophic cardiomyopathy. The septum is large to the extent that the size of the left ventricle is significantly decreased. Dilated cardiomyopathy causes the ventricle to enlarge to the extent that the ventricle is unable to contract effectively. In restrictive cardiomyopathy, the myocardium becomes rigid and loses its elasticity. Ischemic cardiomyopathy is caused by necrosis of the myocardium.

6.3 Vasodilating agents such as nitroglycerin should not be used because they cause an obstruction of the outflow tract, blocking the ejection of blood from the left ventricle. Beta-adrenergic blockers can be helpful in the treatment of restrictive cardiomyopathy. Epinephrine causes vasoconstriction and raises blood pressure, which would increase the cardiac workload. Atropine stimulates heart rate, increasing cardiac workload.

NCLEX CHAPTER 5 ANSWERS—cont'd

Section D

7.2 Group A hemolytic streptococci have been shown to trigger an inappropriate inflammatory response that can cause damage to the heart, skin, joints, and kidneys. This phenomenon has not been documented with other infectious organisms, such as *Staphylococcus aureus, Pneumocystis carinii, or Pseudomonas aureus.*

8.2 An incompetent valve is one that fails to close completely during the cardiac cycle, which allows blood to leak backwards into the heart, causing a build up of blood in the chamber behind the valve. A valve that fails to open appropriately is described as stenotic. Inadequate blood flow within the heart leads to decreased, not increased, cardiac output.

9.4 Blood flow from left atrium to left ventricle decreases, ultimately providing the left ventricle with less blood to eject. Blood backs up from the left atrium into the pulmonary system, causing pulmonary hypertension because of increased pressure. Blood backing into the left atrium causes hypertrophy, not atrophy.

Section C

10.3 Chronic pericarditis is the result of repeated inflammation that causes scar tissue in the pericardium. Chronic pericarditis does not damage the myocardium or cause valve stenosis because pericardial disease involves only the pericardial tissue. Chronic pericarditis does not lead to thinning of the pericardial tissue; recurrent episodes of inflammation lead to thickening and stiffening of the pericardial tissue.

11.2 Scar tissue of the pericardium inhibits ventricles' ability to stretch and fill with blood thus lowering cardiac output. Decreased cardiac output leads to hypotension, not hypertension. Bounding peripheral pulses are not observed with decreased cardiac output. The heart initially beats faster, not slower (as in ventricular tachycardia or ventricular bradycardia) in an attempt to compensate for poor cardiac output.

12.3 Pulsus paradoxus associated with pericardial effusion occurs as a result of decreased filling of the ventricles. Fluid in the pericardial sac interferes with the filling of the ventricles, decreasing it, not increasing filling. An irregular heart rate does not cause changes in blood pressure during inspiration and expiration, nor does stenosis of the coronary vessels.

Section D

13.3 Nitroglycerin is used for ischemic heart disease because it dilates coronary arteries, which decreases preload and afterload. Dilating the coronary arteries and veins decreases the myocardial oxygen demand. Increasing afterload or preload places more stress on the myocardium.

14.2 The patient, NPO for an angiogram, may need to receive medications. The nurse should call the health care provider to determine whether the medications can be given with sips of water. Failure to give cardiac medications can cause acute angina or infarction to develop during a procedure.

15.4 Cardiac pain resulting from an infarction is not relieved by nitroglycerin. Angina does not cause diaphoresis or dysrhythmias. Nitroglycerin relieves cardiac pain resulting from angina.

16.1 Clear liquid diet should be given during acute anginal attacks and for the first 24 hours after an acute MI to decrease the GI tract's demand for oxygen. A low sodium, bland, or regular diet would increase the GI tract's demand for oxygen and is contraindicated.

Section E

17.1 Medications that dilate veins decrease preload. Dilated vessels improve perfusion and oxygenation. Decreasing contractility causes heart failure to worsen.

18.2 Because of the inadequate pumping action of the heart, the weakened ventricle is unable to completely empty the chamber, leading to an increase in left ventricular preload in heart failure.

19.4 During early stages, the heart is able to compensate by increasing the number of contractions (pulse rate). Eventually, the pumping ability of the myocardium declines, resulting in heart failure. With decreased cardiac output, blood flow is shunted away from the kidneys, resulting in decreasing urine output.

20.2 The change in location of the crackles indicates worsening left ventricular failure. Increasing crackles are a reflection of left ventricular failure that is causing congestion of the pulmonary vessels, forcing fluid into the alveoli. Fluids should be restricted in heart failure.

Section F

21.2 Vomiting is a common stimulant of the vagus nerve. Vagus nerve stimulation can lead to sinus bradycardia. No indication that the patient has hypoxemia or myocardial ischemia is present; thus, in this case, these symptoms would not be from sinus bradycardia. Dehydration causes sinus tachycardia.

22.3 Abdominal pain and distention are signs and symptoms of a bowel infarct. Tachycardia, decreased urine output, dark amber urine, weak pulses, and cool skin are characteristics of heart failure. Lower right quadrant abdominal pain and fever are characteristics of appendicitis. Sudden chest pain, difficulty breathing, tachycardia, diaphoresis, and hypoxemia are characteristics of pulmonary embolus.

23.4 In a patient with sinus bradycardia, assessment of patients to determine whether they are symptomatic is imperative. No treatment is necessary if the patient is asymptomatic including absence of hypotension. Atropine is administered only when the patient is hypotensive or symptomatic. Notifying the health care provider and preparing the patient for a pacemaker are premature. Assessment is needed before intervention.

24.1 PVCs may or may not produce a pulse. PVCs are usually not treated if the patient is experiencing no symptoms.

25.3 Patients with atrial fibrillation are at high risk for stroke, bowel infarct, and pulmonary embolus because of thrombus formation. Therefore anticoagulants are the treatment of choice. Sinus bradycardia, sinus tachycardia, and PVCs do not cause clot formation and thus do not need anticoagulant therapy.

NCLEX CHAPTER 6 ANSWERS

Section A

1.3 The term *inter* means between, referring to the membrane or wall between the alveoli. The membranes that cover the lungs and the thoracic cavity are called the visceral and parietal pleura. The pericardium is the outer membrane of the heart.

2.3 Tachypnea is a common sign of pulmonary fibrosis. A productive cough is observed in the presence of an underlying infection. Slow, shallow respirations are more likely to be observed in diabetic coma, neurologic damage, and drug-induced respiratory depression. Pallor is a reflection of inadequate perfusion or anemia.

3.2 Corticosteroids suppress the inflammatory response thereby decreasing scarring and fibrosis of lung tissue. Supporting the immune response is, in this case, causes more scarring and inflammation of lung tissue.

4.4 Any smoker is at increased risk for cardiovascular and pulmonary disease. The risk increases exponentially when the smoker is also exposed to other substances that are harmful to lung tissue, such as air pollution or heavy metals. Therefore a smoker who also works in a steel mill is at an extreme risk for developing pulmonary disease compared with a smoker who works in a boutique.

Section B

5.1 Bronchitis is a result not only of an infectious organism, but also of a chronic irritation from environmental agents, such as dust or smoke. Chronic bronchitis can lead to the development of COPD. Bronchitis usually subsides in 10 days. Bronchitis patients can benefit from inhaling warm moist air.

6.3 Antibiotics are ineffective against viral organisms, such as the common cold. Antitussives, antihistamines, and expectorants help alleviate the discomforts the patient with the common cold experiences.

7.4 Fluid intake should be increased in patients with chronic bronchitis. The patient with chronic bronchitis should be counseled to avoid contact with people who have URI, to avoid smoke and respiratory irritants, and to recognize the signs and symptoms of respiratory infection.

8.3 Immunocompromise decreases the individual's ability to fight off URIs. Obesity, dermatitis, and allergies are not risk factors for developing URIs.

9 2 A sedentary lifestyle, in and of itself, is not a risk factor for pneumonia. An impaired level of consciousness, diabetes mellitus, and cystic fibrosis are all risk factors for pneumonia.

Section C

10.2 Prolonged productive cough lasting 3 months or more for 2 consecutive years is typically observed in the chronic bronchitis patient. A nonproductive cough is highly unusual for a true bronchitis patient. Patients with bronchitis may experience chest pain but only because of repeated prolonged coughing spasms. Most patients with obstructive lung disease lose weight because increased oxygen demands make eating difficult.

NCLEX CHAPTER 6 ANSWERS—cont'd

11.3 Allergies frequently cause asthma in children. Exposure to temperature extremes can cause an asthma attack but does not cause asthma. Airways are blocked as a consequence of asthma. Distal airways are enlarged when patients have emphysema, not asthma.

12.1 Stress has not been directly correlated with the development of bronchitis, although it can precipitate asthma in some individuals. Exposure to respiratory irritants, smoking, and respiratory viruses can cause bronchitis.

13.2 The best oxygen treatment for emphysema patients would be 2 liters per minute by nasal cannula. Oxygen 35% by face mask, 100% by nonrebreather face mask, and 10 liters per minute by nasal cannula decreases the respiratory drive.

Section D

14.2 Surgery is the most effective cancer treatment only when a single lesion is present. Radiation is used in conjunction with surgery or antineoplastic therapy to attempt cure or prolong life. Radiation is especially helpful with metastatic cancers in the bones or brain. Chemotherapy or antineoplastic treatment usually prolongs life only a short time and does not offer opportunity for a cancer cure.

15.2 A 65-year-old smoker who has smoked for 50 years began smoking before the age of 15 and is most likely to contract lung cancer. People who begin smoking before the age of 15 have a greater risk of developing lung cancer than do those who begin after the age of 25. Therefore the 65-year-old person who has been smoking 20 years began smoking well after his teenage years and has less of a chance of contracting lung cancer than does his 65-year-old counterpart who started smoking at age 15. Nonsmoking spouses of smokers have three times the risk of developing lung cancer compared with spouses who live with nonsmokers. Only a small percentage of the population may be genetically predisposed to the development of lung cancer.

16.4 A persistent cough is not necessarily an indicator of lung cancer. Cough can indicate other respiratory diseases, such as bronchitis and asthma. Thick, tenacious, yellow sputum, bloody sputum, and localized chest pain all point to lung cancer.

17.3 A lung cancer tumor large enough to compress the superior vena cava causes the patient's face, arms, and hands to swell. Fluid retention can cause any area of the patient's body to appear swollen. Vascular damage causes swelling only of the face, arms, and hands if the damage is localized to these areas and is not related to lung cancer.

NCLEX CHAPTER 7 ANSWERS

Section A

1.4 A tumor is the most common cause of pituitary dysfunction. Congenital defects can cause many types of conditions affecting all body systems. A drug overdose most likely causes neurological, respiratory, renal, and cardiovascular problems. Head injuries can cause neurological problems.

2.1 Signs and symptoms of diabetes insipidus are related to deficiency of ADH. FSH deficiency reduces growth of ova and sperm. Growth hormone deficiency leads to short stature. Oxytocin deficiency results in lack of uterine contraction and lactation.

3.3 Serum sodium levels less than 120 mEq/L produce signs and symptoms of SIADH. Potassium levels are not directly related to SIADH. A serum sodium level of 150 mEq/L indicates hypernatremia.

4.3 High levels of growth hormone after closure of epiphyses results in increased forehead and jaw size. Alopecia is related to hereditary influences; postpartum hormonal changes; drugs, physical, or psychological stress; nutritional deficiencies; and a number of other diseases and disorders. Growth spurts are found in children and adolescents. Orthostatic hypotension is related to fluid volume deficit.

Section B

5.3 Ingesting iodized salt will help prevent goiter, which is the result of a deficiency of iodine in the system. No relationship between goiter and the use of mouthwash exists. The use of calcium supplements with vitamin D promotes healthy bones and teeth. Restricting caffeine intake reduces the risk of gastric distress, elevated blood pressure, and faculty absorption of calcium.

6.1 Primary hypothyroidism manifests in the absence of thyroid hormones. Congenital absence of the thyroid gland is not a primary cause of hypothyroidism. Excessive iodine intake is not considered to be a significant public health problem in the United States and Canada. Thyroid enlargement is the result of an attempt by the thyroid to increase thyroid hormone secretion.

7.2 The patient with primary hypothyroidism lacks thyroid hormones thus necessitating hormonal replacement for life. The other options (all instructing the patient that treatment time is finite) are not feasible if hypothyroidism is to be adequately treated and adverse effects of the disorder prevented.

8.3 Patients with hypoparathyroidism lack calcium, thus calcium supplements are required. Biphosphates inhibit osteoclastic bone resorption and help normalize serum calcium levels. Antihypercalcemic medications reduce calcium utilization. Intravenous normal saline further reduces serum calcium levels contributing to adverse effects.

9.3 Biphosphates inhibit osteoclastic bone resorption and help normalize serum calcium levels, thus normalizing circulating PTH levels and solving hypoparathyroidism. Vitamin D, calcium, and thiazide diuretics increase serum calcium levels.

Section C

10.1 Glucocorticoids reduce the inflammatory response. Thus the patient may be more ill than is otherwise apparent and in need of evaluation. A minor illness does not increase or decrease the need for mineralocorticoids or glucocorticoids. Lack of glucocorticoids is a life-threatening problem.

11.2 Persons with a recent history of receiving glucocorticoids are at risk for developing Cushing's syndrome. Increased secretion of mineralocorticoids offsets glucocorticoid levels rather than increasing them. Adrenal atrophy reduces the level of glucocorticoids. Cortisol is not found in the hypothalamus.

Section D

12.4 Ninety percent of Americans have type 2 diabetes; 10% of Americans have type 1 diabetes; 50% and 70% are statistically incorrect options.

13.3 Type 1 diabetes is the result of a total lack of insulin production. Insufficient insulin and insulin resistance are associated with type 2 diabetes, as is obesity.

14.3 Birth of a 6-pound infant reduces the risk of GDM. Babies born to a mother with a first-degree relative with diabetes, of Native-American heritage, or with a previous history of GDM is at high risk for developing GDM. Additionally, mothers who have given birth to babies with a birth weight of 9 pounds or more are at risk for GDM in future pregnancies.

NCLEX CHAPTER *8* ANSWERS

Section A

1.4 Genetics has not been shown to be a risk factor for GERD. Asthma, tobacco use, and alcohol use are all risk factors for GERD.

2.4 The patient should be advised to eat small, frequent meals high in protein and low in fat and also to avoid eating within 2 to 3 hours of bedtime to lower pressure on the LES. The patient should avoid alcohol and restrictive clothing and also elevate the head of the bed to decrease pressure on the LES.

Section B

3.1 Patients with burns experience stress ulcers known as Curling's ulcers. A preexisting ulcer does not progress to become a stress ulcer. The patient with severe head injuries may experience stress ulcers known as Cushing's ulcers. Pressure ulcers frequently occur in patients who are bedridden when their positions are not changed on a regular basis and care of skin integrity is not maintained.

Section C

4.3 Abdominal pain is the major clinical manifestation of acute pancreatitis. Cardiovascular hypotension, disseminated intravascular coagulation, and a serum amylase of 100 units are not the major clinical manifestations of acute pancreatitis.

5.4 Resting the GI tract is the major treatment in helping to resolve acute pancreatitis. This approach is accomplished by placement of an NG tube and making the patient NPO. Controlling alcohol intake reduces the likelihood of reoccurrence of acute pancreatitis. Meperidine treats the pain associated with acute pancreatitis but does not cure the underlying disorder. Peritoneal lavage does nothing to treat the acute pancreatitis.

NCLEX CHAPTER *8* **ANSWERS**—cont'd

6.3 The patient with pancreatitis should be monitored for hypocalcemia. Pancreatitis reduces, not increases, calcium levels, thus hypercalcemia is unlikely. Hypoglycemia is unusual; hyperglycemia is more likely. Hyperkalemia requires increased intake of potassium or decreased elimination.

7.2 After recovery from acute pancreatitis, the pancreas should function normally, but the patient may experience future bouts of alcohol-induced pancreatitis. The pancreas will continue to produce insulin following recovery from acute pancreatitis. The pancreas will continue to be inflamed and can become necrotic only when the patient continues to ingest alcohol. Atrophy is not associated with resolution of the inflammatory response.

Section D

8.4 Nutritional deficit is common in both Crohn's disease and ulcerative colitis because of the quick transit of materials through the large intestine. Ulcerative colitis involves the mucosal layer of the intestinal wall and has characteristic fatty stools. Small intestine malabsorption is common in Crohn's disease only because this disease frequently affects the small intestine.

Section E

9.4 Cholecystitis is associated with increased bilirubin levels. Intolerance to fatty foods is more common than jaundice and constipation in cholecystitis.

10.2 Hepatic encephalopathy is a cerebral dysfunction. Ascites, dark urine, and splenomegaly are gastrointestinal and urinary manifestations of liver disease.

11. Helping the patient stop drinking alcohol.

Section F

12.2 Low-fiber, high-fat, high-refined carbohydrate diets and ulcerative colitis are associated with colon cancer. A high-fiber diet is not a predisposing factor to development of colon cancer.

NCLEX CHAPTER *9* **ANSWERS**

Section A

1.4 A minimum of 3000 ml of fluid is required per 24 hours to treat cystitis adequately. 1000 ml, 1500 ml, and 2000 ml are insufficient.

2.4 Because blood pressure is, in part, regulated by kidney function, chronically altered renal function (e.g., chronic pyelonephritis) may contribute to hypertension. Cystitis is a bladder problem unrelated to blood pressure. Acute pyelonephritis is a temporary, not chronic, condition.

3.1 *Staphylococcus aureus, Klebsiella pneumoniae,* and *Proteus* may be found in the urine, but *Escherichia coli* is the most common cause of cystitis or pyelonephritis.

4.1 Urgency and dysuria are the patient's most stressful signs and symptoms of cystitis. Nocturia, incontinence, hematuria, bladder spasms, bladder hesitancy, and cloudy urine may also be present in cystitis but are usually less prominent.

5.1 An acid-ash diet (e.g., cranberry juice, meats, eggs, cheese, prunes, cranberries, plums, whole grains, vitamin C) acidifies the urine and thus reduces symptoms and the risk of chronic cystitis. Tossed vegetable salad, milk, and apple may cause alkaline urine, which can increase symptoms and the chronic nature of the cystitis.

6.2 Wiping front to back is the most important factor to teach. Increasing fluid intake and taking showers rather than baths reduces the risk. An alkaline-ash diet may increase the risk of cystitis.

7.2 A UTI is identified by bacteria in the urine and, occasionally, by red blood cells; however, the cell count is normal. Glucose and ketones in the urine are not associated with infection.

8.3 Phenazopyridine is a urinary tract analgesic. Nitrofurantoin (Macrodantin), phenazopyridine (Pyridium), ciprofloxacin (Cipro) are antibiotics.

Section B

9.4 Excessive production of inhibitors is not a risk factor for calculi formation. Inhibitors prevent kidney stone formation. Calcium is the most common stone-forming substance. Mucoproteins provide the structure for the deposit of crystals, which become trapped and form stones. Struvite is a common stone-forming substance for infection stones.

Section C

10.2 Glomerulonephritis may develop after an untreated beta hemolytic streptococcal infection. Chronic renal failure and nephrosis are not commonly related to streptococcal infection. Pyelonephritis is most commonly associated with *Escherichia coli* infection.

Section D

11.3 Postrenal disease causes obstructions to urinary outflow that elevate BUN and creatinine levels. Prerenal disease is caused by obstruction to blood flow to the kidney. Bacteriuria is the presence of bacteria in the urine. Hypercalcemia is elevated serum calcium levels in the blood.

12.1 BUN levels are increased in chronic renal failure. Oliguria and pruritus are later signs of chronic renal failure. Polyuria is not associated with chronic renal failure.

Section E

13.1 Increased production or reduced clearance IgA in the kidneys is a common cause of IgA nephropathy. IgE is an immunoglobulin found in patients with allergies and is unrelated to IgA nephropathy. IgA nephropathy is an immune disorder unrelated to infection. No known genetic influence on IgA nephropathy exists.

Section F

14.1 Wilms' tumor is uncommon in children over the age of 5 years.

NCLEX CHAPTER *10* ANSWERS

Section A

1.3 The most common symptom of cryptorchidism is an undescended testis. The patient with epididymitis is more apt to experience swelling of the scrotal sac. The patient with an enlarged prostate experiences perianal pain. Infertility is a complaint among adult patients of cryptorchidism but is not the most common.

2.3 Infertility is not a sign of orchitis. Male infertility can be the result of many causes. Severe pain, high fever, and edema are characteristics of orchitis.

3.4 Epididymitis generally occurs in sexually active young men under the age of 35. To find epididymitis in males before they have experienced puberty is rare.

4.3 The four common forms of prostatitis are acute bacterial, chronic bacterial, nonbacterial, and prostatodynia.

5.1 Hypertrophy of prostatic cells is one of the pathophysiologic factors of benign prostatic hyperplasia. Atrophy of prostatic cells does not occur in benign hyperplasia. Stricture of the vas deferens and inflammation of the epididymis are not commonly observed in BPH.

6.2 The risk of developing BPH increases, not decreases, with age.

7.4 The cause of BPH is not related to alcohol consumption, but rather, is related to increased testosterone and estrogen levels, stimulation of the alpha-adrenergic nerve endings, which interferes with the bladder sphincter, and smoking.

8.1 Testicular carcinoma spreads most frequently to the lung. Drainage from the testis enters the interaortic or preaortic lymph nodes. The brain, bladder, and liver are rarely affected by testicular carcinoma metastasis.

9.4 Alcoholics do not appear to be at higher risk for developing prostatic carcinoma than is the general population. African-American men, men who have undergone a vasectomy, and men who work with fertilizer are at risk for developing prostatic carcinoma.

Section B

10.3 Primary dysmenorrhea is pain associated with ovulation but is not caused by any disease process. Increased menstruation is known as either menorrhagia or menometrorrhagia. Absence of menstruation is known as amenorrhea. Dysmenorrhea is not a symptom of pregnancy.

11.4 Urinary tract infections do not cause secondary dysmenorrhea. Secondary dysmenorrhea may be a result of pelvic inflammatory disease, adhesions or fibroids, or endometriosis.

Section C

12.1 Recurrent genital herpes infections result from reactivation of the virus from sacral dorsal root ganglia. Herpes virus does not reside in the genital tissues. Reinfection does not contribute to recurrent infection. The patient already has the virus. Repeated exposure does not produce the immune response. The immune response is already present.

NCLEX CHAPTER *10* ANSWERS—cont'd

13.2 A maculopapular rash on the trunk, palms of hands, and soles of feet characterize the secondary stage of syphilis. Primary syphilis produces a painless chancre at the site of inoculation. Healing of the lesions is characteristic of latent syphilis. Neurologic and cardiovascular disease, soft tumors, auditory or ophthalmic involvement, and cutaneous lesions characterize tertiary syphilis.

14.1 The transition zone of the endocervix is the typical site of chlamydia infection in women. The other structures (intrauterine tissue, ovaries, vulva region) are not typically associated with chlamydia.

NCLEX CHAPTER *11* ANSWERS

1.2 Strong granulation tissue forms from the hematoma in the cellular proliferation stage of bone healing. No callus ossification stage exists in bone healing. The granulation tissue changes into newly formed cartilage during the callus formation stage. The calcium salts and cartilage are deposited in the soft-tissue callus, leading to rigid calcification and permanent callus formation in the cellular consolidation stage.

2.4 Changes for rheumatoid arthritis begin in the joint synovium. Tophi formation is related to elevated uric acid levels, not rheumatoid arthritis. The bursa and cartilage are not initially involved in rheumatoid arthritis.

3.4 The pathophysiologic changes in osteoarthritis involve joint ends repeatedly hitting together, leading to a loss of joint matrix and erosion of cartilage. Faulty purine metabolism and uric acid crystals triggering a phagocytic response by leukocytes are found in the patient with gout. A thick layer of granulation pannus tissue, which covers and invades articular cartilage, is associated with rheumatoid arthritis, not osteoarthritis.

4.2 The pathophysiologic factors of gout involve a uric acid level increase in the blood. Autoimmune lesions of collagen tissue are found in a variety of connective tissue disorders but not gout. Inflammation of the synovial membrane is associated with rheumatoid arthritis. Cartilage and bone erosion is associated with osteoarthritis.

NCLEX CHAPTER *12* ANSWERS

1.4 Determining placement of the feeding tube is the priority nursing action. Not taking this action can lead to aspiration. Measuring intake and output, weighing the patient, and assessing the patient for diarrhea are not directly related to the tube-feeding procedure.

2.4 Leaders of self-help groups are usually not health care professionals. Self-help groups by definition are characterized as a group designed to serve people who have a common problem in which people with similar problems are able to help others and provide support to each other.

3.4 The nurse realizes that this behavior indicates the patient is fearful of discharge. This behavior is not normal. The patient already has an altered or distorted body image by virtue of her diagnosis. Her behaviors do not reflect regression to previous symptoms of her disorder.

4.2 The patient who is identifying healthy ways to handle anxiety indicates that she has progressed. Conversations focusing on food, spending time alone after eating, and vigorously exercising are all signs that she will continue to practice bulimia.

5. Kwashiorkor is associated with protein deficiency. Marasmus is a severe deficiency of all nutrients.

NCLEX CHAPTER *13* ANSWERS

Section A

1.2 In macular degeneration, peripheral vision remains intact. Macular degeneration is neither prevented nor cured. The disorder is not easily diagnosed.

2.3 Scleral buckling is used to correct retinal detachment. Iridectomy and trabeculectomy promote outflow of humor thus reducing intraocular pressure. Keratoplasty redesigns the cornea.

3.4 Remaining in a head-down, lateral position facilitates reattachment of the retina and prevents further problems. This postoperative care is appropriate for a patient treated for detached retina. Miotic eye drops will constrict only the pupil and may worsen the detachment. Allowing the patient to ambulate can cause further detachment. Covering only the affected eye does nothing to help but adds stress because the eyes work in tandem.

4.2 Your neighbor should be referred to an ophthalmologist. An ophthalmologist is the only person qualified to treat a retinal detachment. An oculist, optician, or an optometrist cannot treat retinal detachment.

Section B

5.2 Anything that blocks the external ear canal can cause conductive hearing loss. Disease or trauma to the inner ear may cause balance problems, as well as hearing loss. Disease or trauma to the external ear may cause conductive hearing loss, depending on the situation. Damage to the nerve pathways causes a sensorineural hearing loss.

6.4 The most common problem of the external ear is infection. The external ear may be invaded by insects and foreign bodies, be subject to injury or trauma, or suffer allergic reactions, but these situations are less common compared with infection.

7.2 The pinna is pulled down and back in a child, up and back in an adult. Pulling the pinna forward and down or forward and up will obstruct the canal.

Section C

8.2 The usual transmission route for type 2 herpes is by sexual encounter, not kissing and touching. Contaminated food and water and coughing do not spread the herpes virus.

Section D

9.4 Thick, scaly, erythematous plaque lesions indicate psoriasis. Nonscaling, violet-colored, pruritic papules are associated with a number of disorders, the most common of which is Kaposi's sarcoma. Black comedones are associated with acne. Pruritic vesicles are associated with itching and allergic response.

10.1 Oily skin causes acne vulgaris. That poor diet and hygiene causes acne vulgaris is a misconception. Excessive melanocytes cause a darkening of the skin.

11.2 Alcohol and hot drinks cause vasodilation of the skin thus making the face appear red. Body temperature (hypothermia and hyperthermia) and vasoconstriction are not associated with rosacea.

Section E

12. Most melanoma lesions are slightly raised and black or brown. The borders are irregular and the surfaces uneven. Periodically, melanomas ulcerate and bleed. Surrounding erythema, inflammation, and tenderness may be present. Dark melanomas are frequently mottled with red, blue, and white shades.

13.2 An ulcerated, hyperkeratotic nodule with dermal invasion is characteristic of squamous cell carcinoma. Irregular pigmentation of the skin is associated with vitiligo. A slightly elevated, pearl-colored nodule may reflect basal cell carcinoma. Multifocal brown macules are known as nevi or freckles.

14.3 Malignant melanoma metastasizes the earliest. Basal cell carcinoma rarely metastasizes. Kaposi sarcoma is confined to the skin and subcutaneous tissues, although it may become widespread to include the viscera.

15.3 Untreated basal cell carcinoma ulcerates and involves local tissues. Untreated basal cell carcinoma grows slowly, does not involve regional lymph tissues, or metastasizes.

NCLEX CHAPTER *14* ANSWERS

1.2 Endorphins reduce pain sensations; they do not increase them. Endorphins are not related to transmission of painful impulses or their interpretation.

2.1 Increased blood pressure and pulse are sympathetic responses to acute pain. Pink skin, muscle tension, constricted pupils, dry skin, and decreased or normal blood pressure are representative of parasympathetic nervous system activity.

3.4 Decreased or normal blood pressure and pulse are parasympathetic responses to chronic pain. Increased blood pressure, increased pulse, pallor, skeletal muscle tension, dilated pupils, and diaphoresis are sympathetic nervous system responses and are characteristic of an acute pain response.

4. Factors influencing a patient's response to pain include previous experience with pain; family and occupational roles; spiritual belief system; physical influences, such as sleep or stress; pain threshold; pain quality, location, duration, and type; patient personality; and communication skills.

5. The sensation is known as phantom pain—pain felt in an absent body part. The patient "thinks" the body part is still present because of the continued transmission of afferent nerve impulses.

Index

Page numbers followed by *f* indicate figure; *t*, table; *b*, box.